dr. susan lark's
hormone
revolution

dr. susan lark's
hormone
revolution

Yes, You Can Naturally Restore & Balance Your Own Hormones

---

by Susan M. Lark, MD
with Kimberly Day

PORTOLA
PRESS

Published in the United States by Portola Press, LLC
www.portolapress.com

Library of Congress Control Number: 2007933399
"Dr. Susan Lark's Hormone Revolution"

ISBN-13: 978-0-9795409-0-5 hardcover
ISBN-10: 0-9795409-0-9 hardcover

Printed in the United States of America

Cover and interior design: Deborah Mills Thackrey
Cover photo of Dr. Lark: Jim Douglas, courtesy of Healthy Directions, LLC
Kimberly Day's photo: Jennifer Greenwald
Typesetting: Janis Reed

10   9   8   7   6   5   4   3   2   1

First Edition

acknowledgements

Many people, both directly and indirectly, contributed immensely to the writing of this book. We would like to thank everyone who helped in this complex process. Many of them are long term friends and colleagues of Susan's. Their assistance and advice were relied upon heavily in the creation of *Hormone Revolution*.

A very special thank you goes to the following:

Jacquelyn Aldana • Brooke Baggett • Kathy Blair • Lewis Connor, D.C. • Tammie Donnelly • Sierra Dunn • Chandra Giovanni • Karen Hoxeng • Kerry Jacobson • Jennifer Lamb • Marcus Laux, N.D. • Cathy Lewis • Yana Mocak • Evelyn Oliver • Shiva Pourizima, N.D. • Bill Ralph • Jim Richards • D. Graeme Shaw, M.D. • Sandra Smith • Katie Spidell • Deborah Thackrey • Bill Todd • Dave Weiner • Barbara White • Artemas Yaffe • All of our friends at Healthy Directions, LLC • All of our friends at Portola Press, LLC

Susan would like to give a very special acknowledgment, lots of love, and a huge thank you to Kimberly Day without whose tremendous capability, persistence, and perseverance this book could not have been written.

Kimberly would like to send a huge hug and profound gratitude to Susan. Without her love, insights, and amazing advice, Kimberly would not be who she is today. Kimberly would also like to thank her husband Trip for his never-ending support and understanding throughout this project.

table of contents

Introduction **1**

Section One: Healthy Hormones **13**

    Chapter 1: How Hormones Work **15**

        How Sex Hormones Are Produced Within the Body 16

        How Hormones Deliver Their Messages 17

    Chapter 2: Estrogen **18**

        The Chemistry of Estrogen 19

        How Estrogen Affects the Body 21

        How Diet, Health, and the Environment Affect Estrogen Levels 21

    Chapter 3: Progesterone **24**

        The Chemistry of Progesterone 24

        How Progesterone Affects the Body 26

        How Lifestyle and Health Affect Progesterone Levels 26

    Chapter 4: Testosterone **27**

        The Chemistry of Testosterone 27

        How Testosterone Affects the Body 28

        How Diet, Health, and the Environment Affect Testosterone Levels 28

    Chapter 5: Pregnenolone **30**

        The Chemistry of Pregnenolone 31

        How Health and Lifestyle Affect Pregnenolone Levels 31

    Chapter 6: DHEA **32**

        The Chemistry of DHEA 32

        How DHEA Affects the Body 33

        How Diet, Health, and the Environment Affect DHEA Levels 33

Chapter 7: Hormone Balance Through the Years 35

The Normal Menstrual Cycle 36

The Menopause Transition 37

Menopause: The Change of Life 39

Section One: Summary 40

Section Two: Create a Healthy You 43

Chapter 8: Fool's Gold 45

Women as Human Guinea Pigs 45

The Heart-Wrenching Reality of HRT 46

Chapter 9: Safe, Natural, and Effective Options 54

Restore Your Own Hormones 54

Natural Hormone Substitutes 55

Understanding Bioidentical Hormones 55

Section Two: Summary 56

Section Three: Restoring the Balance 57

Chapter 10: Estrogen Dominance: The Premenopause 59

Estrogen Dominance and Your Health 59

The Cosmetic Effects of Estrogen Dominance 64

Testing for Estrogen Dominance 68

Chapter 11: Reversing Estrogen Dominance 71

A Better Way 73

Modulate Estrogen with Hormone Mimics 74

Create an Estrogen Breakdown 78

Balance Excess Estrogen with Progesterone 82

Chapter 12: Menopause and Estrogen Deficiency 95

What is Menopause 95

Menopause by Any Other Name 95

The Physiology of Menopause 96

The Dark Side of Menopause 98

Testing for Menopause 103

The Cosmetic Effects of Menopause 105

The Lure of Fools' Gold 113

A Better Option 114

Chapter 13: Treating Estrogen Deficiency **115**

Hysterectomy—Surgical Menopause 116

Restore Your Own Hormones 120

Fend Off a Breakdown 132

Protect Your Health with Hormone Safeguards 134

Benefit from Estrogen-Like Hormone Substitutes 137

Estriol: Your Body's Natural Estrogen 145

Using Biochemically Identical Estrogen 147

Chapter 14: Health-Promoting Progesterone **150**

What is Progesterone 150

Progesterone's Role in Your Body 151

How Progesterone Deficiency Occurs 152

Symptoms of Progesterone Deficiency 153

Testing for Progesterone Deficiency 160

Chapter 15: Restoring Progesterone **162**

Stimulate Progesterone Production 162

Ovarian Progesterone Production 170

Supplement with Progesterone 172

Chapter 16: Feminine Benefits of Testosterone **181**

What is Testosterone 181

Testosterone's Role in Your Body 182

How Testosterone Deficiency Occurs 182

Symptoms of Testosterone Deficiency 183

Testing for Testosterone Deficiency 189

Chapter 17: Restoring Testosterone **191**

Restore Your Own Hormones 191

Testosterone Production in the Ovaries and Adrenals 199

Slow Down the Breakdown 202

Support the Effects of Testosterone with Hormone Mimics 202

Promote Nitric Oxide Production 204

Supplementing With Testosterone 207

The Proof is in the Research 209

Chapter 18: Pregnenolone: the Mother Hormone 212

What is Pregnenolone 213

Pregnenolone's Role in Your Body 213

How Pregnenolone Deficiency Occurs 214

Symptoms of Pregnenolone Deficiency 214

Testing for Pregnenolone Deficiency 217

Chapter 19: Restoring Pregnenolone 219

Boost Adrenal and Ovary Function 219

Maintain Adrenal Health with Amazing Herbs 226

The Benefits of Bioidentical Pregnenolone 229

Prove It to Me 230

Supplementing With Pregnenolone 234

Chapter 20: The Unsung Benefits of DHEA 238

What is DHEA 238

DHEA's Role in Your Body 239

How DHEA Deficiency Occurs 239

Symptoms of DHEA Deficiency 240

Testing for DHEA Deficiency 246

Chapter 21: Restoring DHEA 248

Boost Your Adrenal Function 248

Beneficial Bioidentical DHEA 258

Using DHEA 263

Supplementing With DHEA 264

Section Three: Summary 267

Section Four: Energy Medicine for Healthy Hormones 269

Chapter 22: Understanding Acupuncture 271

The Rivers of Life 272

Overwhelming Medical Support 274

Performing Acupressure for Healthy Hormones 275

Exceptional Healers 281

My "Heal the World" Exercise 285

Chapter 23: Chakras—Your Spinning Wheels of Wellness **289**

A Western Take on an Eastern Practice 289

Reading the Chakras 290

Promote Healthy, Balanced Chakras 293

Chapter 24: A Rainbow of Healing **296**

Make Color Work for You 296

A Colorful Exercise 298

A Colorful Meditation 299

Chapter 25: Light Your Way to Hormonal Health **300**

The Early Research 301

The Twentieth Century 301

Research Today 302

How Colored Light Works 303

Healing Benefits of Red Light 303

Healing Benefits of Blue Light 310

Applying Colored Light to the Body 313

Self-Treating With Colored Light 314

Choosing a Light Device 315

Benefits of Sunlight 316

Chapter 26: Feel the Vibration of Great Health **319**

The Sound Frequency 319

Exceptional Healers 323

The Benefits of Biofeedback 327

Electromagnetic Frequencies 337

The Father of Bioelectrical Medicine 337

The Research Continues 340

Section Four: Summary 345

Section Five: The Optimum Lifestyle for Healthy Hormones **347**

Chapter 27: Your Perfect Diet **349**

Understanding pH 349

Eating for Your Type 361

Inflammation and Hormone Health 378

Common Saboteurs for All Hormone Types 381

Chapter 28: Healing Foods for Hormonal Health 386

    The High Enzyme Diet 386

    Healing Sugars 390

    Green Foods 393

    Making the Transition 396

Chapter 29: Eating Made Easy 399

    The Dining Out Dilemma 399

    Dining With Your Opposite 401

    Easy Meals for the Non-Cooker 402

    The Culinary Dabbler 406

    The Healthy Gourmet 408

    Recipes 409

Chapter 30: Reduce Stress, Maintain Hormonal Health 432

    What is Stress 432

    What is Your Body Trying to Tell You 433

    How Stressed *Are* You? 435

    The Physiology of Stress 438

    The Stress–Adrenal Connection 439

    The Stress–Neurotransmitter Connection 440

    Stress and Your Hormones 441

Chapter 31: My Program for Stress Reduction 444

    Practicing Deep Breathing and Meditation 444

    General Relaxation Exercises 445

    Stress Reduction for Different Hormonal Types 449

    Create Female Health with Positive Emotions 453

    Five Exceptional Healers 474

Chapter 32: Exercise Your Right to Great Hormonal Health 484

    Walk (or Run) Your Way to Health 484

    Before You Start, Be Prepared 492

    Bone-A-Fide Reasons for Strength Training 497

    Stretch Your Body and Your Mind 498

    Section Five: Summary 506

Conclusion 509

Resource Guide 510

Bibliography 520

Index 534

introduction

Dear Friend,

Every woman I know wants to live a life filled with energy, vitality, and vigor. We all want to maintain a zest for life and to be able to participate in our favorite activities, including an active and satisfying sex life. We also want to be able to think clearly and remember facts and events. No one relishes the idea of becoming infirm or losing the faculties needed to fully participate in favorite activities.

This central, common desire to get the most out of life led me to study the crucial role that hormones play in our physical, emotional, and even spiritual health and well-being, beginning more than 30 years ago. In fact, you could even say that hormones have been a personal hobby for me. From my late 20's and into my early 60's, I've worked to keep myself in as good a hormonal balance as possible. In fact, I am currently in my early 60's and still have menstrual periods!

This hobby quickly turned into a passion, and I began to share this knowledge with my friends, family, patients, and readers like you. I am always amazed by people's response. Most women who have come to me with a hormonal issue complain about the traditional therapies that are offered—not only their ineffectiveness, but also the dangerous side effects that many can cause.

"Renata" is a typical example of this. When she came to me for a menopause consultation, she placed a newspaper article on my desk that discussed conventional hormone replacement therapy (HRT) and the risk of breast cancer. She was 54 years old and had moderately severe menopause symptoms, including five to six episodes of hot flashes a day, night sweats two to three times per week, anxiety and jitters, and difficulty concentrating on her work. Clearly she needed help.

Her regular physician recommended that she begin a course of conventional HRT, but she was not enthusiastic about this treatment option. She found it quite upsetting to read about the increased risk of breast cancer with the use of HRT. Her own mother had died of breast cancer at age 60 and she herself had a long history of benign breast disease.

Clearly, women need a different approach from what traditional medicine has to offer. They need and deserve safe, effective options for balancing and restoring their hormones. This became my mandate, my calling in life.

Over the years, I've discussed different aspects of my philosophy in a variety of books, newsletters, magazine articles, and the like. However, this is the first time I've put all of the information I've studied for more than three decades into one place.

I am immensely proud to be able to offer this book as my gift to you. By putting all of the research, solutions, and fabulous sources I've gathered into one book, I am able to lead you by the hand throughout this journey toward great hormone health, and subsequently great overall health and well-being.

A Bit About My Background

I have worked very hard throughout my career to ensure that I have the educational, clinical, and practical experience that patients and women all over the world could depend on and trust. I received my medical degree from Northwestern University Medical School in Chicago, and became Board Certified in Family Practice.

While I did have a very busy family practice in the early years of my career in the San Francisco area, more and more of my practice became focused on my female patients and their specific health needs, which was a very strong personal as well as professional interest of mine.

From the day I entered clinical practice, my emphasis has been on how complementary and alternative health care could greatly improve a person's health, especially that of women. I also spent many years educating my peers (including other physicians, nurse practitioners, nurses, and physicians' assistants) so they could better integrate complementary medicine into their respective fields.

I served on the clinical faculty of Stanford University Medical School from 1981–1983, and taught women's health care in Stanford's Primary Care Associate Program in the Division of Family and Community Medicine from 1991–2002. I have also taught women's health care and complementary medicine to other health care professionals and consumers through institutions such as the California Academy of Family Physicians, North American Menopause Society, Stanford Research Institute, Kaiser Hospitals, Foundation for New Options, CorText Seminars for Continuing Medical Education, New Hope Communication, University of California Santa Barbara, and many other organizations.

In 1978, I founded one of the first clinics in the United States dedicated to women's health care and preventive medicine, as well as one of the first clinics specializing in family practice and preventive medicine. Throughout my 33 years of clinical experience, I was fortunate enough to be one of the first physicians in the U.S. to pioneer the use of self-care treatments such as diet, nutrition, exercise, and stress management therapies in both the fields of women's health care and family medicine.

Beyond my clinical experience, I have a great passion for research and education. This led me to write 13 different books on women's health and the critical role that hormones play in female health, including the *Premenstrual Syndrome Self-Help Book,* the *Menopause Self-Help Book*, and *The Estrogen Decision*. These and other books that I have authored have been sold in their English language versions in the U.S., Canada, U.K., Australia, New Zealand and South Africa. Many have even been translated into foreign language editions such as Chinese, Russian, French, German, Portuguese (Brazil) and Spanish.

Since 2000, I have also authored *Women's Wellness Today* (formerly *The Lark Letter*), a monthly women's health newsletter, published by Healthy Directions, LLC. I also offer a free bi-weekly eLetter on a wide variety of women's health conditions that you can receive electronically.

My Own Hormone Journey

Like most women I know, I struggled with hormonal issues early in life. When I was in my late teens, I began to suffer from PMS symptoms, including food cravings, bloating, and weight gain of five to eight pounds and extreme breast tenderness. My hair started to get oilier and little red pimples began to break out on my nose and chin. I also suffered from excruciating menstrual cramps, irregular periods, and breast cysts.

At the time, my mother (also a physician) could only offer me aspirin and sympathy. She told me I'd likely outgrow the PMS, but instead it got worse. During medical school, the pain would be so extreme for one week every month that I couldn't even do my work properly. There was many a time that my nausea and pain were so severe that I had to leave the medical ward and go lie down in the medical student on-call room.

To make matters worse, my moods fluctuated terribly. I was my normal calm and relaxed self most of the time, but just before my period, I'd become more irritable and difficult to deal with. I was very sensitive, emotionally speaking, and would frequently steal away and cry, wondering how I would ever complete my medical training. I also craved sugar almost uncontrollably and would often go on junk-food binges.

About this same time, I was diagnosed with benign breast disease. When my period would come, the cysts in my breasts would become so large and tender that I couldn't bear to bump up against anything.

As a doctor-in-training, I had access to the best medical care. I tried virtually every medication—mild tranquilizers for my moods, antispasmodics for the cramps, diuretics for my bloating—but nothing worked particularly well or for very long.

Then, in 1974, during my internship, everything changed. I was training in obstetrics and gynecology and read in one of the medical journals about work being done by doctors in Europe using high doses of vitamins to treat breast cysts.

I had never been taught that what I ate could affect my health! The concept took a hold of me and never let go. I ended up spending the entire next year hunting through journal after journal in the medical library looking for more information on how you could treat menstrual and other female hormonal disorders and general health with nutrition and supplements. It was amazing how much research I found, even in those early years, that was not being utilized to help female patients improve their hormonal status.

I searched for anything I could find related to regenerating and balancing your hormones, including conventional, Eastern, and alternative medicine; nutrition; and the emotional and spiritual perspective. These included natural treatments such as acupuncture/acupressure, energy, diet, supplements, exercise, yoga, and prayer.

Since there were no guideposts or programs in existence at that time, I had to pioneer and create my own nutritionally based plan and tested it on myself. On the diet front, I cut out sugar, fat, and caffeine. This was no small feat for a busy doctor-in-training who depended on fast food, cola, coffee, and the sandwiches and sweet rolls available in the hospital cafeteria. I also began to eat more whole grains and fresh fruits and vegetables, and put myself on a vitamin and mineral program, initially high doses of vitamin B-complex, vitamin E, and other nutritional supplements.

I was amazed with the results. My PMS symptoms and menstrual cramps that had plagued me for years began to diminish on a month-by-month basis. My menstrual periods become regular, monthly occurrences, which would come and go without fanfare or any discomfort. My quality of life significantly improved as my symptoms receded more and more each month.

I then added in regular exercise and implemented the stress reduction therapies I had been studying, including yoga, acupressure, meditation, and biofeedback. In no time, my PMS, menstrual cramps, irregular periods, and benign breast disease were a thing of the past, never to be revisited again.

I was, in essence, my first successful PMS and menstrual cramps patient. But it's not just younger, menstruating women who can benefit from my program. Women of all ages and hormonal profiles can find success with my plan as well. My own hormonal health has remained very stable over the years. My program sustained me beautifully, and I literally had perfect menstrual periods well into my mid-40's.

At this time, my hormones appeared to shift, and I noticed that I had skipped two menstrual cycles. I realized that this was reflecting changes in my brain and reproductive chemistry that are typical of the normal aging pattern that I have seen in many thousands of women entering mid-life.

I decided to see if I could reestablish my normal hormonal balance and bring my estrogen and progesterone levels back to normal. I began to rethink my own program and made the changes in my regimen in order to rebalance and support the chemistry in my brain that regulates healthy female hormone production. I also found the use of energy medicine therapies to be very helpful.

Fortunately, I was able to rebalance my hormones and get myself back on track. All of my perimenopausal symptoms quickly disappeared and I started to have normal, healthy menstrual periods once again.

I maintained virtually perfect menstrual periods into my late 50's, until my mother became seriously ill at the age of 84. She had been extremely healthy up to that time, but then suddenly developed a very serious pneumonia. At this same time, my mother-in-law, who was in her late 80's, also became seriously ill. This took a toll on my hormonal health. I began to feel very tired, and noticed that my normal stamina had evaporated. I knew that stress was very debilitating to hormonal and overall health, and I had clearly allowed these intensely stressful situations to impact me. For the first time in my life, I actually experienced what a hot flash felt like!

As always, I went back to the drawing board and looked for a way to balance and support my hormones once again. I instituted a few simple, yet very powerful, changes to my program, and was thrilled to find that, over a period of months, my symptoms dramatically disappeared. I could literally feel my own estrogen begin to "turn on" again as my hot flashes went away, my sleep pattern began to normalize, and I started to regain my normal level of energy.

To my delight, I even started to have regular, monthly menstrual periods again, and they have continued to this day. The benefits to me are that I keep producing so much of my own hormones that my energy is terrific. I have a very positive and joyful mood and attitude towards life. I also have great resistance to illness. This allows me to be extremely busy and productive in my work and really enjoy a full life.

Plus, my program has helped to keep my skin and hair healthy and shiny, so much in fact that most people cannot believe that the photo on the cover of this book was taken the year I turned 60. I also still have the same dark brown hair that I had when I was in my 20's, and thanks to my program, it has never shown any sign of turning gray. (I am also blessed with good hair genes, which I have to thank my mother for.) Additionally, I'm very proud of the fact that I have never used any hormonal therapy, except for the very brief use of a progesterone mini-pill in my early 30's. I have always simply supported and balanced my own hormones naturally.

In the years since I first put together my own PMS and menstrual cramps treatment program, I have greatly expanded my treatment programs, and have worked with tens of thousands of women of all ages—from teens to those in their 80's and 90's—who have benefited from this self-care approach. My programs have greatly helped them to enjoy improved hormonal and overall health, which, in turn, has dramatically enhanced their overall quality of life.

In my experience, once a woman realizes that her hormonal symptoms can originate in, or be worsened by, bad habits of diet, exercise, and stress management (as well as the wear and tear of life that we all experience), she is willing to do almost anything to change. She just needs a bit of guidance. And that's what this book is all about.

Kimberly's Hormone Journey

I've worked with Kimberly since 2001, when she was the editor of my monthly newsletter. Kimberly is like so many of the estrogen dominant women I've treated over the years.

Since she was a teenager, Kimberly suffered with infrequent periods and horrendous cramps that would often leave her in a fetal position on the bathroom floor alternating between diarrhea and vomiting for hours on end. When she was in college, the pain was so severe that one of her friends almost called an ambulance when Kimberly collapsed on the bathroom floor in agony.

Unfortunately, her doctors didn't offer much in the way of treatment. While they did tell her that she had multiple cysts on both ovaries, it was through her own research that she realized she had polycystic ovary syndrome. At that point, her doctors wanted to put her on the birth control pill, but she has a blood clotting disorder and cannot take the pill (thank God!). They then prescribed the painkiller Anaprox for her menstrual cramps, but since she couldn't predict her menstrual periods, it didn't do her any good.

The pain and irregularity of her periods continued well into her early 30's, but now they were eclipsed by a different concern—she and her husband had decided to try to conceive. However, with infrequent ovulation, their chances were slim.

I suggested that Kimberly make a few dietary changes—no sugar, no alcohol, no wheat, no caffeine, and no dairy. I also suggested that she begin taking a few key nutrients, including lutein, beta-carotene, and flaxseed that would help to promote more regular ovulation and menstrual periods. Within six months, she began having regular monthly periods for the first time in her life, experienced significantly less pain during menstruation, and even lost weight!

After two years on this program, Kimberly and her husband decided to consult a fertility expert. After previously hearing time and again that her hormone levels were totally unbalanced, she was pleasantly surprised to hear that her hormones were now perfect! In fact, the doctor was concerned about overstimulating her and placed her on the lowest possible dose of medication and even changed their previously discussed protocol.

Clearly, those 24 months of diet and supplement changes based on my recommendations not only helped to bring her progesterone and estrogen levels back into balance, but, more importantly for her, she is better able to predict her now much more frequent and regular ovulations. Let's hope conception is not far behind!

Creating Your Own Personal Journey

My goal for you as you read this book is to learn a bit about how your body works and what you can do to keep your hormones healthy and balanced. Specifically, you'll discover how maintaining the five key sex hormones (pregnenolone, DHEA, estrogen, progesterone, and testosterone) impact every area of your life and even play a major preventive role in such debilitating conditions as cardiovascular disease, osteoporosis, arthritis, and even Alzheimer's disease. They can also play an important role in helping to sustain your productivity and physical vigor.

You'll also learn why women who go off balance and are no longer on the healthy course tend to show three patterns: estrogen dominance, estrogen deficiency–slow processor, or estrogen deficiency–fast processor.

A woman with estrogen dominance is usually younger and menstruating. She often produces too much estrogen (which has an expansive and growth-stimulating effect on the body) and too little progesterone, which is more contractive and has a growth-limiting effect. She will frequently suffer from conditions such as PMS, menstrual cramps, irregular menstrual periods, heavy menstrual bleeding, bloating, oily skin and hair, fibroid tumors, endometriosis, and/or mood swings.

After working with many thousands of patients going through menopause, I noticed that most of their complaints related to losing their healthy middle ground, which I define as that optimal place where the brain and body chemistry, nervous system, and other functions within the body are in good balance, and therefore, not producing any uncomfortable symptoms. However, when a woman enters menopause (even if she had previously been in healthy physical and chemical balance), her body and brain chemistry starts to become more unbalanced.

Additionally, during menopause, I've found that things aren't as simple as just too much or too little of any given hormone. Instead, my patients tended to experience a total shift in their entire physical, chemical, and energetic makeup that manifested as one of two distinct patterns. Their body and brain chemistry tended toward becoming either too fast or too slow. For this reason, I call the first pattern estrogen deficiency–fast processor. The second is its mirror image—estrogen deficiency–slow processor.

An estrogen deficiency–fast processor woman is in menopause with too little estrogen. She will frequently appear more anxious, wiry, with thin, dry skin and tissues. Her health complaints often include hot flashes, night sweats, insomnia, vaginal dryness, sore joints, and increased risk for heart disease and osteoporosis. Her brain and body chemistry is imbalanced towards the more excitatory chemicals like dopamine, norepinephrine, and epinephrine that stimulate, speed up, and overheat her body processes and body chemistry. She tends to show more of a deficiency in chemicals like serotonin, GABA, and taurine, which slow down or inhibit the body's chemical and physiological processes. In essence, she has too much "speed up" and not enough "slow down."

An estrogen deficiency-slow processor woman is also in menopause, but she has the opposite body type and temperament. On the surface, she appears to still have good estrogen production, as she tends to be plumper, have a more difficult time losing weight, may have more fluid retention, stronger bones and connective tissue, thicker skin and hair, and a more placid temperament. (Remember, estrogen is a growth-stimulating hormone, so it causes tissues to thicken and expand.) All of these traits are supported, in part, by estrogen in younger women and even, to some degree, after menopause, but they are also supported by many other chemicals and substances within the body that are not related to sex hormone production, but still provide benefits for these women.

However, the estrogen deficient-slow processor is definitely hormone deficient and, as such, will often suffer from symptoms typical of women in menopause. However, because she tends more toward the production of inhibitory chemicals like serotonin, taurine, and GABA that calm and slow down the body, and is deficient in the stimulating and excitatory chemicals like dopamine and norepinephrine, she tends to lack energy, sex drive, mental acuity, and zest for life. (This is described in more detail in Chapter 13.)

In addition to the Western medical model detailed above, which describes these two opposing and complementary menopausal types in chemical and physiological terms, they can also be described energetically using the traditional Chinese model. In this model, health and well-being are believed to be a balance of two equally important, but opposing, principles—yin and yang. Yin is associated with attributes such as femininity, receptivity, calmness, coolness, and moisture. Yin also regulates the fluids, blood, and tissues of your body, as well as its structural components, including flesh, tendons, and bones. Yang, on the other hand, is associated with masculinity, aggression, heat, and dryness. It also regulates your body's energy, which acts as the spark plug to your structural elements. Its effect on tissues such as your muscles, tendons, and joints tends to be contractive. This is particularly true for estrogen deficient women who are fast processors.

Therefore, an estrogen deficient-fast processor tends to be more yang and has a yin deficiency. Conversely, an estrogen deficient-slow processor has excess yin and a yang deficiency. For more information on this concept, see **Section Four: Energy Medicine for Healthy Hormones**.

WHAT'S YOUR TYPE?

As you follow through the book, you'll notice that all of the recommendations are based on whether you are estrogen dominant, an estrogen deficient-fast processor, or an estrogen deficient-slow processor. Use the checklist below to determine your type so you can get started on your journey to healthy hormonal balance.

Estrogen Dominance
✓ PMS
✓ menstrual cramps
✓ irregular menstrual periods
✓ heavy menstrual bleeding
✓ bloating
✓ oily skin and hair
✓ fibroid tumors
✓ endometriosis
✓ increased risk of breast cancer
✓ mood swings

Estrogen Deficiency–Fast Processor
✓ menopausal
✓ more anxious
✓ wiry
✓ thin and dry skin, hair, and other tissues
✓ hot flashes
✓ night sweats
✓ insomnia
✓ vaginal dryness

✓ sore joints
✓ rheumatoid arthritis
✓ increased risk for heart disease
✓ increased risk of breast cancer
✓ osteoporosis

Estrogen Deficiency–Slow Processor
✓ menopausal
✓ excess weight and/or a more difficult time losing weight
✓ fluid retention
✓ thicker bones and connective tissue
✓ beautiful skin and hair
✓ placid temperament
✓ lack of energy
✓ low libido
✓ poor mental acuity
✓ lack of zest for life
✓ osteoarthritis
✓ increased risk of breast cancer
✓ increased risk for heart disease

My objective is to help bring you back into the mid-range, naturally and effectively, no matter which of these categories you fall into. When you reach this place of greater balance, you will notice that your symptoms will begin to recede and eventually disappear altogether. You'll have renewed energy, great skin and hair, optimal weight, mental focus, and improved overall health and well-being. In short, you will feel fantastic when you reach this nirvana and start feeling the way a person in balance feels—happier, cheerier, and in love with life.

That is what every chapter in this book is designed to accomplish. The first section provides an overview of the five major sex hormones (estrogen, progesterone, testosterone, DHEA, and pregnenolone), and how they should work in a healthy balance.

The second section takes a look at the current conventional and usually dangerous treatment options and why you should take great care to avoid them. I then discuss my program in general terms, and explain why it is the safest, healthiest, most effective way for you to bring your hormones back into proper balance.

The third section takes a look at each of the individual sex hormones and lays out my three approaches to bringing them into balance. The first is to restore your own hormones. In fact, everything in the book is designed toward helping you restore your own hormones and bring you into balance. Next, you'll learn about a wide variety of nutrients that provide hormonal support and even act as hormonal mimics. Finally, we'll discuss the use and benefit of chemically bioidentical hormones.

The fourth section discusses the use of energy medicine therapies to help restore your hormones back to the healthier middle range. I'll discuss acupuncture and acupressure; chakra and color therapy; light therapy; electrotherapy; biofeedback; and frequency and sound therapy. With each of these therapies, I have customized programs for you so that you can use them to help correct your specific hormonal imbalance profile.

Finally, the fifth section discusses the role that diet, exercise, and stress reduction play in hormonal health. You'll learn how to "eat for your type," discover the best kind of exercise regimen for your hormonal profile, and encounter wonderful and effective stress reduction techniques that will make you feel happier, joyful, peaceful, and full of light and love.

Plus, you'll have an easy-to-use Resource Guide that has every supplement, device, food, beverage, CD, DVD, and piece of exercise equipment mentioned throughout the book all in one location for your convenience. I've even included a few additional suggestions for you! And, if you are curious about any of the research studies I reference, there is a vast and complete bibliography for you as well.

How to Use This Book

The true beauty of my program is that you get to pick and choose from all of these different therapies and decide how you want to start your own program. If you're interested in learning about the chemistry and physiology of hormone production, you can. Conversely, if you are not interested in the physiological material and want to skip those chapters and go right to the therapy sections of the book, that is fine too. There is no right or wrong way to use this book.

Similarly, not every woman will use the program to accomplish the same goal. I have used the program to delay menopause and support healthy menstruation, as well as maintain excellent general health and well-being, energy, and stamina. Kimberly uses it to keep her estrogen and progesterone levels in proper balance so she can have healthier menstrual periods, ovulate regularly, and eventually conceive. I've had patients use my program to successfully relieve menopause symptoms, reduce their risk of heart disease, alleviate arthritis, strengthen their bones and reverse osteoporosis, lose weight, restore the health and beauty of their skin and hair, tone their body, treat insomnia, melt away fibroid tumors and endometriosis, regulate their menstrual cycles, correct heavy and irregular menstrual bleeding, and eliminate breast cysts and tenderness.

The key is that everyone's goals are different. Whether you are in your 30's and 40's and have fibroids, PMS, and perimenopause; are into your 50's and 60's and have hot flashes, insomnia, and low libido; or are in your 70's, 80's, or 90's and want to prevent senility, maintain good cognitive function, enjoy a strong heart and bones, and ease arthritis, my program will go a long way to help you. For this reason, some information is repeated in a couple of areas to ensure that important data and recommendations are not missed.

Finally, you don't have to follow the recommendations in any particular order. If you want to start with diet and exercise, you can skip ahead to those chapters. If the supplement recommendations appeal to you, you can start there. And if the energy therapies I discuss sound particularly intriguing, by all means, give them a try first.

Whatever you decide, start slowly and choose those therapies that most appeal to you. I've found that it's better to start with a few changes you feel will have a powerful and positive effect on your hormonal health than to try to do too much all at once.

Next, put together a plan that utilizes a few more of the other treatments that I discuss. This may include changing your diet, the type of exercise you do and how often you do it, the techniques you practice to handle stress, or taking different types of nutritional supplements, as well as trying some of the energy therapies you feel are important and may help to correct your own personal hormonal issues.

Most importantly, it is crucial that you keep your program as easy to implement as possible. Be realistic about your available time and financial resources. Putting together a program that is too complicated, time-consuming, or expensive is a setup for failure.

Once you have mastered making a few positive changes in your life and have seen their benefits, you can then go on to institute additional changes. I have personally been thrilled and very proud of myself over these many decades when I have seen my own hormonal issues and imbalances resolve. I know you will too.

Lots of love to you,

Susan

healthy hormones

Every woman I know wants to enjoy strength, vitality, and vigor. She wants to maintain optimum health, radiant skin, and luxurious hair. She also wants to stay physically active and vital, and still be able to think clearly and remember facts and events. That's where hormones come in.

Thousands of research studies and decades of clinical experience have confirmed that the maintenance of sex hormones can go a long way toward helping women remain strong, healthy, and beautiful for years to come. Of all the hormones in your body, five are particularly important: estrogen, progesterone, testosterone, DHEA, and pregnenolone.

In this section, we'll take a look at the role each of these hormones play in helping you maintain virtually every aspect of health. Specifically, I'll address the individual chemistries of each hormone, how it affects your body, and how health and lifestyle affects the levels of the hormone. We'll also discuss how all of these hormones need to be in proper balance in order to create and maintain optimum health.

continued

Finally, we'll explore the four distinct phases of a woman's life: normal menstruation, premenopause, perimenopause, and menopause. As we travel this hormonal path of life, I'll define each phase so you can identify where you are in nature's cycle.

I've been researching hormones and their effect on the body for more than three decades. After the thousands of research studies I've read, paired with decades of clinical experience, I have confirmed that the maintenance of sex hormones can go a long way toward helping most people remain vital, strong, and healthy well into old age.

Research also suggests that the maintenance of sex hormone levels can play a major preventive role in such debilitating conditions as cardiovascular disease, osteoporosis, and even Alzheimer's disease. It can also play an important role in helping to sustain your productivity and physical vigor. Sufficient levels of sex hormones support the balance you need to extend your career well beyond the normal retirement age, or to maintain your sexual vigor.

Of the various steroid hormones made by the adrenal glands and the reproductive organs, five have a profound effect on the quality of a person's life: the two precursor hormones pregnenolone and DHEA; and the three sex hormones estrogen, progesterone (the two primary female sex hormones), and testosterone (the primary male sex hormone). For optimal health, a person needs adequate levels of all five. In the following chapters, we'll discuss these important hormones in detail, as well as how you can maintain them either through replacement therapy, nutritional therapies, or techniques that help to sustain your own hormone production.

how
hormones
work

Hormones are powerful substances that function as the chemical messengers of the body. They are primarily secreted by your glands and released into the bloodstream, where they circulate either to a target gland or to various tissues of the body. Hormones either stimulate a target gland to release its own hormone or directly trigger chemical reactions in the tissues.

The glands of the body (also referred to as the endocrine system) secrete dozens of hormones, which have a multitude of physiological effects on target tissues. Working in concert, hormones initiate and coordinate cellular events, as well as balance and pace various physiological processes. As an integral part of many bodily functions, hormones enhance cognitive abilities, help stabilize mood, and are essential for health, promoting growth, healing, and repair. They play a crucial role in preventing the onset of many ailments, such as cardiovascular disease, Alzheimer's disease, and osteoporosis. Considering all the functions that hormones influence, it is no wonder that achieving optimum health is not possible without an optimally functioning endocrine system.

What Are Sex Hormones?

Sex hormones belong to a classification called steroid hormones, which are all derived from cholesterol, a waxy, white, fatty material found in all cells of the body. Other steroid hormones are the stress hormones, the glucocorticoids, and the mineralocorticoids. The steroid hormones are made in the adrenal glands, as well as the ovaries. Within these tissues, cholesterol is converted to hormones through a number of intermediary steps, leading to the final production of three major sex hormones—estrogen, progesterone, and testosterone.

While women produce all three major sex hormones, estrogen and progesterone predominate, supporting normal functioning of the reproductive tract and menstrual cycle. The ovaries and adrenals also make small amounts of male hormones, or androgens. Although they are only secreted in tiny amounts, androgens play a vital role in the female libido, or sex drive, as well as helping to maintain bone mass. The sex hormones also help to determine the physical characteristics, such as skin texture, muscle tone, and body shape.

How Sex Hormones Are Produced Within the Body

Sex hormones are produced through a series of chemical reactions, beginning with cholesterol. Of the total cholesterol in the body, about 75 percent is produced in the liver. The remaining 25 percent is supplied in the diet by foods such as meat and dairy products. On average, a person's body contains about one-third of a pound of cholesterol (150 g), mostly as a component of cell membranes. There are also about seven grams of cholesterol that circulate in the blood.

Both the overproduction and the underproduction of cholesterol can lead to hormone imbalances. People who go on stringent low-fat diets may lower their levels of cholesterol to such a degree that they don't have enough to make sufficient amounts of hormones. For

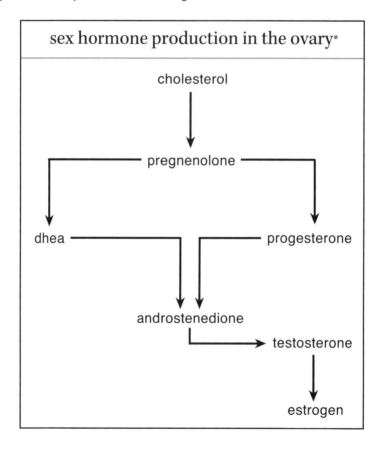

*For women in their active reproductive years, the DHEA pathway occurs during the first half of the menstrual cycle and the progesterone pathway normally occurs during the second half. Women in menopause normally go through only the DHEA pathway.

Sex hormone production in men occurs primarily in the testicles. The main male sex hormone, testosterone, is produced from cholesterol or acetyl coenzyme A. Male sex hormones are also produced by the adrenal glands.

example, teenage girls who go on crash diets often have irregular menstrual cycles, as their body's production of estrogen and progesterone, which regulate the cycle, diminishes. At the other extreme, people who are obese and eat the high-fat foods of the standard American diet have the opposite risk: Their bodies make too much cholesterol, making them prone to diseases and disorders for which elevated levels of estrogen are a risk factor, including premenstrual syndrome (PMS), fibroid tumors, fibrocystic disease of the breast, heavy menstrual bleeding, and uterine cancer.

In the hormonal pathway, cholesterol is first converted into pregnenolone, a steroid hormone that is the precursor to all the other sex hormones. Because of its precursor role, pregnenolone is considered the mother sex hormone, thus inspiring its name. Pregnenolone is then converted into a variety of other hormones, following two pathways. By one route, pregnenolone leads to DHEA, which is then converted into testosterone and subsequently estrogen. This pathway is operative in women during the first half of the menstrual cycle, when estrogen is the dominant hormone. In the second pathway, pregnenolone is converted into progesterone. The progesterone is then converted into testosterone and, finally, into estrogen. In females, this second pathway predominates during the second half of the menstrual cycle, when progesterone and estrogen are dominant.

How Hormones Deliver Their Messages

Each hormone is coded to bind only to certain tissues. The cells in these hormone-sensitive tissues contain specific receptors. When a hormone reaches its target tissue, it binds to these receptors like a key fitting into a lock. When binding occurs, the hormone then transmits its chemical message to the target tissue, causing a change in the tissue. For example, estrogen is a growth-stimulating hormone that causes tissues to grow and thicken, while progesterone is a growth-limiting hormone. Some hormones can cause rapid changes in a target tissue, occurring literally within seconds, while other reactions may take several days, but may then have a continuing influence for days or even years.

2 estrogen

Estrogen is the "queen bee" of the female sex hormones. As one of the two major female sex hormones, it is an especially important factor in health for women. When many women enter their menopausal years, it's as if they cross over an invisible line in their lives. As a result of the decline in their estrogen levels, these women find that many of the functions needed for peak performance, which had formerly been effortless, seem to evaporate or diminish. While women often do complain of menopausal symptoms that are strictly physical—such as vaginal dryness, more frequent bladder and vaginal infections, and dryness of the skin—they complain just as often about menopausal symptoms that impair their job performance, social relationships, and even their ability to take pleasure in day-to-day activities.

Many of the long-term consequences of estrogen deficiency during the menopausal years, such as osteoporosis and an increased risk of heart attacks and strokes, do not initially produce symptoms. It is important that women check their risk of these conditions at the time of menopause with tests such as lipid panels and bone density studies as well as routine blood cell counts and blood chemistry. Many of these tests provide sensitive and very helpful indicators of early risk and are particularly important for women who do not want to use conventional hormone replacement therapy. For a description of these laboratory tests of estrogen levels, see page 104.

I have always been amazed by the number of female patients I have worked with who reach menopause and begin to complain of forgetfulness and memory loss. Small details of life, such as remembering someone's name or where they put the car keys, suddenly become an issue. Competent performance at work is a real concern for some of these women. They report going from one office to another with no idea of why they went there. They may even complain about an inability to recall important work data. Virtually all of my patients who suffer from forgetfulness and memory loss are concerned about this problem. Some of them wonder if they are in the early stages of senility or even Alzheimer's disease. Fortunately, this is rarely the case. However, the brain is loaded with hormone receptors, and your normal mental and emotional functions depend, in part, on the abundant production of female sex hormones.

While memory loss can affect a woman's competence at work, frequent hot flashes can be downright embarrassing. Women with more severe symptoms may have as many as 10, 20, or even 40 episodes a day. Hot flashes cause a woman to turn pink and either perspire profusely or simply generate a lot of heat within the body. In any case, women often feel like shedding clothes, which is often not possible in a professional setting.

Hot flashes are triggered by stress and often occur at the worst possible times. Some of my patients report having hot flashes and starting to sweat profusely when presenting a report in front of a professional audience, in meetings with important customers, or when going for a job interview. Hot flashes also frequently occur at night, waking the woman, and sometimes even her bedmate, from a deep sleep. Frequently interrupted sleep can cause any-one to be tired, irritable, and relatively unproductive the next day.

In addition, the ability to experience joy in life can be blunted by the onset of menopause. The hormones produced within the ovaries as well as within the adrenal glands are crucial for maintaining sexual pleasure, a sense of emotional well-being, optimism, and many other qualities that many women regard as essential for an exciting and satisfying life.

The negative effects of the natural decline in female sex hormone production during menopause are not uncommon. Menopausal symptoms are so common in the United States that 80 to 85 percent of American women experience them to some degree. A small num-ber of these women are lucky enough to have mild symptoms, such as occasional hot flashes over a period of a few months to a year. However, the majority of women have symptoms that are bothersome enough to cause them to seek the help of physicians or complementary health care practitioners, or to seek solutions on their own by reading books and articles and exploring the use of natural hormones, vitamins, and herbs to relieve their symptoms.

The Chemistry of Estrogen

Estrogen, along with progesterone, is one of the two major hormones that support the func-tioning of the female reproductive organs and the menstrual cycle. The ovaries and adrenal glands produce substantial amounts of estrogen during a woman's active reproductive years and continue to produce small amounts after menopause. While we are accustomed to using the term *estrogen*, this term actually refers to several different types of estrogens made within the body. At least six types of estrogen have been identified and are classified according to their potency. The term *potency* refers to the time that estrogen is bound to the estrogen receptor within a specific tissue. The higher the estrogen potency, the more time it remains bound to the receptor and, therefore, the more pronounced are the physiological effects that estrogen promotes within that tissue. For example, estrogen is a growth-stimulating hor-mone, causing tissues to grow and thicken; it also causes water and salt to be retained within the tissues of the body. The more potent and powerful forms of estrogen cause these effects to occur in a more pronounced fashion.

The three main types of estrogen produced within the body are estradiol, estrone, and estriol. Estradiol is the most potent form of estrogen. It is the primary type of estrogen produced by the ovaries during a woman's reproductive years. Estrone is an intermediate-potency form of estrogen, 12 times weaker than estradiol. It is mainly produced within the fatty tissue of the body from precursor hormones made by the adrenal glands. Obviously, the more weight a woman carries, the more adrenal estrogen she is capable of making. Small amounts of estrone are also produced by the ovaries after menopause, when production of estradiol ceases.

As estradiol and estrone circulate through the body, they pass through the liver. It is the liver's job to detoxify and metabolize these two estrogens to a weaker form, which can then be eliminated from the body. Since estrogen is constantly being produced by the ovaries and adrenal glands, the liver helps to prevent its accumulation to toxic levels. Estriol, the liver metabolite of the other two estrogens, is the weakest form of estrogen produced by the body. It is 80 times weaker than estradiol.

ESTROGEN AND AGING

The amount of estrogen a woman produces changes during her lifetime. The normal output of estradiol is 100 to 300 mcg a day. Estrogen is also produced in pregnancy by the placenta (a spongy structure in the uterus, from which the fetus derives oxygen and nourishment). The placenta produces estrogen in great quantity, as much as 100 times the amount normally made by the ovaries.

Levels of estrogen also fluctuate during the month because of menstruation, reaching peak levels during the first half of the menstrual cycle. During the second half of the cycle, both estrogen and progesterone predominate, though estrogen production does decline somewhat from its levels earlier in the month.

With the onset of menopause, after menstruation has ceased entirely, ovarian production of estrogen is greatly reduced, and levels of circulating estrogen decline by as much as 75 to 90 percent. However, after menopause, one-fourth to one-third of all American women continue to make enough ovarian and adrenal estrogen in its weaker form, estrone. While the quantity produced is not enough to cause a monthly menstrual cycle, it is sufficient to support the health of tissues such as bone, skin, and the vaginal lining. Although being overweight is a liability for many health conditions, those women who have more fatty tissue are better able to convert androgens to estrone after menopause. Consequently, they tend to have stronger bones and more youthful-looking skin. These women who maintain estrogen production after menopause probably do not need to consider hormone replacement therapy for ten to fifteen more years. The majority of women, however, have an abrupt decline in their estrogen production to the point that uncomfortable symptoms will lead these women to seek medical care.

How Estrogen Affects the Body

The effect that estrogen has on a woman's body begins even before birth, since estrogen plays an important role in the development of female sexual characteristics. During childhood, a girl's body produces only small amounts of estrogen. Then, at puberty, when estrogen production increases twenty-fold or more, these higher levels stimulate the female sexual organs of young girls to begin to mature into those of an adult woman.

Estrogen causes the uterus and vagina to increase in size. It stimulates the vagina and urinary tract linings to thicken and become more resistant to trauma and infection, thus preparing a woman to eventually become sexually active and bear children. In addition, estrogen causes an increase in overall body fat, contributing to the softly rounded female contours that we associate with sexual maturation. Firm, youthful-looking skin is also attributable to estrogen, which stimulates collagen, a protein that makes up 90 percent of the skin. Estrogen promotes the growth of pubic hair and coloration of the nipples and also stimulates bone growth. Beginning at puberty, when estrogen production soars, a young woman's height also rapidly increases.

The various actions of estrogen are balanced by the complementary effects of progesterone. These two hormones, working together, help regulate a notably wide range of physiological processes. For instance, estrogen decreases the level of oxygen in cells, and progesterone restores oxygen to normal levels. While estrogen increases body fat, progesterone helps the body burn fat for energy. Estrogen also promotes salt and fluid retention, whereas progesterone is a natural diuretic, increasing the flow of urine. Estrogen promotes blood clotting, while progesterone normalizes clotting. Furthermore, estrogen impairs blood sugar control, and progesterone normalizes blood sugar levels. When these hormones are in balance, they provide a host of health benefits.

BENEFITS OF ESTROGEN

- Prevents menopausal symptoms
- Protects against heart disease and stroke
- Prevents osteoporosis and joint disease
- Increases physical vitality and stamina
- Enhances mental clarity and acuity

How Diet, Health, and the Environment Affect Estrogen Levels

While estrogen production declines with age, the amount of estrogen in the body will also be influenced by a range of other factors, including diet, digestive capabilities, liver function, enzyme levels, and exposure to environmental toxins—a topic that has not received sufficient attention to date.

Diet

Meat, poultry, and dairy foods contain estrogens that have been injected into the animals to fatten them for market. One of the synthetic estrogens routinely given to livestock was DES (diethylstilbestrol). DES was also given to women to prevent miscarriages and symptoms of menopause, until it was associated with birth defects in their offspring and was finally banned in 1979. However, today poultry and livestock, especially dairy cows, are still given other forms of estrogen compounds. Hormones such as estrogen accumulate in fatty tissue in the animals we eat as well as in us, and high-fat diets have been associated with changes in human estrogen levels.

Caffeine and alcohol consumption can also influence estrogen levels. Excessive alcohol intake can affect the liver's ability to break down estrogen for excretion, thereby elevating the body's blood estrogen levels, particularly of the more chemically active forms of estrogen. A three-year study appearing in the *American Journal of Epidemiology*, involving 728 white, postmenopausal females aged 42 to 90, found that caffeine intake had an effect on estrogen levels. Having more than two cups of coffee or four cans of caffeinated soda per day increased blood levels of this hormone. Another research study suggested that a diet high in sugar may impair liver function, affecting its ability to metabolize estrogen. Even the public water supply may contain estrogens, if that water is recycled at treatment plants and still contains traces of excreted synthetic estrogens such as those contained in birth control pills and excreted from the bodies of women using these products.

Physiological Factors

Poor digestive function can prevent hormone precursors such as fat molecules from being absorbed. Problems with the liver can also lead to low levels of hormones. Persons with functional disorders of the liver have been shown to have low levels of estrogen. When liver enzyme systems are impaired and the detoxification function is inadequate, the quantity and quality of hormone formation is reduced. Depressed levels of HDL cholesterol can also lead to lower levels of estrogen, as this deficiency blocks the biochemical pathway required for the production of the primary precursor hormone, pregnenolone, and all the consequent sex hormones.

Environmental Estrogens

Pollutants that have estrogen-like activity when they are taken into the body (xenoestrogens) are found in an enormous range of products for the home and workplace. They are present in cosmetics, detergents and dishwashing liquids, and bug spray. Pesticides and industrial chemicals such as organochlorines, dioxins, and PCBs (polychlorinated biphenyls) also contain substances related to estrogen. A study from Stanford University, published in the *Journal of the American Medical Association*, noted that when polycarbonate plastics are heated, they release bisphenol-A, a substance that is known to have estrogenic activity. Microwaving foods in plastic containers or using a plastic cup for hot coffee can cause estrogen substances to shed into the food.

There are many suspected health consequences of our wide exposure to xenoestrogens, including an increased risk of PMS and breast cancer. This problem has also affected male reproductive health, and has been implicated in lowering sperm counts in men all over the world.

According to a study published in the *British Medical Journal*, there has been a clear decline in the average sperm count worldwide during the last 50 years. The researchers conducted an analysis of 61 papers that involved a total of 14,947 men. When the results were compared, the researchers found that the average sperm count had decreased by nearly half from the late 1930's to the early 1990's. A further study, published in the *Lancet*, found that the multiplication of Sertoli cells, which are responsible for sperm production, is inhibited by estrogen.

3 progesterone

Progesterone is the yang to estrogen's yin. While estrogen is a growth-stimulating and expansive hormone, progesterone tends to limit the growth of tissue, therefore having a more contractive or yangizing effect on the body. Often a "silent partner," progesterone is produced in the ovaries in women, with some production in the adrenals. During pregnancy, as the fetus matures, the placenta produces large amounts of progesterone (the name actually means "for gestation"). In women, progesterone works in tandem with estrogen, in many cases acting to balance the effects of that hormone. Low levels of progesterone can contribute to a number of health conditions and can negatively affect one's outlook on life, energy level, and emotions.

BENEFITS OF PROGESTERONE
- Helps control excessive and irregular menstrual bleeding during perimenopause
- Helps prevent health problems related to high estrogen levels, such as endometrial hyperplasia and uterine fibroids
- Reduces hot flashes
- Helps prevent uterine cancer
- Helps prevent osteoporosis
- Increases libido
- Aids in the healing of certain types of nerve disease
- Improves sleep patterns
- Enhances mental clarity and acuity

The Chemistry of Progesterone

The chemical structure of progesterone is similar to that of the other sex hormones, such as estrogen and testosterone, and like the other sex hormones, it is converted from the precursor hormone pregnenolone.

The progesterone used in replacement therapy today, whether described as synthetic or natural, is all produced by commercial laboratories. The terms *natural* and *synthetic* refer to the actual structure of the progesterone molecule. Progesterone that is natural has the same structure as the hormone the body produces. In contrast, while synthetic progesterone has the same function as the progesterone produced by the body, its structure differs slightly. In the United States, most prescriptions are for the synthetic form, called a progestin. The most common progestin is Provera, or medroxyprogesterone.

Natural progesterone became available in the early 1980's, but initially only as a rectal or vaginal suppository. Although many women found the use of natural progesterone to be helpful, using it as a suppository was messy, since it tended to leak from the rectum or vagina. Progestin remained the preferred form because it was easy to take as a pill and also more absorbable. However, a natural progesterone was subsequently developed in a micronized form (pulverized into tiny particles) that is readily absorbed and is taken orally. Today, many women prefer using natural progesterone, as it produces fewer side effects.

The Role of Progesterone in Menstruation and Pregnancy

The purpose of the menstrual cycle is to prepare the female body for conception and possible pregnancy. The process depends on the balanced interaction of several hormones, especially estrogen and progesterone. Working together, they prepare the lining of the uterus (the endometrium) to receive a fertilized egg, should pregnancy occur. The surge of progesterone after an egg is released from the ovarian follicle greatly stimulates the libido, which increases the likelihood that a sperm will enter the female and unite with the egg.

The increase in production of progesterone at mid-cycle causes a rise in body temperature of about 0.5° to 1°F, which many women monitor to identify when ovulation is most likely to occur and therefore the days when they are fertile. If the egg does not unite with a sperm, progesterone output declines. This stimulates the cells of the uterine lining to slough off and be excreted, which is experienced as menstruation. A rapid decline in progesterone triggers the monthly menstrual bleeding.

During a woman's monthly cycle, the level of progesterone rises and falls dramatically, from 2 to 3 mg per day in the first half of the month, to 22 mg per day in the second half of the month. Production in some women a week after ovulation may be as high as 30 mg per day.

Should pregnancy occur, the placenta also begins to produce progesterone, greatly adding to the amount in circulation. By the fourth month of gestation, a woman produces 10 times her normal amount. During the last months of pregnancy, daily production can be as high as 300 to 400 mg a day. To appreciate the significance of this quantity, consider that the various hormones produced within the body are usually measured in micrograms (a thousand-fold less).

How Progesterone Affects the Body

While estrogen causes tissues to grow and thicken, progesterone has a maturing and growth-limiting effect on these tissues. For example, progesterone prevents the uterine lining from becoming too thick during the second half of the menstrual cycle and even, over time, from becoming cancerous. Progesterone also prevents menstrual bleeding from becoming too profuse or long lasting.

Progesterone and estrogen have a balancing effect in other ways as well, affecting many physical and chemical functions in the body. For example, progesterone acts as a sedative on the nervous system, and high levels of progesterone can cause depression and fatigue. In contrast, estrogen has a stimulatory effect on the nervous system. In fact, increased levels of estrogen can trigger anxiety, irritability, and mood swings. Progesterone tends to elevate the blood sugar level, while estrogen lowers it. Thus, the healthy balance between these two female sex hormones is crucial.

How Lifestyle and Health Affect Progesterone Levels

Progesterone production diminishes with age, but its output is influenced by lifestyle factors as well. Digestive capability and liver function will also influence progesterone levels. Following is a discussion of how all these factors affect progesterone production.

Exercise

Women who exercise a great deal and consequently have low levels of body fat may eventually no longer ovulate once a month. This is most frequently seen in female athletes, dancers, and other extremely physically active women. When this happens, the body does not have sufficient levels of cholesterol to manufacture the hormones needed to cause ovulation to occur. And when a women is anovulatory, the ovaries cease making progesterone.

Stress

Physical, emotional, and mental stress can inhibit the production of progesterone. When the body is put through long-term physical stress, as is true of athletes, the daily rhythms of hormone production, including progesterone, can be disrupted.

Physiological Factors

People with poor digestion are unable to absorb certain hormone precursors, which limits hormone production. Poor liver function, with reduced activity of liver enzyme systems, can also lead to lower levels of progesterone, as the conversion of pregnenolone to DHEA and progesterone is impaired.

testosterone 4

I've always felt that testosterone is often misunderstood by women. While most often associated with men, muscles, and aggression, testosterone is a critical hormone for women as well. It plays a key role in drive and assertiveness. It also supports your energy, mental agility, mood, outlook on life, and sex drive.

Admittedly, most women I know forget about testosterone when they think about their unique set of hormones. And although they produce much smaller amounts of testosterone, it is just as important for hormonal balance as the more feminine hormones estrogen and progesterone.

BENEFITS OF TESTOSTERONE

- Relieves menopausal symptoms such as hot flashes, nervousness, and vaginal dryness
- Helps prevent osteoporosis
- Balances mood
- Restores energy
- Enhances libido

The Chemistry of Testosterone

Testosterone is the predominant male sex hormone, or androgen, a substance that stimulates the development of male sexual characteristics. All androgens, including testosterone, are steroid compounds and share a similar structure. They can all be synthesized from cholesterol or made directly from acetyl coenzyme A, a chemical produced in the liver and made from fatty acids and amino acids.

The use of testosterone to increase libido has a long history. Traditional healers have used the sexual organs and glands of male animals to restore potency in men. These medicines probably contained small quantities of animal testosterone. The search for a male elixir continued into modern times. In France, in the late 19th century, physiologist Charles-Edouard Brown-Sequard injected himself with fluid extracted from animal testicles and pronounced the substance rejuvenating. The use of such substances to treat male impotence became a fad in the first decades of this century; however, it is questionable whether these contained active ingredients or only had a placebo effect. Then in 1934, scientists synthesized testosterone from cholesterol, preparing the way for the development of present-day testosterone replacement therapy.

The Production of Testosterone in Women

Women make small amounts of testosterone in the ovaries and adrenal glands. The precursor to testosterone is androstenedione. Like estrogen and progesterone, the level of androstenedione varies throughout a woman's menstrual cycle. The level rises at midcycle, when androstenedione is secreted from the ovarian follicle (a structure in the ovary containing a female reproductive cell), and during the second half of the menstrual cycle, when it is produced by the corpus luteum (a structure that develops within the ruptured ovarian follicle after ovulation or the release of the egg from the ovary and that secretes progesterone and estrogen).

How Testosterone Affects the Body

Testosterone plays an important role in normal female sexual development. The initiation of menstruation and puberty is, in part, triggered by testosterone production. Testosterone stimulates libido in women. Levels of the hormone rise and decline during the menstrual cycle to insure that sexual desire increases just before ovulation, when a woman is fertile and chances are greatest for conception. Testosterone also restores vitality and energy levels, helps reduce depression, and (in part) engenders in women the attributes of assertiveness and aggressiveness usually associated with male behavior. Testosterone also benefits female health by helping to strengthen bones and minimize the symptoms of menopause.

How Diet, Lifestyle, and Health Affect Testosterone Levels

The aging process affects testosterone levels in both men and women, but testosterone levels are also sensitive to various environmental factors such as diet, alcohol use, lifestyle habits such as smoking, stress levels, and a person's general state of health. Poor lifestyle habits can negatively impact testosterone production.

Diet

Eating a typical American high-fat diet can alter testosterone levels. This correlation was demonstrated in a study published in *Modern Medicine*. Eight healthy men, ages 23 to 35, were given a daily milk shake containing 800 calories, 57 percent of which was fat. The researchers found that following the high-fat meal, blood levels of testosterone dropped by about 30 percent. How much caffeine and alcohol a person consumes will also affect testosterone levels. The effect of caffeine on testosterone levels in women was investigated in a large study published in the *American Journal of Epidemiology*. Women who had more than two cups of coffee or four cans of caffeinated soda per day experienced a decline in testosterone levels.

Stress

Stress is also associated with diminished hormone levels, as evidenced in a study appearing in the *Journal of Internal Medicine*. The study examined 439 men, all aged 51, and found that chronic psychosocial stresses such as tense, difficult working conditions, painful thoughts, and sad feelings were associated with a low testosterone level. The researchers suggested that chronic stress contributed to premature aging.

Physiological Factors

Having a low level of HDL cholesterol, which performs the function of transporting hormones, can impair the body's ability to produce testosterone. Poor digestive function can also be a limiting factor. The ability of the body to absorb certain substances such as fat molecules and fragments of protein from which hormones are manufactured affects the quantity of testosterone that the body can produce. How well the liver is able to break down toxins and metabolize hormones will also impact testosterone levels.

5 pregnenolone

If you are like the majority of people, you have most likely never heard of the hormone pregnenolone. Ironically, it's the most important of the five primary sex hormones. In fact, it is often referred to as the "mother hormone," due to its pivotal role in the production of all the others.

As a precursor to all the major sex hormones, pregnenolone has a widespread effect throughout the body. However, pregnenolone offers health benefits far beyond being a precursor. In animal and human studies, pregnenolone has been shown to increase energy, improve cognitive function, and stabilize moods. Other studies suggest that pregnenolone may be useful in reducing symptoms due to inflammation in cases of rheumatoid arthritis, spinal cord injuries, and possibly Alzheimer's disease.

BENEFITS OF PREGNENOLONE
- Helps to lessen symptoms of arthritis and other autoimmune diseases
- Useful in speeding recovery from spinal cord injuries
- Helpful in the treatment of Alzheimer's disease and multiple sclerosis
- Helps treat PMS and menopause transition symptoms
- Helps balance mood

Pregnenolone was first synthesized in Germany in 1934, and by the 1940's, researchers had begun to study its many uses, including reducing fatigue, increasing physical and mental endurance, and in treating various inflammatory conditions. However, this research came to a halt in the 1950's when synthetic cortisone became the therapy of choice for such diseases as rheumatoid arthritis. Cortisone relieved symptoms quickly, while pregnenolone sometimes required weeks to produce results. Furthermore, synthetic cortisone could be patented, turning it into a highly lucrative drug, so pharmaceutical companies were far more motivated to develop cortisone as a product, and research on pregnenolone was abandoned. Subsequently, patients on cortisone began to suffer its harmful side effects, including a weakening of the immune system and a deterioration of bone mass leading to osteoporosis. Unfortunately, by the time these side effects were fully known, cortisone was established as a widely accepted treatment, and pregnenolone therapy, although known to be nontoxic, was forgotten.

Today pregnenolone is again being studied, thanks to the widespread renewed interest in natural therapies. Researchers are investigating pregnenolone in relation to a wide range of topics, including memory, mood, enzyme activity, joint function, premenstrual syndrome, and the aging process. Given the exciting results of these studies, the potential benefits that pregnenolone can provide in the health arena deserve greater attention.

The Chemistry of Pregnenolone

Pregnenolone is made primarily in the adrenal glands, but it is also produced in the cells of the liver, skin, ovaries, and brain. It is manufactured in the mitochondria, the energy-producing factories of the cells. In the mitochondria, nutrients from your diet are converted into usable energy, and cholesterol is converted into pregnenolone. The pituitary gland regulates the amount of pregnenolone produced. A study published in the *Journal of Steroid Biochemistry and Molecular Biology* found that pregnenolone accumulates in the brain, independent of sources in other areas of the body. This may have great significance, given the beneficial effects that pregnenolone seems to have on maintaining physical energy as well as stabilizing mood.

Pregnenolone levels are assessed by measuring the amount of pregnenolone sulfate in the blood. Pregnenolone sulfate is more water-soluble than pregnenolone itself, and is therefore more easily transported through the circulatory system. In adult men, blood levels of pregnenolone sulfate are about 10 mcg per 100 ml. Average daily production of pregnenolone is about 14 mg a day, a relatively small amount (30,000 mg equals about 1 ounce). However, these amounts may vary significantly among individuals.

How Health and Lifestyle Affect Pregnenolone Levels

A variety of factors can decrease pregnenolone production, as noted in an article published in *Biochemical Pharmacology*. In particular, stress and disease can lower levels of pregnenolone throughout the body and in specific tissues.

6   dhea

I first became aware of DHEA as a medical student more than 30 years ago while reading my textbooks on reproductive medicine. However, it was barely mentioned since no one seemed to know what it actually did. And when it was mentioned, it was always described as a hormone produced abundantly by the adrenal glands, the production of which appeared to diminish significantly with age.

During my early years in the medical field, I thought it odd that the body would produce so much of a hormone that seemed to have no purpose. As subsequent research studies on DHEA began to receive attention, both in the medical literature and in the popular press, it became apparent that my skepticism was well-founded. As you'll discover, DHEA is critical for maintaining many aspects of health.

BENEFITS OF DHEA
- Decreases the risk of heart disease
- Strengthens the immune system
- May be useful in the treatment of autoimmune diseases such as rheumatoid arthritis, lupus, ulcerative colitis, and multiple sclerosis
- May help prevent cancer
- Reduces body fat
- Lessens symptoms of menopause and osteoporosis in women
- May be useful in the treatment of diabetes, asthma, and burns
- Enhances mental clarity and acuity
- May enhance libido

The Chemistry of DHEA

DHEA is the abbreviation for dehydroepiandrosterone, one of the primary steroid sex hormones. Until about 20 years ago, scientists thought that DHEA had little use beyond its role as a precursor for other hormones. Only recently have studies begun to reveal its many physiologic activities that benefit both performance and health. Most DHEA is produced by the adrenal glands, with smaller amounts made in the brain and skin tissue. As discussed in the previous section, pregnenolone is converted to many other hormones via two pathways; the first stage in one of these pathways is the creation of DHEA. Curiously, not all animals make DHEA in significant amounts. It is produced in abundance by just the primates, which include humans, monkeys, apes, and gorillas.

Once DHEA is produced by the adrenals, it travels through the bloodstream to cells throughout the body. Within the glands and sex organs, it is converted to testosterone and estrogen. Some DHEA is also converted in the liver to a sulfur compound when a molecule of sulfate, which is sulfur plus oxygen, is added to it. This new substance is referred to as DHEA-S. It is thought that DHEA is predominantly produced in the morning. This form of the hormone is rapidly excreted through the kidneys. In contrast, DHEA-S is eliminated slowly, so levels remain more constant in the body. Because of the two different rates of excretion, of the total amount of this hormone in the blood, 90 percent is DHEA-S.

How DHEA Affects the Body

DHEA travels through the bloodstream to cells throughout the body. DHEA has been shown to enhance psychological well-being. A study cited in *Lancet* found that 70 percent of volunteers who were given 50 mg of DHEA per day reported increased feelings of well-being. A similar research study on DHEA found that individuals with higher DHEA levels handled stress better, were more optimistic, and seemed to lead fuller lives.

Additionally, other studies suggest that DHEA may lessen the effect of stress hormones like cortisol, thereby reducing the impact of stress on your body. Constant triggering of the stress response eventually leads to adrenal imbalance and finally exhaustion. One of the common consequences of this state of affairs is that cortisol and DHEA become unbalanced, with cortisol levels often rising too high while DHEA levels diminish. This imbalance is aggravated in perimenopause and menopause, since our production of DHEA normally drops significantly at this time.

How Diet, Health, and Lifestyle Affect DHEA Levels

In addition to the aging process, a poor diet, excessive stress, and lack of exercise can all lower DHEA levels.

Diet

Avoid or reduce your intake of caffeinated beverages, products made with refined sugar and white flour, alcohol, excessive amounts of fruit juice, MSG, aspartame (Nutrasweet), and foods to which you are allergic, since they all can stimulate the release of stress hormones, thereby reducing DHEA levels.

Stress

One study I found fascinating was done at the Institute of HeartMath in Boulder Creek, California. Researchers took DHEA samples from 28 volunteers, then asked them to listen to music specifically designed to promote a sense of peacefulness and emotional balance every day for one month. At the end of the month, researchers took a second DHEA sample from the volunteers. The results were impressive. Among all volunteers, DHEA levels increased, on average, 100 percent; for some, the levels tripled and even quadrupled. And since DHEA is a precursor hormone, this means that the hormones that arise from DHEA, such as testosterone and estrogen, are also more likely to increase with the use of the Heart-Math program.

Exercise

A study highlighted in *Age and Ageing* showed that regular moderate aerobic exercise and a physically active life enhanced higher production of DHEA in older people. Because of research such as this, I particularly recommend doing physical activities at least 4 to 5 days a week in order to help restore your DHEA levels. Aim for 30 minutes to an hour per session, outdoors if possible.

hormone
balance
through the years

As you can see, each and every one of your hormones has a significant and profound impact on your health. But the amazing thing is how they work together to help you maintain optimum health and vibrant energy. They perform this beautiful and intricate dance throughout your life, working together in perfect complement to keep you hormonally balanced.

While all five hormones play key roles in this dance, for the purpose of explaining how hormone levels fluctuate throughout your life, I'm going to focus on the two primary female sex hormones—estrogen and progesterone.

When estrogen and progesterone are produced in normal amounts, they have opposing and complementary effects on your body. For example, estrogen increases body fat while progesterone helps you burn fat for energy. Estrogen promotes salt and fluid retention, while progesterone acts as a natural diuretic. Similarly, estrogen hinders blood sugar control, while progesterone normalizes it. And on the flip side, estrogen lifts your mood while progesterone is more calming.

However, when these hormones are out of balance, your body and your health can pay a dear price.

It's a Balancing Act

Optimal hormone balance is achieved in two ways—producing complementary amounts of both estrogen and progesterone, and getting rid of excess hormones by metabolizing and excreting them from the body. Since we've already discussed hormone production, let's talk a bit about their breakdown and removal from the body.

Once a hormone has done its job in your body, it is no longer necessary. In a healthy body, the hormone is metabolized and broken down by your liver. In the case of estrogen, your liver will transform the strongest, most chemically active and efficient form of estrogen—estradiol—into other weaker forms of estrogen, namely estrone and estriol.

When your liver is working properly, it breaks estradiol down into estrone, then into estriol. However, if your liver cannot properly metabolize estradiol, it stays in your body for too long, wreaking havoc along the way. Research has shown that excess estradiol may be a risk factor for breast and uterine cancer, as well as a host of other adverse health conditions.

You may be asking yourself, "Why is estradiol so dangerous, but not the other two forms of estrogen?" That's because estradiol is 12 times more potent than estrone and 80 times more potent than estriol. This makes the total "estrogen effect" of estradiol several times greater than either of the other two forms. Therefore, smaller amounts are needed.

Two of the best ways to balance out estrogen is with proper breakdown and excretion of this hormone, as well as optimal progesterone production, which I'll discuss in more detail in Chapter 10.

For now, what you need to know is that proper balance between estrogen and progesterone is the key to a balanced mood, healthy sex drive, ideal body weight, and soft, firm skin. They can also offer protection against heart disease, stroke, osteoporosis and even Alzheimer's disease.

Estrogen and progesterone produce these positive effects in your body by binding to hormone receptors in tissues in your uterus, breasts, blood vessels, brain, bones and heart, as well as many other tissues. When a hormone reaches its target tissue, it binds to these receptor cells like a key fitting into a lock. When binding occurs, the hormone transmits its chemical message, causing a change in the tissue. In fact, the health of all of the tissues in your body is very sensitive to the healthy balance between estrogen and progesterone. And nowhere is this balance more evident or more critical than your menstrual cycle.

For example, hormones are at their peak during your younger years, when you are menstruating regularly. However, as you reach your 40's, your hormones often go haywire, either producing too much or too little estrogen. This is a key sign that you are entering the menopause transition. Eventually, every woman ends up with diminished hormone levels, signaling the end of her periods and the start of menopause.

To better understand this natural transition from menstruation to menopause, let's take a look at each stage individually.

The Normal Menstrual Cycle

To fully understand a normal menstrual cycle, you should first know why menstruation even occurs. Menstruation refers to the monthly shedding of the uterine lining. Every month, as your uterus prepares a home for a new baby, it creates a thick, blood-rich lining in which to cushion the fertilized egg.

If conception occurs, the egg will implant itself in this cushion within a week or so. If pregnancy does not occur, the cushion is no longer necessary, and your uterus cleanses itself of the unnecessary lining, making room for a new cushion to be created the next month. This monthly build up and break down of the uterine lining is controlled by hormones.

To trigger the start of your menstrual cycle, your hypothalamus and pituitary glands secrete a hormone (called FSH) that stimulates the follicle surrounding each egg in your ovaries and causes an egg to mature. During this process, the follicle produces increasingly high levels of estrogen. Your ovaries then produce estradiol, while your adrenal glands, triangular shaped organs resting atop each kidney, produce the weaker estrone form of estrogen.

At midcyle, a second hormone called the luteinizing hormone (LH) is produced by the pituitary gland. LH triggers the expulsion of the egg from the ovarian follicle. It also increases the synthesis of prostaglandins, short-lived hormones that are needed for this process to occur. Once ovulation has occurred, the egg leaves the ovary and travels down the fallopian tube to the uterus, where pregnancy can occur.

Both estrogen and progesterone are produced during this second half of the cycle by the corpus luteum. This is the structure that develops from the ruptured ovarian follicle after the egg is released from the ovary. If the egg isn't fertilized, both estrogen and progesterone production decline rapidly, triggering menstruation. It can take three to five days for your body to completely shed the uterine lining. Once it is complete, the hormone cycle starts all over again, with estrogen being produced during the entire menstrual cycle, and progesterone only produced during the second half of the cycle.

The Menopause Transition

As you enter your 40's, you may notice that the symptoms preceding your periods, as well as the length of the menstrual cycle and the amount of blood lost, will begin to change. This often signals the beginning of the menopause transition.

There are several variables associated with the menopause transition. It can occur as early as the mid-30's or as late as the upper 50's. Plus, it can last anywhere from one year to as long as five or six years. But what remains consistent is the wild hormonal fluctuations that occur. These fluctuations are the hallmark of the menopause transition.

Phase One: Premenopause

The first phase of the transition is premenopause. This phase is often marked by PMS symptoms such as irritability, anxiety, and bloating, as well as weight gain, fibroid tumors, endometriosis, breast tenderness, difficulty conceiving, and even mental fog and concentration problems.

During this time, your estrogen levels can fluctuate. For some women, their levels are too high, while other women will have normal to even lower levels of estrogen production. You also ovulate less frequently, which means that you are also producing less progesterone. Often, the progesterone levels are relatively deficient and unbalanced in relationship to the estrogen levels.

During this same time, your ovaries are beginning to age, actually undergoing physical and structural changes. They begin to shrink and become less responsive to the hypothalamic-pituitary signals. Additionally, you have much fewer eggs available to mature, and the eggs you do have left are older and less functional. This situation often prevents a follicle from maturing enough to expel an egg. When this happens, the second half of the menstrual cycle never kicks in properly, so progesterone isn't adequately produced. As a result, you often are left with too much estrogen and not enough progesterone—or estrogen dominance.

Estrogen dominance is often the cause of symptoms women experience during the pre-menopause phase of the transition. Estrogen dominance is marked by periods of heavy and/or irregular bleeding when the uterus sloughs off a lining that has been thickened by too much estrogen. This can occur either as a pattern of heavy, prolonged menstrual bleeding or irregular bleeding and spotting. Some women also have mid-cycle bleeding and pain during this time, depending on their underlying gynecological issues.

Some women also develop fibroid tumors during this time. Fibroid tumors are benign growths that usually form on the uterine wall. They can grow so large that in addition to causing heavy or irregular bleeding, they may also put pressure on the bladder or intestines, causing discomfort, frequent urination, or changes in bowel routines in some women. In some cases, they can become so large that a woman can appear to be in her second trimester of pregnancy! Other problems during premenopause include worsening of endometriosis-related pain, as well as the appearance of ovarian and breast cysts, tenderness, fluid retention, and bloating—all due to the shift towards estrogen dominance.

Eventually, this irregular and/or heavy bleeding will begin to taper off, signaling the start of phase two of the menopause transition—perimenopause.

Phase Two: Perimenopause

Some women may skip phase one altogether and only experience perimenopause. Like premenopause, perimenopause can also be marked by wildly fluctuating hormones, weight gain and irregular periods. Because estrogen levels are starting to decline significantly during this phase, you may also start to experience some menopause symptoms, such as hot flashes, insomnia, night sweats, decreased libido, and fatigue, even if you are still having menstrual periods.

However, unlike premenopause, your production of estrogen and testosterone are definitely diminishing. This can occur over several years. Additionally, you have less and less frequent ovulation, which means lower and lower levels of progesterone. This creates a state of hormone deficiency (especially estrogen), rather than a relative excess of estrogen as compared to progesterone, as seen with estrogen dominance.

And, instead of the heavy menstrual bleeding that occurs during premenopause, perimenopause is marked by fewer and fewer periods. Often, they will be spaced further and further apart, with less bleeding during each occurrence. Eventually, menstruation ceases entirely as you complete your transition into menopause.

Menopause: The Change of Life

Some lucky women—about 10 percent—make this transition easily. They simply have fewer and fewer periods, mild to no symptoms, a couple of hot flashes and their periods stop. However, you aren't officially in menopause until you have not had a period for at least one year. For 95 percent of women, this takes place between the ages of 45 and 55, with most women reaching menopause right around age 50 or 51.

When a woman enters menopause, her levels of estrogen, progesterone, and testosterone decline to levels that no longer support menstruation. While women after menopause can occasionally experience a bleeding episode, essentially menstruation ceases. In addition, other more wide-ranging shifts occur in her physical, chemical, and energetic makeup.

As I mentioned in the Introduction, even if a menopausal woman previously enjoyed healthy physical and chemical balance, her body and brain chemistry now starts to become more unbalanced. She also tends to manifest one of two distinct patterns. She either becomes an estrogen deficient–fast processor or an estrogen deficient–slow processor. The brain and body chemistry of an estrogen deficiency–fast processor is imbalanced towards the more excitatory chemicals like dopamine, norepinephrine, and epinephrine that stimulate, speed up, and overheat her body processes and body chemistry. Conversely, an estrogen deficiency–slow processor tends more toward the production of inhibitory chemicals like serotonin, taurine, and GABA that slow down the body's processes.

Regardless of which category a woman falls into, the patients I've seen in my practice who have the easiest transition into menopause are those who are already on a strong preventive nutritional program. But frankly, most doctors don't usually see this healthy transition. Unless a woman is one of the lucky 10 percent or is on a strong preventive nutritional program, she is more likely to begin experiencing health problems due to estrogen–progesterone imbalances.

By the time menstrual periods stop, estrogen production has diminished by as much as 75 to 90 percent, progesterone production has virtually ceased, and the production of androgens—male hormones that stimulate sex drive—are up to 50 percent lower. Simply put, menopause is a state of hormone deficiency.

This life change is due to normal aging of ovaries and egg follicles. Previously, the medical textbooks indicated that a woman was born with a set number of eggs and that over time, as the ovaries aged and shrank and there were fewer eggs that could be utilized, a woman would eventually just naturally slip into menopause. But new research from the journal *Nature* has shown just how wrong this is.

Researchers at Massachusetts General Hospital in Boston have discovered that special stem cells that, until now, have been overlooked, allow women to continue to produce eggs throughout their life. The eggs derived from these cells also form new follicles (where the eggs ripen and mature). It is these follicles within the ovary that, together with the adrenal glands, are responsible for hormone production. This may be a partial explanation for why the exciting approach that I am sharing with you in this book can offer so much potential to better optimize your hormone production and balance, no matter what your age, and allow you to enjoy a much more vital and healthy life.

During menopause, the ovaries and adrenal glands continue to produce estrone (a lower potency estrogen) and the liver produces some estriol (another weak form of estrogen). And while their action is not nearly as strong as the hormones produced before menopause, these hormones do continue to provide some support for the bones, breasts, brain, heart, and vaginal tissues.

The problems that often accompany menopause—hot flashes, insomnia, vaginal dryness, painful intercourse, loss of libido, vaginal and bladder infections, loss of muscle and skin tone, achy joints, brittle bones, fatigue, and mental confusion—are unpleasant, distressing, and can prevent us from living life to the fullest. Some naturally disappear in a few years; others do not. The good news is that with my program you don't have to accept these as a "natural" part of the life cycle.

Section One: Summary

Hormones, primarily secreted by the glands, or endocrine system, are the chemical messengers of the body. They perform myriad functions and are divided into several categories. The series of chemical reactions that produce the sex hormones begins with cholesterol. The three major sex hormones are estrogen, progesterone, and testosterone. The two precursor hormones, from which these and all other sex hormones are made, are pregnenolone and DHEA. An adequate, balanced supply of all five sex hormones is necessary for optimal health.

Defining where you are in the four distinct phases of a woman's life—menstruation, premenopause, perimenopause, or menopause—will help you better understand your own hormonal makeup, and help you decide which hormones you need to focus on to achieve great health and well-being.

In Section Two of *Hormone Revolution*, you'll learn why the days of conventional medicine blindly leading women down the HRT path are over. You'll also discover the gentle, safe, and effective natural options Mother Nature has provided.

create a
healthy
you

When I began my medical training nearly 40 years ago, synthetic hormone replacement therapy (HRT) was available only through a doctor's prescription or administered by injection in a medical office. Very few types of HRT were available, and the use of precursor hormones like DHEA and pregnenolone was virtually unknown.

What's worse, women were uninformed about the benefits and risks of hormone therapy. This situation has changed dramatically over the last three decades. Books and articles on this subject have proliferated, and hormone therapy is now discussed constantly in the media.

But even with all of this attention on HRT, many women are still confused or uninformed about their choices of hormonal therapy. The scariest part of this is that they are often unaware of—or do not understand—the possible side effects and long-term risks of HRT, especially estrogen and progesterone replacement.

In this section, we'll focus on conventional HRT for estrogen and progesterone, their inherent dangers, and the natural alternatives that are not only safe, but extremely effective.

fool's gold

8

With all the buzz surrounding hormone replacement, it shouldn't surprise you to learn that most women are going without HRT. According to a study conducted by an HMO back in 1996, of the 2,000 some women who had been given a prescription for HRT, 75 percent either ceased using the hormones entirely or had significantly cut their originally prescribed dosage within one year. Most surprising is that the majority of the women never told their doctor about their decision.

A separate study presented in *Family Practice News* stated that there has never been a time in the United States when more than 35 percent of menopausal women have opted to use HRT. In fact, the most recent statistics show that HRT use has dropped substantially, with numbers as low as 8 percent in some parts of the country.

Many women who choose not to take estrogen say that their decision is based on the fact that HRT could intensify serious pre-existing health problems, such as uterine cancer, heavy bleeding from fibroids, severe migraine headaches, or blood-clotting problems. Other women fear that the long-term use of estrogen may accelerate the onset of a disease, such as breast cancer. Still others state that they would like to use estrogen, but experience terrible side effects, such as depression, anxiety, breast tenderness, weight gain, and fluid retention—regardless of their dosage.

And the research shows that their concerns are right on the money.

Women as Human Guinea Pigs

If you've read my newsletter or any of my other books, then you are undoubtedly aware of my strong concern regarding physicians' continued persistence in using HRT.

For years, conventional physicians prescribed animal-based and synthetic HRT to women to help stave off hot flashes, night sweats, irritability, and other menopausal symptoms. Additionally, the medical establishment has long believed that HRT—in the form of estrogen alone or estrogen combined with progestin—lowered postmenopausal women's risk of heart disease and osteoporosis.

Available studies showed a 35 to 50 percent reduction in risk for CHD (coronary heart disease) among women taking HRT. The risk reduction was even higher among women known to have CHD before starting HRT.

One of the best-known studies of this time was the Postmenopausal Estrogen/Progestin Intervention (PEPI) trial, published in 1995 in the *Journal of the American Medical Association*. This study examined how HRT use impacted risk factors for CHD. In other words, the researchers simply monitored factors associated with increased and decreased risk of heart problems. The actual incidence of heart problems, such as heart attacks, was not monitored.

A total of 875 postmenopausal women received estrogen alone, estrogen and the progestin medroxyprogesterone (Provera), estrogen with micronized (oral) progesterone, or a placebo. The authors noted improvements in blood lipid profiles among all women receiving hormones, including lower LDL (low density lipoprotein) levels and higher HDL (high density lipoprotein) levels. Based on these results, they endorsed the use of HRT to reduce CHD risk.

A few critics pointed to flaws in these early studies. All of the early studies were observational—meaning that the researchers simply observed and analyzed what happened to women who did or didn't take HRT. Skeptics noted a strong possibility that the two groups of women weren't matched with respect to their habits and lifestyles.

Critics argued that the women who chose to take HRT and stuck with it for the entire study period are likely to take a more active role in promoting their overall health than the women in the non-HRT group. Thus, if the women taking HRT were at lower risk of heart disease, it might have been because of their general healthy habits and lifestyles, not the HRT. Skeptics also noted that any women who stopped taking HRT because of negative side effects were usually dropped from the studies and their experiences were not included in the final analysis.

And, in the case of the PEPI study, there was an extremely problematic finding from the study that was downplayed by the researchers. All of the women taking hormones experienced increases in their C-reactive protein levels. C-reactive protein, an indicator of inflammation, is now known to be a very strong predictor of future heart attacks, superior to LDL or HDL levels.

Of course, this finding and the concerns of alternative medicine physicians were largely ignored. The numbers were good and the medical profession believed, overall, that it had struck gold in the fight against postmenopausal heart disease. Soon, a prescription for HRT came to be considered the equivalent of "heart disease insurance policy."

The Heart-Wrenching Reality of HRT

But now the research tide has turned in the other direction. The newest studies are randomized controlled trials—far more scientifically rigorous than the older observational studies.

Not surprisingly, these new studies are showing a very different outcome: Estrogen plus progestin doesn't protect women against postmenopausal CHD. In fact, recent studies show that this therapy actually increases cardiac risk. This appears to be true not only for healthy women, but also for women who already have a history of CHD.

The HERS study

One of the largest randomized placebo-controlled trials of postmenopausal HRT to date is the Heart and Estrogen/Progestin Replacement Study (HERS) trial. A total of 2,763 post-menopausal women with a known history of heart disease received either estrogen plus medroxyprogesterone (Provera) or a placebo. The incidence of heart attacks and of other problems related to cardiac disease (such as bypass surgeries and hospitalizations for unstable angina or heart failure) was monitored. Data on other health problems were also collected.

The results clearly cast doubt on HRT. Researchers discovered that during the first year of use, women taking the hormones had significantly *more* heart attacks and other heart problems than those receiving the placebo. While the HRT group did eventually experience a decline in CHD risk, this did not occur until the third year of therapy. In fact, it wasn't until an average of 4.1 years of use that women enjoyed a significantly reduced risk for heart disease in general or for specific heart problems.

Interestingly, the women receiving hormones did show improved blood lipid profiles, just like the women in the PEPI study. Yet those improvements were not associated with reduced risk of heart attack.

The conventional interpretation of the HERS results is that the increased risk of cardio-vascular disease during the first year of HRT indicates that women with known heart disease shouldn't start taking it. However, if they have been taking HRT for more than a year, they are into the reduced-risk phase and it could be appropriate for them to continue.

I find this conclusion astounding. Clearly, a prescription drug affects the *entire* body, not just some isolated organ system. Moreover, the women in the HERS study that took HRT were found to have three times as many blockages of blood vessels by blood clots and a 40 percent increase in gallbladder disease, when compared to the women taking the placebo. For me, this is enough to raise concern about *any* woman using HRT at *any* point.

The ERA Trial

Results from another study put one more nail in the HRT coffin. Like the HERS study, the Estrogen Replacement and Atherosclerosis (ERA) trial followed 309 women with heart disease, which was determined by atherosclerotic narrowing of one or more arteries feeding the heart.

Participants received estrogen alone, estrogen plus medroxyprogesterone (Provera), or a placebo for an average of three years. Results revealed that neither hormone treatment slowed the progression of the blockage. Once again, the women taking hormones showed lower LDL levels, but as in the HERS study, the improved blood lipids weren't linked to a decrease in actual heart problems.

Neither the ERA nor HERS studies investigated the relationship between HRT and heart disease risk in *healthy* postmenopausal women. But the Women's Health Initiative did, and the news isn't good.

The Women's Health Initiative

In April 2000, preliminary results of the Women's Health Initiative (WHI) study involving 27,000 healthy postmenopausal women were released—and they were troubling.

The participants received either estrogen plus progestin, estrogen alone if post-hysterectomy, or a placebo. Despite the fact that the participants had no history of heart disease, those who received hormones experienced more cardiac problems, including heart attacks, during the first two years of the study.

Now, you may be wondering why the study wasn't stopped. The answer is that the researchers anticipated a drop-off in cardiac risk at the point where the preliminary results were released, similar to the one seen in the HERS study. As you'll see on page 50, they were deadly wrong.

HRT Warnings Finally Go Mainstream

Soon, influential organizations such as the American Heart Association and the American College of Cardiology began to issue warnings about starting HRT in postmenopausal women with a history of heart disease.

Similarly, the Food and Drug Administration (FDA) made drug manufacturers strengthen the warnings on package inserts and patient information sheets for HRT. They were now to read that women who take HRT are more likely to suffer from clots in their blood vessels than women not taking the drug.

Still, physicians continued to prescribe HRT. Only they now claimed that it helped prevent osteoporosis.

HRT's Brittle Side

The use of HRT for the treatment of osteoporosis is so blindly accepted that a physician actually told one of my friends that he would not order her a bone density test unless she agreed to use HRT. I have heard similar stories from thousands of women for whom HRT was the only treatment offered by their physicians.

While some studies do support the use of HRT for osteoporosis, sadly, this benefit is also contested. According to a study from the *American Journal of Medicine*, HRT is not effective for either the prevention or treatment of osteoporosis. The study highlights the results of the HERS study (yes, the same one that tested HRT and heart disease) on osteoporosis-related fractures. After following some 2,700 post-menopausal women for more than four years, researchers found that HRT use in women over the age of 60 is unlikely to be beneficial for the treatment of osteoporosis. In fact, HRT was found to be no more effective in protecting women from osteoporotic fractures than the placebo.

Even the Food and Drug Administration (FDA) has questioned the true effectiveness of HRT. In 1999, they limited the claims manufacturers could make regarding estrogen replacement therapy, citing that definitive proof was lacking in regard to the effectiveness of either estrogen or combined HRT to treat osteoporosis.

The HRT—Breast Cancer Connection

Not so long ago, conventional HRT's impact on breast cancer risk was still the subject of heated debate. This debate essentially ended when an article described by a Harvard Medical School professor as "close to being the final word" on HRT and breast cancer was published in the *Lancet*. Fifty-one studies involving more than 161,000 women were reviewed. The conclusion: Conventional HRT increased the risk of breast cancer with each year of use. Women using HRT for five or more years were at 35 percent greater risk.

Another study revealed that after 10 years of use, ERT (hormone replacement therapy using estrogen alone) increased a woman's risk of dying from breast cancer by 43 percent. Other similar studies indicate that combined estrogen-progestin therapy, the kind used by most women, increases breast cancer risk even more than ERT does!

Concerns about combined estrogen-progestin hormone replacement treatment were identified by a large National Cancer Institute study and were reported in the *Journal of the American Medical Association*. The study concluded that women who took the combined treatment for five years were 40 percent more likely to develop breast cancer than women taking estrogen alone or no hormones.

Similarly, other studies have confirmed an even higher 60 to 70 percent increase in breast cancer risk with the long-term use of HRT.

While the figures vary from study to study, the evidence is clear, compelling, and consistent—*conventional HRT increases a woman's risk of developing breast cancer, and with each additional year of use, that risk gets higher.*

The Landmark *JAMA*-HRT Study

Reports on the risks associated with conventional HRT have filled medical journals for more than 20 years. There was clear evidence that conventional HRT use increased a woman's risk for heart disease and breast cancer. And yet, many physicians were still insisting on prescribing HRT. And many women were still taking it. But the summer of 2002 forever removed the curtain of doubt surrounding the dangers of HRT.

On July 17, 2002, the *Journal of the American Medical Association (JAMA)* reported on the findings from one part of the Women's Health Initiative (WHI), an 8.5 year project funded by the National Institutes of Health. As I indicated earlier, the WHI involved 161,809 postmenopausal women between the ages of 50 and 79, and outlined the benefits and risks of a variety of treatments designed to lower the incidences of several diseases, including heart disease, breast and colon cancer, and fractures in postmenopausal women. Of this group, 16,608 women who were healthy and had an intact uterus participated in one part of the WHI, which tested the effectiveness of estrogen/progestin therapy.

According to the findings, women taking estrogen/progestin for five years or more had an increased risk for blood clots, coronary heart disease (CHD), strokes, and breast cancer. The researchers concluded, "The results indicate that this regimen should not be initiated or continued for primary prevention of CHD."

The data indicated that if 10,000 women took the drugs for a year and 10,000 did not, women in the first group would have eight more cases of invasive breast cancer, seven more heart attacks, eight more strokes, and 18 more instances of blood clots.

In fact, researchers felt so strongly about the negative implications of long-term combined HRT, especially the unacceptably high risk for breast cancer, that they ended the study *three years early*! Participants were contacted and instructed to stop taking the drug—immediately.

The Post-*JAMA* Aftermath

As you can imagine, the *JAMA* findings turned the world of hormone replacement on its head. For alternative and complementary doctors such as myself, there was no surprise. It's what we have been telling our patients for decades. For conventional physicians, the race was on to prove the study wrong.

They claimed that the Women's Health Initiative (WHI) did, in fact, prove that women taking HRT enjoyed greater bone mass density and fewer fractures. The study found that taking combined estrogen/progestin for at least three years yielded a 3.7 percent increase in bone density, and reduced hip fractures by 33 percent.

But that's about all they could say. Subsequent studies have served to reinforce the deadly truth revealed by the July 2002 *JAMA* data. Continuing research from the WHI has shown that women who take combined estrogen/progestin replacement for at least five years have increased incidence of invasive breast cancer, as compared to women who don't take HRT. Additionally, the tumors are larger and more advanced.

They also found that women who took the combination for just one year had more abnormal mammograms than those who didn't take the drugs. And taking estrogen didn't help. Research indicated that taking estrogen for more than seven years also increases the risk of abnormal mammograms, and the need for subsequent follow-up.

Additionally, studies have shown that women who have had a hysterectomy and are taking combination HRT are at increased risk for stroke. In fact, if 10,000 women took the drugs for a year and 10,000 did not, women in the first group would have 12 more cases of stroke than the second group.

This correlation is not just conjecture. According to a study reported at the San Antonio Breast Cancer Symposium, U.S. breast cancer rates plunged 7.2 percent in 2003. With 200,000 cases of the disease projected for 2003, this means that 14,000 fewer women were diagnosed with breast cancer. This drop in cancer rates comes just one year after millions of women stopped taking conventional HRT, thanks in large part to the abovementioned findings that HRT is conclusively associated with an increased risk of breast cancer and heart disease. Researchers found that the largest decline was among women aged 50–69, the exact age group most likely to use HRT. In fact, the drop was three times greater than that of any other age group.

PREMARIN—AN ETHICAL DISGRACE

Many of the active hormones in Premarin are chemically different than human estrogen—they're a combination of several different estrogenic compounds gathered from horse urine that are fine for a horse, but unhealthy and biologically foreign to a human female.

Even if the hormones were identical to humans and completely safe, the practice is an ethical disgrace. The mares used to produce Premarin are impregnated, then confined to stalls for months for urine collection. Their foals are a "by-product" and are usually sent to slaughter. If the mares don't conceive when they're rebred, they're sent to slaughter as well.

This truly horrifies me. I love horses, as do most people I know. They are beautiful, intelligent animals and don't deserve this disgraceful treatment—especially for the gathering of a dangerous drug.

The Research is Clear

The research leaves no room for doubt about HRT and its negative effects on women's health.

- **It does not reduce a woman's risk of heart disease.** While it can improve HDL and LDL cholesterol levels, these improvements are not associated with fewer heart attacks or other heart problems.
- **It increases a woman's risk of heart attack, stroke, and blood clots.** In fact, it places healthy women and women with a history of cardiac disease at increased risk of heart attack within the first year or two of usage.
- **It does not reverse pre-existing heart disease.**
- **It raises levels of C-reactive protein,** an indicator of inflammation that is a strong predictor of a future heart attack.
- **It increases the risk of invasive breast cancer.**
- **It increases the likelihood of an abnormal mammogram after just one year of use.**
- **It increases risk of gallbladder disease by 40 percent.**

Even though the HERS study suggests that long-term HRT use (four to five years or longer) might be beneficial for prevention of heart disease, I still don't believe that this is compelling enough evidence to recommend its use—especially since we know that HRT begins to increase a woman's risk of breast cancer just when the cardiovascular benefits seem to kick in.

Why Some Physicians Are Still Dragging Their Feet

Given the strength of the evidence that HRT increases the risk of heart disease and estrogen-positive breast cancer, you might wonder why most physicians haven't reduced the number of prescriptions they write for HRT or urged women to stop using it.

Until recently, mainstream physicians had a plausible excuse for sticking with conventional HRT. They still viewed it as the best thing they could offer a post-menopausal woman to protect her from two of her greatest health threats—heart disease and osteoporosis—and to relieve her menopausal discomforts. They weighed HRT's ability to defeat these common problems against its tendency to increase the risk of breast cancer as well as heart disease, and decided that the benefits of HRT outweighed its risks.

As we now know, this line of reasoning doesn't hold water. Still, I simply cannot explain why most conventional practitioners are still so slow to act on the latest findings. But even if the research doesn't make the doctors change, their patients just might.

Where Do We Go From Here?

While many physicians and researchers are still hoarding the "fool's gold" known as HRT, complementary medicine is busily mining the mother lode of *real* gold—and women are taking notice.

Large numbers of American women are either abandoning their HRT or deciding to never start taking it. Many are rejecting physicians unfamiliar with or unsympathetic to natural health supports. They are also realizing the power and wisdom of using natural medicines and herbal remedies for easing menopausal discomforts, and are very interested in natural solutions for heart disease and osteoporosis.

Before changing your HRT regimen, be sure to discuss your plans with your physician. Chances are, you will be able to eliminate your conventional HRT or dramatically reduce the dose you require for symptomatic relief. Either way, you win: Recent research indicates that breast cancer risk returns to normal within a few years of stopping HRT, and it's likely that lower-dose HRT has less of an adverse impact on estrogen-positive breast cancer risk.

In the next chapter, we'll explore the natural hormone replacement options available to you. I'll also introduce you to the cutting-edge concept of restoring your own hormone production.

9

safe, natural, & effective options

Now that you are aware of the dangerous side effects associated with conventional HRT, you may be wondering what options you do have. Let's face it, hot flashes, insomnia, lapses in concentration, mood swings, anxiety, night sweats, and the idea of thinning bones is something no woman should have to endure. Fortunately, you don't. There are several safer and less risky nutritional and dietary therapies that have been proven to be very effective.

In the 33 years I've been a physician, I've been astounded by the effectiveness of these safe, natural hormone replacement options. Many thousands of women I've treated have breezed through menopause risk-free and symptom-free by using a combination of natural therapies.

Specifically, there are three main approaches to replacing and enhancing your own natural hormones. The first is to restore your own "brand" of hormones. In fact, the primary focus of my program is to help you restore your own hormones and bring you into better hormonal balance.

The second involves the use of natural substances such as phytochemicals, herbs, and vitamins that provide hormonal support and even act as hormonal mimics. These are non-prescription, self-care treatment options that can be acquired in health food stores and pharmacies without a doctor's prescription. The third option involves the use of biochemically identical hormones, which are prescribed by your physician from a compounding pharmacy.

Regardless of which option you select, all of these complementary treatments are gentle, yet highly effective. Let's take a quick look at each category so you can have a better understanding of how each of them works.

Restore Your Own Hormones

To help a woman reverse any hormonal issue she may have, the first thing I do is work with her to restore and balance her own hormones. Over the years, I have had wonderful success using my safe, gentle, and effective program to accomplish this goal.

My hormone restoration program involves the use of several different modalities, including nutritional supplements, energy medicine therapies, dietary changes, stress reduction, and exercise. In terms of nutrients, I focus on those that either support your own production and levels of hormones or stimulate hormone production. To *support* production, it's critical to increase your levels of key nutrients that sustain your own hormone levels. Examples of these nutrients are wheat germ oil for estrogen and lutein and beta-carotene for progesterone production.

In order to *stimulate* hormone production, you also need to boost the health and vitality of those body systems that play key roles in the creation and regulation of the hormones themselves. These include the central nervous system, hypothalamus, ovaries, pituitary and adrenal glands, and your liver, as well as other organs. Over the years, I've found energy medicine to be particularly helpful in this arena. During my own particular hormonal journey, I've learned and mastered many different types of energy medicine, all of which I share with you in Section Four. Specifically, we'll take a look at how acupuncture and acupressure, chakras realignment, color and light therapy, sound therapy, frequency medicine, and other types of energy therapies all work to bring your hormones back into balance.

Lastly, I'll show you how lifestyle choices can support the nutritional and energy therapies, as well as how they individually impact your hormone health. In addition to your diet, I'll explain how reducing stress and doing the right kind of exercise for your hormonal type can go a long way to restoring your hormones safely, naturally, and effectively.

Natural Hormone Substitutes

In addition to restoring your own hormones, you can also gain a hormone-like effect from certain foods, nutrients, and herbs. Foods such as soybeans and flaxseed contain phytoestrogens, which are chemically and functionally similar to estradiol—a woman's most prominent natural estrogen.

Nutrients such as bioflavonoids and vitamins A and C have also been shown to mimic estrogen in the body. These compounds are particularly beneficial in relieving hot flashes and vaginal dryness, as well as headaches and irritability.

Finally, herbs like black cohosh and dong quai have been used for centuries to treat abnormal menstruation and alleviate menopausal symptoms. These and other similar herbs—both Western and Chinese—work by stimulating receptors in the pituitary gland and the hypothalamus.

Understanding Bioidentical Hormones

Lastly, if you need that extra push toward hormonal balance, I recommend the use of biochemically identical hormones. Biochemically identical hormones are molecularly identical to the hormones found in the human body. Moreover, they are produced in the laboratory from natural ingredients such as soy and wild yam, derived from plants, not horse urine.

Since bioidentical hormones are biologically similar to the hormones your body produces, they do not appear to have the grave risks associated with conventional HRT.

The bioidentical estrogen that I typically recommend is estriol. Of the three types of estrogen produced within your body, estriol is the weakest and least potent. More importantly, several research studies have found that it is as effective as the stronger, more potent estrogens for treating menopause symptoms.

One study published in the *Journal of the American Medical Association* found that estriol was particularly effective in treating vaginal atrophy, mood swings, and hot flashes. Researchers selected 52 symptomatic, postmenopausal women and separated them into four groups, giving each group either 2 mg, 4 mg, 6 mg, or 8 mg of estriol per day for six months. On average, women in every group experienced a decrease in their menopausal symptoms after one month of treatment. Furthermore, in the groups with the three highest dosages, women who had ranked their symptoms as severe now felt that their symptoms were very mild.

Section Two: Summary

The days of conventional medicine blindly leading women down the HRT path are over. From increased risk of blood clots and heart disease to more invasive and advanced stage breast cancer, science has shown that traditional hormone replacement has dangerous, and often lethal, repercussions.

The good news is there are gentle, safe, and effective natural options. Whether you use bioidentical hormones, hormone substitutes, or restore your own levels of hormones, Mother Nature has provided a solution.

In Section Three of *Hormone Revolution*, you'll learn how each of these three therapy options applies to the five main sex hormones, starting with estrogen.

restoring the
balance

Up to now, we've been discussing hormones in their healthy, balanced state. I've defined what each hormone is, its chemistry, how it affects your body, and how your health and lifestyle affect the hormone itself.

We've also taken a look at the hormone replacement options available to women. In the past, those choices have been pretty grim. Often, women had to choose between dangerous, potentially lethal drugs or else suffer with unpleasant and often debilitating menopausal symptoms such as hot flashes, anxiety, and low libido.

In Section Three of Hormone Revolution, *we'll switch gears and look at hormone imbalance. I'll tell you how to determine if you are producing too much or too little estrogen, and whether you are suffering from a deficiency of progesterone, testosterone, DHEA, and pregnenolone.*

I'll also give you safe, natural, effective solutions to restore the balance. Specifically, you'll learn how to use a wide variety of plants, foods, herbs, and other types of nutrients to restore your own healthy hormone levels and function.

We'll start this discussion with excess estrogen production—the hallmark of premenopause.

estrogen dominance: the premenopause

10

For many women, the mid- to late-30's and 40's often signal a major shift in their hormonal life. Some women simply produce fewer and fewer of all five sex hormones. However, most will experience hormonal fluctuations, usually marked by normal to excess estrogen and decreased progesterone. This is known as estrogen dominance, and often marks premenopause.

Estrogen dominance is most common during the seven to 10 years preceding the cessation of your menstrual periods, although for some women, this condition may only last for a few years. During this time, you will likely produce normal to elevated levels of estrogen, while progesterone is produced in low amounts, due to less frequent ovulation (this occurs when the egg is released from the ovary at the middle of your cycle, allowing for the production of progesterone during the second half of the menstrual cycle).

With normal to excess estrogen production and too low progesterone levels, your body cannot offset estrogen's negative effects. This often leads to symptoms such as increased body fat, salt and fluid retention, and poor blood sugar control.

This imbalance can also lead to health problems such as headaches, irregular or heavy menstrual bleeding, sleep difficulties, anxiety, irritability, weight gain, lowered sex drive, brain fog, and/or pre-menstrual swollen breasts. Worse yet, elevated estrogen levels can over-stimulate the growth of the uterine lining and the outer muscular tissue of the uterus, causing the growth of benign tumors called fibroids, as well as an inflammatory condition called endometriosis. Both of these conditions can cause heavy and irregular menstrual bleeding. If left untreated, fibroids can even lead to severe anemia. Elevated estrogen levels can also stimulate a potentially pre-cancerous condition called endometrial hyperplasia.

Estrogen Dominance and Your Health

As I indicated, there is a wide variety of negative health conditions that can often result from estrogen dominance. In addition to the discomfort of premenstrual syndrome, estrogen dominance can trigger more severe and possibly life-threatening conditions.

PMS

Premenstrual syndrome (PMS) is thought to be a result of hormonal changes, diet, and lifestyle. Studies have shown that women with PMS tend to have relatively high levels of estrogen and relatively low levels of progesterone. This imbalance results in physical and emotional symptoms that can start a few days or as much as two weeks prior to menstruation. They often include:

- swelling and tenderness in the breasts
- abdominal cramping
- backaches
- bloating
- headaches/migraines
- irritability
- anxiety and/or depression
- mood swings
- food cravings

Living with these symptoms can be very difficult. Fortunately, increasing progesterone levels and decreasing estrogen through proper diet, exercise, and the right combination of nutrients (and in severe cases, the use of natural progesterone) can ease most, if not all, PMS-related symptoms.

Fibroid Tumors

About 40 percent of women between the ages of 30 and 50 have fibroids—benign tumors that are found in the smooth muscle layers of the uterus. Occasionally, fibroids occur through and beyond menopause.

The word fibroid is actually a misnomer, because it implies that these tumors arise from fibrous tissue. In actuality, fibroids consist of smooth-muscle cells of the uterus.

There are three main ways fibroids can develop within your uterus. They can grow on the inside of the uterus and extend into the uterine cavity from the interior lining of the uterus (the endometrium). They can also grow within the uterine wall itself, or on the outside of the uterus, in the exterior lining between the uterus and the pelvic cavity.

While fibroids may sometimes be asymptomatic, they often cause heavy menstrual bleeding and spotting. In extreme cases, the blood loss may be so pronounced that women may have the fibroid tumor (myomectomy) or even the uterus itself removed (hysterectomy). However, in the minority of cases (30–40 percent), symptoms can include bloating, pain during sex, frequent urination due to the pressure caused by the fibroids on neighboring organs like the bladder, and abnormal bleeding. While we are unsure of what causes fibroids, we do know that they are estrogen dependent. Therefore, if you are estrogen dominant, you are at greater risk for fibroid tumors.

Endometriosis

Endometriosis occurs when cells lining the uterus (the endometrium) break away and grow where they don't belong—on the ovaries, cervix, appendix, bowel, bladder, or inside the uterus. On rare occasions, these cells can travel and invade areas as far away as the lungs or armpits.

One theory for endometriosis was proposed by researcher John A. Simpson. He suggested that instead of exiting through the vagina during menstruation, small pieces of the endometrium "back up" into the fallopian tubes and pelvic cavity, eventually implanting themselves onto nearby pelvic organs.

Since these implants are comprised of endometrial tissue, they respond to fluctuations in the level of estrogen and progesterone just like the endometrium itself does within the uterus. In other words, these implants will bleed slightly at the time of menstruation. During menstruation, this blood cannot exit the body through the vaginal opening and remains trapped in the pelvis, where it can cause severe cramps, pain during sexual intercourse, and other menstrual irregularities.

These implants can also invade and injure pelvic tissue, cause pain during intercourse and bowel movements, and even cause infertility. They can also cause irregular bleeding. Fortunately, reducing excess estrogen can reduce your risk for this painful condition.

Ovarian Cysts

An ovarian cyst is a result of a follicle malfunction. A follicle is the fluid-filled structure that houses an egg (or ovum) before it's released into the fallopian tube and then trails down into the uterus—this process is called ovulation. During normal ovulation, a follicle grows to a certain size and then ruptures, releasing the egg. It's then converted into a larger structure, the *corpus luteum*—which produces both estrogen and progesterone needed to promote proper growth and maturation of your uterine lining during the second half of your menstrual cycle. This ensures that either menstruation takes place in a normal, healthy fashion, or that your uterus is prepared to sustain a baby, should pregnancy occur.

An ovarian cyst forms when the follicle continues to grow, instead of releasing the egg and dissolving like it's supposed to. In other words, the cyst is a failed ovulation, and as such, you aren't producing the progesterone needed to balance your estrogen levels.

Ovarian cysts are so common that conventional medicine considers them normal. In fact, most go away on their own within a couple months. In the event they don't go away, your treatment options aren't so positive—surgically draining, cauterizing, or removing the cyst (along with a section of the ovary); removing the ovary; and/or taking synthetic hormones—all of which only treat the symptoms, not the cause.

PEGGY'S STORY

When I first met "Peggy," she was in her mid-40's, and was about 30 to 40 pounds overweight. She had a history of ovarian cysts, and had already undergone one surgery to remove them. She had heavy menstrual bleeding, incredibly painful menstrual periods that put her out of commission for several days at a time, uncomfortable PMS symptoms, and depression.

However, what was most concerning to me was that she did not have the usual support systems and health knowledge that I see in a lot of my patients. In fact, I found her to be aloof and guarded, and she didn't seem to want to connect with me at all. But as I began to learn more about her, I could understand why. She didn't have any family or social support to speak of. Her father had died years earlier, and she was completely estranged from her alcoholic mother. She had an office job that didn't provide a lot of contact with other people and, although she had some acquaintances, she didn't seem to have any close friends. In other words, she didn't have any strong personal connections, which can be a problem for many women. A big part of healing is having a solid support system around you.

What Peggy *did* have was a strong desire to be well.

Although her gynecologist recommended that she have a hysterectomy, she didn't want to go through another surgery. So she and I started working together to help her avoid going under the knife.

One of the first things I addressed was her lack of a support system. She made a commitment to herself that she would start attending services at her local church more regularly, and that she would join a women's group, so she would have more personal contact and support.

In addition, she immediately started to make the important dietary changes, such as cutting way back on cheeseburgers, and following the nutritional supplement program I put together for her. That's when I *really* started to see the health benefits of her strong desire and commitment to change.

Peggy became very motivated, and she made a lot of major growth steps in a short period of time. She quickly lost 10 pounds, and started to pay more attention to her appearance. She became more interested in nutrition, and even bought a few books on the subject. Her demeanor changed as well—she became much warmer and more positive. She made friends, developed a social life, and even took on a roommate. As she made these changes, a truly beautiful woman started to emerge.

Best of all, her physical symptoms started to improve. Not only was she shedding weight, but her crippling menstrual cramps and heavy bleeding started to diminish within a few months. The PMS symptoms that had previously ruled her life started to recede and shorten in duration. She slowly eased her way into a more normal menstrual pattern.

By the end of the year, Peggy was quite a different person. A beautiful swan had emerged—and she never had to have the hysterectomy.

Heavy Menstrual Bleeding

During a normal menses, a woman typically bleeds every 21 to 35 days, with a norm of 28 days. The bleeding usually lasts an average of three to seven days.

If your period is more frequent than every 21 days or lasts longer than seven days, you are likely suffering from menorrhagia, or heavy menstrual bleeding. Some women will even "spot" between periods.

Heavy menstrual bleeding is also marked by a blood loss of more than 80 ml (just over three ounces) during menstruation. That's at least double the amount a woman loses during a healthy cycle. The flow often includes large blood clots, and even the highest absorbency pad or tampon quickly becomes saturated and has to be changed frequently.

Menorrhagia can put a real dent in your life, making you constantly concerned about embarrassing "breakthrough bleeding." It can leave you feeling weak, fatigued, and drained of energy for a day or two each month. Of even greater concern, it can lead to anemia or severe blood loss.

Benign Breast Disease

Benign breast disease is a catch-all term for changes in the breast that aren't *cancer*. According to the American Cancer Society, nine out of 10 women have some type of benign breast disease at some point in their lives. Often, it manifests as breast swelling, pain, and engorgement that can last several days to two weeks each cycle. In many cases, women complain that their breasts are so tender they can't bear to have them touched. Some women even have to stop running during this period because of the pain.

Like fibroids and endometriosis, benign breast disease is also linked to excess estrogen. Once you reduce estrogen and/or increase progesterone, odds are the symptoms will disappear and benign breast cysts will shrink.

Hyperplasia and Endometrial (Uterine) Cancer

Endometrial hyperplasia usually affects women between the ages of 50 and 70. In some women, this can be a pre-cancerous condition, in which there is an overgrowth of the cells of the uterine lining, or endometrium (a precursor to endometrial or uterine cancer). In the early stages, there may not be any symptoms, but as the condition progresses, more common symptoms like abnormal vaginal bleeding may occur.

Both hyperplasia and endometrial cancer are estrogen dependent. In fact, researchers have found that using an estrogen treatment regimen without the addition of progesterone increases the incidence of endometrial cancer four to eight times in women with an intact uterus. Clearly, women with estrogen dominance are at an increased risk for these conditions.

The Cosmetic Effects of Estrogen Dominance

Women who are producing excessive amounts of estrogen and other chemicals often have increased fat deposition in the body, which can cause them to gain as much as 10 to 50 pounds. Additionally, the overproduction of estrogen can also cause fluid and sodium retention in the tissues. This can lead to abdominal bloating, weight gain, and puffiness around the face, particularly the eyes.

Women with an allergic tendency may find that intake of wheat and dairy products can worsen bloating and weight gain. And the overuse of salt in the diet can worsen symptoms of edema as well.

GREAT EXERCISES FOR PUFFY EYES

You can use a wonderful acupressure exercise to reduce the appearance of swollen eyes. Using the tips of your fingers, stimulate the pressure point just below the base of your skull, a finger-width away from the spine, with gentle to medium pressure.

For eyes that are overworked and overfocused, I recommend the following eye exercise to promote the relaxation response within your eyes and the tissues surrounding them, thereby supporting the beauty of your eyes safely and naturally. Over time, this exercise (adapted from Paul Scheele's groundbreaking work on Photo Reading) will also help to soften the fine lines and wrinkles around your eyes.

1. Close your eyes and rest your arms at your sides.
2. Touch your eyes gently with the tips of your fingers. See if your eyes feel tense or even hard. Are you noticing a feeling of tightness or tension in the muscles that surround your eyes? If so, you need to soften your gaze.
3. Take several slow, deep breaths.
4. Open your eyes, but instead of gazing intensely at the fine print of the page or monitor, soften your gaze by widening your field of vision to focus on the entire page or screen. You should be able to see all four-corners of what you are looking at. Look at the white space of the margin and the areas between the paragraphs. As you do this, you will begin to feel the tension in your eyes melt away. You can also do this step if you are watching television by looking at the empty spaces on the screen.
5. Close your eyes again, continuing to breathe slowly and effortlessly.
6. Open your eyes. Repeat the process of softening your gaze while looking at the white spaces on the page.

Both excessive fat deposition and fluid retention greatly impact the appearance of the skin in this group. These women have skin that actually appears overhydrated. The skin is overly moist and plump and may hang loosely on the body. The underlying musculature beneath the skin layers does not provide good support since it tends to be flabby and lacking in tone. Often, microcirculation to the skin is poor and the skin may be pallid and pasty. All of this can be a recipe for pronounced cellulite.

Getting Rid of Cellulite

When it comes to cellulite, estrogen dominant women can be particularly vulnerable. Because they are more prone to excess weight, they are also more prone to cellulite. But with so many different options and products on the market, it's tough to know whether you're losing inches from your waist or wallet! But before you can fight cellulite, you need to know exactly what you are up against.

The first three layers of your skin are the epidermis, dermis, and subcutaneous layer. The subcutaneous layer consists of separate compartments that contain fat cells. As women age, the dermis becomes thinner and thinner, thus allowing fat cells from the subcutaneous layer to enter the dermis layer. At the same time, the fat cells in the subcutaneous layer increase in size, causing the compartments to bulge, thus producing the dimples and pitting known as cellulite.

Like anything with health, prevention is the best medicine. And cellulite is no exception. Slender women and female athletes have far less cellulite than their heavier and less active counterparts.

If you already have some cellulite, I would recommend working to reduce the size of the fat cells, improving circulation in the affected areas, and increasing the integrity of your connective tissues. I have found that exercise, diet, massage, and certain nutrients can go a long way in helping you get rid of cellulite.

Diet and Exercise

I know you already know this, but yes—you'll need to lose excess weight to truly reduce cellulite. Just be sure to do it slowly and gradually. Rapid weight loss can make the appearance of cellulite even worse.

To accomplish this goal, I recommend eating a diet that is high in complex carbohydrates and lean protein, and low in saturated fat. You'll also want to reduce your intake of condiments and beverages that worsen fluid retention, including products with salt and caffeine. Additionally, try to increase the amount of water you drink. This will help to flush fats and toxins from your system.

If you are not already exercising regularly, you should include 30 minutes of aerobic activity at least five days a week.

Massage

Studies have shown that massage and/or dry brushing helps to remove toxins and improve circulation in the affected area. One of the best remedies I've seen for using massage to treat cellulite involves coffee grounds and plastic wrap. And since you are reducing your caffeine intake—you should have plenty of extra grounds on hand! The grounds not only work themselves into the dimples and pockets commonly associated with cellulite, but the caffeine helps to tighten your skin and tissues by constricting your superficial blood vessels.

First, warm about ½ cup of coffee grounds. You can do this by heating them up in a microwave or running them through your automatic drip coffee maker. Next, massage the warm coffee grounds into the affected area, then secure with plastic wrap. After 10–15 minutes, simply rinse the grounds off.

> **MY LATTÉ LATHER**
> For a more luxurious, spa-like experience, try my special latte. I love it!
>
> - ⅓ cup raw brown sugar
> - 1½ tablespoon fresh coffee grounds
> - 1½ tablespoon ground almonds
> - 2 teaspoons peppermint oil
> - 4 teaspoons flaxseed oil
> - 1 teaspoon BioMarine Squalane (*www.drlark.com* or 800-941-1997)
> - 9 drops peppermint oil
> - ¼ teaspoon cocoa powder
>
> 1. Mix all ingredients in an air-tight container (preferably plastic).
> 2. Use in the shower, rubbing all over your body in a circular motion. (You can use as much or as little as you want.)
> 3. Store remaining mixture in the refrigerator until your next at-home spa experience!

Cellulite-Blasting Nutrients

There are three nutrients that are particularly effective for reducing the appearance of cellulite by working to increase the integrity of your connective tissues by strengthening the collagen fibers in the subcutaneous layer. They are gotu kola, glucosamine sulfate, and grape seed extract.

One study from as far back as 1975 found that 58 percent of patients who took gotu kola every day for three months reported very good results in their cellulite reduction, while another 20 percent said they were satisfied with their results. **If you are interested in using gotu kola, I recommend taking 500–1,000 mg twice a day in capsule form.**

Glucosamine sulfate and grape seed extract also work to strengthen the collagen fibers.

Grape seed extract offers the added benefit of also improving circulation. **I recommend taking 1,000–1,500 mg of glucosamine sulfate a day, in two to three divided doses, as well as 50 mg of grape seed extract twice a day.** Gotu kola, glucosamine, and grape seed extract are available in most health food stores and Whole Foods Markets.

Is It Estrogen Dominance?

If the health conditions and cosmetic issues I discussed earlier in this chapter sound like you, you can use the following checklist to help you determine if you are estrogen dominant. If you answered yes to four or more of these questions, you are very likely in estrogen dominance.

- ✓ Are you over age 35?
- ✓ Do you suffer from premenstrual syndrome (PMS)?
- ✓ Do you have heavy, irregular periods?
- ✓ Do you suffer from anxiety, irritability, and mood swings?
- ✓ Have you gained more than 10 pounds?
- ✓ Do you have noticeable cellulite?
- ✓ Do you have puffiness around your eyes or face?
- ✓ Do you have a decreased interest in sex?
- ✓ Are you experiencing sleep difficulties?
- ✓ Are you retaining fluids?
- ✓ Are you having headaches?
- ✓ Do you have bouts of brain fog—forgetting your friend's first name, where you put your car keys, or the point of a text you recently studied?
- ✓ Have you recently discovered cysts in your breasts?
- ✓ Have you been told you have fibroid tumors?
- ✓ Do you have symptoms of endometriosis?
- ✓ Have you been diagnosed with either hyperplasia or endometrial cancer?
- ✓ Have you been diagnosed with ovarian cysts?

If you are concerned that this sounds like you, then the next step is to get your hormone levels tested.

Testing for Estrogen Dominance

Until the 1990's, the method for checking women's hormone levels had severe limitations. A single blood sample was taken and analyzed, though the results of this one-time check were disgracefully unhelpful. In addition, the stress of having blood drawn was enough to throw off a woman's hormone levels and skew the results.

Fortunately, there are saliva female hormone tests that are both non-invasive (no needle sticks!) and highly accurate. These tests can take the guesswork out of making a proper diagnosis and make it possible to design individualized treatment that delivers maximum benefits with minimum risk of side effects.

Best of all, saliva hormone testing is accessible. Even physicians who still don't routinely order saliva hormone testing will usually do so if a patient requests it. You can even order a limited saliva hormone test kit on your own directly from a laboratory, without a doctor's prescription.

Saliva Versus Blood

Most women are surprised when I suggest saliva testing over blood testing. Let me explain.

Like blood, saliva closely mirrors hormone levels in your body's tissues. However, saliva is a particularly accurate indicator of free (unbound) hormone levels. This is the key, as only free hormones are active, meaning that they can affect the hormone-sensitive tissues in your breasts, brain, heart, and uterus. Saliva testing therefore provides a superior measure of the levels of hormones that actually affect vital body systems, mood, tissue levels of sodium and fluid, and many other important functions.

Additionally, blood testing only provides a one-time "snapshot" of hormone levels, whereas saliva testing provides a dynamic picture of hormonal ebb and flow over an entire menstrual cycle. In fact, 11 samples are collected during the month, all at the same time of day, then sent to a laboratory. The lab measures and charts your progesterone and estradiol (your most prevalent and potent form of estrogen) levels. These results are compared to normal patterns.

Finally, saliva testing is easy, stress-free and non-invasive. You can collect your own saliva samples, which means you don't have to go to your doctor's office or a lab. Plus, there's no need to draw blood.

Get Tested

If you think saliva hormone testing is right for you, consider consulting your physician. Having your doctor order the test has two advantages: The profile is more extensive, and your insurance may cover the cost. Several laboratories perform the test; in the event your physician does not have a preference, I recommend Genova Diagnostics—formerly Great Smokies Diagnostic Laboratory—(*www.gdx.net* or 800-522-4762), as well as ZRT Laboratory (*www.zrtlab.com* or 866-600-1636). If your doctor doesn't order the test, or you simply want insight to help you develop your own self-care regimen, you can order a test kit from several sources. Aeron Laboratories has a wonderful Life Cycles saliva test kit (*www.aeron.com* or 800-631-7900).

When you are tested, they will be looking to determine your estradiol and estriol levels. Levels of estradiol normally fluctuate during the menstrual cycle and variability is rather broad among individuals. Estriol production is uniformly low throughout a woman's life, except in pregnancy, when high levels occur.

The following measurements are for blood levels of the hormones. If you opt for saliva testing, keep in mind that salivary levels are approximately one percent of the total blood concentration.

Ranges of estradiol in women:

Follicular phase:	< 2 to 4 pg/ml
Early luteal phase:	4 to 10 pg/ml
Mid luteal (peak) phase:	2 to 4 pg/ml
Women taking oral contraceptives:	< 1 pg/ml

Ranges of estriol:

Nonpregnant women:	< 15 pg/ml
With estriol supplementation:	20 to 500 pg/ml

If your results show that you are estrogen dominant (or if you scored high on the questionnaire), you are far from alone. I have treated thousands of women with this condition, and hardly a day goes by that I don't get calls or emails from women all over the country looking for relief. Thankfully, relief is possible.

reversing
estrogen
dominance

11

Throughout my many, many years in the field of women's health, I've seen several remedies aimed at helping women reduce their estrogen levels and/or increase their progesterone production. I have had wonderful success over the years using safe, gentle, effective nutritional and other therapies to accomplish this goal. This has been terrific for my patients, because they have been able to reduce and even eliminate health issues such as fibroid tumors of the uterus, endometriosis, adenomyosis, PMS, fibrocystic breast disease, and endometrial hyperplasia without resorting to conventional therapies and their many side effects.

Conventional medicine often uses dangerous drugs and even surgery to treat the symptoms of estrogen dominance—both of which have a host of nasty side effects. Plus, these treatments never address the underlying hormone imbalance.

One common conventional therapy is low-dose birth control pills, which can commonly cause a worsening of PMS symptoms and even increase your risk of a stroke. Another conventional option is a prostaglandin inhibitor. While these are effective for treating pain and bleeding due to endometriosis, they can cause gastrointestinal bleeding, peptic ulcers, heartburn, nausea, vomiting, and diarrhea.

Some physicians even prescribe a synthetic form of testosterone called Danazol to help depress the output of the follicle-stimulating hormone (FSH) and luteinizing hormone (LH) from the pituitary and hypothalamus, which then works to lower estrogen production in the ovaries. Unfortunately, this can decrease estrogen levels so much that your natural male hormone response is accentuated, leading to acne, abnormal hair growth, decreased breast size, and possibly a deepening of your voice.

Other conventional doctors prescribe synthetic forms of the gonadotropin-releasing hormone, such as Lupron and Nafarelin, which work to inhibit the secretion of FSH and LH by the pituitary. As a result, estrogen levels decrease. While these drugs don't have the masculinizing side effects of Danazol, they do produce typical menopausal symptoms, such as hot flashes and migraines, and can increase your risk of osteoporosis by lowering estrogen levels and increasing the excretion of calcium from your body.

Finally, the extreme option is hysterectomy or other gynecologic surgeries, which are often performed needlessly on women, when much safer and less invasive natural therapies could be used instead. As far as I'm concerned, removal of your uterus, and especially your ovaries, is often unnecessary when treating estrogen dominance-related problems. However, women facing possible surgery for conditions like endometriosis or fibroid tumors need to institute changes that I describe in this chapter, and stick with them in order to navigate through their premenopause years comfortably and in good health.

FACING HYSTERECTOMY

Nearly 600,000 hysterectomies are performed every year in the United States, many of which are a result of a variety of medical problems typically seen in women suffering from estrogen dominance-related conditions, including fibroid tumors, endometriosis, and prolonged heavy menstrual bleeding. In fact, fibroid removal accounts for nearly one-third of all hysterectomies performed annually in the United States, many of which are completely unnecessary. The fact is, many fibroids will likely shrink and may even disappear with menopause.

If you have had a hysterectomy due to fibroid tumors, endometriosis, or heavy menstrual bleeding, you very likely had only your uterus removed, but may still have your ovaries. In this case, the surgery will not necessarily trigger menopausal symptoms such as hot flashes and vaginal dryness, although your hormone levels may fluctuate or even diminish due to the stress of the surgery. Hopefully, your own hormone production will then stabilize for a while, and you will resume production of your own normal complement of hormones until you would normally have entered menopause. And even though you will no longer menstruate, you can still expect to go through the normal chemical and physical changes associated with perimenopause and menopause as your ovaries begin to show the normal signs of aging.

Because hormone replacement requires a delicate balance of estrogen, progesterone, and testosterone, I recommend saliva testing within six to 12 months after the surgery to determine your baseline levels. If you find that you do need to boost your hormone levels, I suggest using my natural hormone restoration program (and even biochemically identical hormones, if necessary), as described in later chapters of this book, depending on your symptoms and their severity. This will help to bolster the levels of these hormones still being produced by your ovaries and adrenal glands.

Not only do these treatments have a host of nasty side effects, they don't help women get back into balance. Fortunately, there is a better, safer way to ease through premenopause and estrogen dominance with minor or diminished symptoms. I've used the following program to help thousands of women go through the menopause transition in a much more comfortable way, allowing them to avoid drugs and surgery and find relief safely and effectively.

A Better Way

With my program, you'll use nutrients to help you decrease estrogen production; increase the breakdown, metabolism, and elimination of estrogen; increase progesterone production; or use supplemental progesterone. The end result is that both the production of hormones and their elimination from your body is improved, helping to bring your estrogen and progesterone levels back into a much healthier balance.

You can decrease estrogen production at both the adrenal level and the ovarian level by using weakly estrogenic herbs and nutrients to bind to key enzymes, thereby preventing the male hormones testosterone and androstenedione from being converted into estrogen. These enzymes are aromatase in the adrenals and estrogen synthetase in the ovaries. By blocking your body's own more potent estrogen from binding to the enzyme itself, you can hinder complete estrogen production from taking place. At the same time, you are providing the body with less potent, safer, and healthier estrogen-like chemicals from nutrients to support your body's needs during the transition into menopause.

In order to effectively break down, metabolize, and eliminate estrogen, you need to ensure that your liver, gallbladder, and intestinal tract are working properly and effectively. If these organs are not performing to optimum capacity, they cannot adequately metabolize and eliminate estrogen. Without proper deactivation of estrogen, there is more free-floating hormone circulating in your body.

This is how the whole system works: As estrogen goes through the detoxification process in your liver, it is inactivated by being bound to sulfuric and glucuronic acid and converted from the more potent form of estrogen—estradiol—to the less potent forms of estrone and estriol. This process of binding hormones with other chemicals makes them unable to attach to the specific hormone receptor sites within the cells. Once the hormone has been detoxified by the liver, it is then secreted with the bile into the small intestine and eliminated through the intestinal tract in your bowel movements.

Another way to offset excess estrogen is to increase progesterone production by stimulating ovulation. To do this, you need to stimulate the production of the pituitary's luteinizing hormone (LH) so that it is properly balanced with the production of the pituitary's follicle-stimulating hormone (FSH). The imbalances in these hormones in the pituitary upset the normal production of estrogen, progesterone, and testosterone by the ovaries and adrenal glands, disrupting the healthy balance between all three of these sex hormones. Additionally, increasing the production of the different types of neurotransmitters in the brain—those linked with energy and alertness, as well as those associated with relaxation, calm, and sleep—are necessary for healthy menstruation, as they regulate hormone output from the hypothalamus and pituitary, the master hormone-regulating glands in your brain. In turn, these hormones help to stimulate ovulation from your central nervous system.

Finally, you can use biochemically identical progesterone to increase hormone levels and counterbalance excess estrogen. Studies have shown that women who took progesterone for less than 10 days a month had more than double the risk of endometrial cancer than those who took progesterone for 10 days or more each month. I'll talk more about the benefits of supplemental progesterone in Chapter 12.

Modulate Estrogen with Hormone Mimics

As I indicated above, certain plants and nutrients curb estrogen production by binding to the estrogen receptor sites and blocking the enzymes that convert testosterone into estrogen. The key plant foods in this process are soy, flaxseed, and bioflavonoids (mainly from citrus fruit sources).

Thanks to its weak estrogenic activity, soy reduces the production of more potent estrogens within your body. It does this through its phytoestrogens genistein and daidzein, which belong to the class of chemicals called isoflavones. Soy isoflavones were first discovered during the 1930's, but their potency was not assayed until the 1950's. At that time, genistein was found to be a natural plant estrogen that's 50,000 times weaker than any strong, synthetic form of the hormone.

According to a study from the journal *Cancer*, women who took 40 mg of the soy isoflavone genistein for 12 weeks had a 53 to 55 percent reduction in their estrogen levels. Several similar studies have shown the same results.

To enjoy these types of estrogen-reducing advantages at home, take in 50 to 100 mg of soy isoflavones each day, either through soy foods, isoflavone capsules, or a combination of both.

ISOFLAVONE CONTENT OF SOY PRODUCTS
½ cup tofu=35 mg isoflavones
½ cup tempeh=35 mg isoflavones
1 cup soy milk=35–40 mg isoflavones
½ cup edamame (whole soy beans)=150 mg isoflavones

Flaxseed is unusual since it contains a double source of plant-based estrogen. Both the oil and the flax lignan (a substance contained within the cellulose-like material that provides structure to plants) contained within the seed have been researched for their estrogenic effect. Once plant lignans are eaten, intestinal bacteria convert them to weakly estrogenic substances that are absorbed into the body.

Lignans also inhibit the production of estrogen, as seen in a study conducted at the University of Minnesota, and published in the *Journal of Clinical Endocrinology and Metabolism*. Eighteen women with normal menstrual cycles ate normally for three cycles and then added 10 grams of flaxseed powder per day to their diet for an additional three cycles. During the time that the women did not eat flaxseed, there were three cycles when no ovulation occurred. But when flaxseed was included, all of the women in the study ovulated every menstrual cycle. Thus, ground flaxseed was found to improve the estrogen-to-progesterone ratio favoring the levels of progesterone within the body.

Flaxseed also contains fatty acids, from which short lived, hormone-like chemicals called prostaglandins are created. Prostaglandins are essential for the process of ovulation to occur. Each of your ovaries contains thousands upon thousands of follicles. These structures contain an ovum (or egg). During each menstrual cycle, one of these follicles becomes the dominant one for that month. At mid-cycle, this dominant follicle will burst or rupture, thereby releasing the egg into the fallopian tube and down into the uterus, where it can then be fertilized and pregnancy can occur. In order for the follicle to rupture and release the ovum, prostaglandins must be present.

To help rebalance estrogen levels and increase ovulation, I recommend taking 1–2 tablespoons of cold-pressed flaxseed oil or 4–6 tablespoons of ground flaxseed daily. Flaxseed oil is sold in opaque containers in the refrigerator section of most health food stores, as it is very sensitive to heat, light, and oxygen. Whole flaxseed is also available, as is pre-ground and capsule form. If you purchase the whole seed, be sure to grind it into a fine meal before consumption in order to release the beneficial lignans.

Finally, bioflavonoids are often used to balance hormone levels. These mildly estrogenic antioxidants, found in the pulp and rind of citrus fruit, are also antiestrogenic. Though bioflavonoids have weak, estrogen-like properties, they have also been shown to interfere with the production of estrogen by competing with estrogen precursors such as androstenedione and testosterone for binding sites on an enzyme called estrogen synthetase. In essence, this blocks the male hormones from being converted into estrogen in the ovaries as well as fatty tissues.

In this way, bioflavonoids work to normalize estrogen balance, bringing excessively high estrogen down to more normal levels. In a related mechanism, bioflavonoids also bind to estrogen receptor sites in the uterus and breasts, blocking your body's own high-octane estrogen from doing damage.

Additionally, studies have shown that bioflavonoids, in combination with vitamin C, also help to reduce heavy menstrual bleeding in transitioning menopausal women, as well as women suffering from bleeding due to fibroid tumors.

Other research indicates the same benefit from flavonoids alone. According to a study from the *Journal of Gynecology and Obstetrics*, flavonoids not only reduce heavy menstrual bleeding, but also ease menstrual cramps. Of the 36 women who took 1,000 mg a day of a flavonoid-based nutritional product for just under 12 months, 70 percent of them enjoyed a 50 percent reduction in their bleeding, and the duration of the bleeding was one-third less. Seventy-five percent of the women also saw a 50 percent reduction in the severity of their menstrual cramps.

I suggest taking 1,000–2,000 mg of citrus bioflavonoids per day. Bioflavonoids are considered very safe and have virtually no side effects. *Note:* In addition to the citrus variety, other specific bioflavonoids such as quercetin and rutin also have anti-estrogen properties. In fact, research studies are finding that quercetin may also help reduce your risk of ovarian cancer. And rutin has been shown to be particularly helpful in strengthening capillaries and reducing heavy menstrual bleeding.

Vital Vitamins for Estrogen Modulation

There are also key vitamins that work to regulate the effects of estrogen on menstrual bleeding and PMS symptoms, as well as promoting healthier menstrual function. These include vitamins C and vitamin E. Vitamin C helps strengthen and fortify blood vessels, thereby reducing heavy menstrual bleeding, particularly when taken with bioflavonoids. According to a study from the *American Journal of Obstetrics and Gynecology*, women who received 600 mg each of both vitamin C and bioflavonoids daily, in divided dosages, for two months experienced less blood loss, as compared to those taking a placebo.

Similarly, a study from *Fertility and Sterility* found that vitamin C improved hormone levels and increased fertility in women with luteal phase defect. As I indicated earlier, your menstrual cycle has two phases. The first is the follicular phase, which begins on day one of your period and ends at ovulation. The second luteal phase starts with ovulation and ends on the first day of your period. Estrogen levels rise during the follicular phase, while progesterone levels increase in the luteal phase.

Several factors can prevent adequate progesterone production in the luteal phase, including oxidative stress. That's where vitamin C comes in. A recent study found that women who received 750 mg of vitamin C every day for three months enjoyed increased progesterone levels. Interestingly, those women who did not receive vitamin C not only had lower levels of progesterone, but also showed increased levels of estrogen. One reason for this is that vitamin C is necessary to convert essential fatty acids into prostaglandins. Remember, progesterone can only be produced in the ovary during the second half of your menstrual cycle, after ovulation has occurred.

To help lower estrogen levels in your body, I suggest taking 1,000–4,000 mg of mineral-buffered vitamin C per day, in divided doses to prevent diarrhea.

Another key nutrient is vitamin E. Vitamin E helps to relieve the symptoms of PMS, including menstrual cramps, as well as benign breast disease. Although it is unclear exactly how vitamin E works to relieve PMS symptoms, it is widely believed that either its antioxidant properties or its modulation of prostaglandin production are involved. Research conducted at Johns Hopkins University Medical Center also found that vitamin E helps to reduce discomfort from fibrocystic breasts.

Early research has also shown that vitamin E was useful to reestablish healthy menstrual cycles in young women. Living under the stress of war is often associated with widespread disruption of menstrual cycles. This was true of women living in an internment camp in Manila during World War II. Doctors who treated these women observed that menstruation had stopped abruptly after the first bombing of Manila, before a nutritional deficiency would have been experienced. These physicians conducted a small study, published in the *Journal of the American Medical Association*, in which 10 women with amenorrhea (a lack of menstruation) were given 20 drops of wheat germ oil (a great source of vitamin E). The doses were taken orally, three times a day, for a period of 10 days, preceding the onset of each woman's expected menstrual flow. Of the 10 women, eight began to menstruate.

I suggest taking 400–1,000 IU of natural vitamin E a day, in an oil-based capsule. If you cannot tolerate oil-based products, there is a dry form of vitamin E available. Start with the lower dose and increase by 400 IU every two weeks until the desired effect is achieved. *Note:* Vitamin E is considered extremely safe and is commonly used by millions of individuals. However, women with certain medical problems, such as hypertension, insulin-dependent diabetes, and menstrual-bleeding problems, should begin taking vitamin E at lower dosages, starting with 100 IU per day and slowly increasing the dosage. If you have any of these health conditions, check with your doctor before supplementing with vitamin E.

Magnificent Minerals for Estrogen Dominance

In addition to vitamins C and E, certain minerals have been shown to be especially useful in regulating the effects of estrogen. These include magnesium and calcium.

Magnesium has been shown to significantly mitigate PMS symptoms, including mood changes, pain, inflammation, and breast cysts. According to a study conducted at the University of Reading in England and published in the *Journal of Women's Health and Gender-Based Medicine*, 200 mg of magnesium a day eased water retention and bloating in women suffering from PMS. A follow-up study also suggested that the same amount of magnesium, taken with 50 mg of vitamin B_6, eased PMS-related anxiety.

Like vitamin C, magnesium and vitamin B_6 are also critical to convert essential fatty acids (like those found in flaxseed, cold-water fish, walnuts, soy, and green leafy vegetables) into beneficial, inflammation-fighting prostaglandins. **I suggest taking 600–750 mg of magnesium with 50–100 of vitamin B_6 per day.**

Another critical mineral—calcium—is also quite successful at alleviating PMS-related symptoms. A study from the *American Journal of Obstetrics and Gynecology* looked at the effect calcium had on reducing PMS symptoms such as mood swings, bloating, food cravings, and menstrual cramps. They divided 466 women into two groups. The first received 1,200 mg of calcium a day and the other received a placebo over the course of three months. By the end of the third month, those women taking the calcium saw a 48 percent decrease in their PMS symptoms. **To enjoy relief from your PMS symptoms caused by excess estrogen, I recommend taking 1,200–1,500 mg of calcium carbonate a day.**

* * *

While plant-based nutrients, vitamins, and minerals all work to reduce your estrogen production, you should also increase the metabolism and elimination of the hormone. Let's take a look at the best ways to accomplish this.

Create an Estrogen Breakdown

The best way to tell you how to create an estrogen breakdown is by showing you how your liver and digestive tract help to metabolize and eliminate estrogen from your body, thereby helping to keep estrogen levels balanced and healthy. This occurs through a process called the enterohepatic circulation of estrogen.

During this process, estrogen circulates in the blood throughout your body and passes through your liver. Your liver then metabolizes it from its more potent forms, estradiol and estrone, to a more chemically inactive and safer form, estriol. When the liver is healthy, this occurs efficiently. The estrogen metabolites are then secreted into the bile and, from there, into your digestive tract.

There are several substances that help to facilitate this process. These include the well-known B vitamins, as well as the lesser-known but powerful combination of DIM, calcium-d-glucarate, d-limonene, fiber, and probiotics.

The vitamin B complex is a group of 11 separate, water-soluble nutrients: B_1 (thiamine), B_2 (riboflavin), B_3 (niacin), B_5 (pantothenic acid), B_6, B_{12}, biotin, folic acid, para-aminobenzoic acid (PABA), choline and inositol. In addition to regulating mood and restoring energy, B vitamins have been shown to help your liver inactivate estrogen. According to a 1942 study published in *Endocrinology*, a lack of B vitamins negatively affects your liver's ability to detoxify estrogen. Specifically, researchers found that women with several health problems related to excess estrogen levels (heavy menstrual flow, benign breast disease, and PMS) who received vitamin B-complex supplements enjoyed relief of their symptoms.

Additionally, like magnesium, B vitamins also help convert essential fatty acids taken in through your diet into inflammation-fighting prostaglandins. This anti-inflammatory effect helps relieve muscle cramps and reduces the symptoms of endometriosis, and possibly even retards the spread of the disease.

Finally, a study conducted by Guy Abraham, M.D., at UCLA Medical School found that women who took 500 mg of vitamin B_6 for three months enjoyed a reduction in PMS symptoms, including menstrual cramps, pain, and weight gain. According to Dr. Abraham, vitamin B_6 helped to change the blood levels of both estrogen and progesterone and bring them into balance.

To help neutralize estrogen and ease symptoms of excess estrogen, I suggest taking 50–100 mg of a vitamin B-complex a day. Be sure it includes 50–100 mg of vitamin B_6.

DIM the Lights on Estrogen

Diindolylmethane, or DIM, is a plant-compound found in *Brassica* veggies such as broccoli, bok choy, cauliflower, cabbage, and Brussels sprouts. Researchers have found that this interesting little compound is quite beneficial in promoting estrogen metabolism.

During estrogen metabolism, the most potent form of estrogen (estradiol) is converted into estrone. Estrone then becomes either 2-hydroxyestrone—a "good" estrogen metabolite—or 16-alpha-hydroxyestrone—a "bad" estrogen metabolite. The good metabolite (2-hydroxyestrone) is then converted into 2-methoxyestrone and 2-methoxyestrodial.

This is where DIM comes in. Research has shown that when DIM is ingested, it not only encourages its own metabolism, but that of estrogen. While it is not an estrogen or even an estrogen-mimic, its metabolic pathway exactly coincides with the metabolic pathway of estrogen. When these pathways intersect, DIM favorably adjusts the estrogen metabolic pathways by simultaneously increasing the good estrogen metabolites and decreasing the bad 16-alpha-hydroxyestrone.

The research confirms this action. In a study from *Epidemiology*, American researchers took urine samples from 34 healthy postmenopausal women. They then added 10 grams of broccoli a day to the women's diets. After taking another urine sample, researchers found that this dietary change significantly increased the 2-hydroxyestrone to 16-alpha-hydroxyestrone ratio.

In addition to eating more *Brassica* vegetables like broccoli and cauliflower, I recommend taking 30 mg of DIM a day with meals.

Detoxify With D-Glucarate

Glucuronidation, a detoxification process that occurs in the liver, depends on glucuronic acid, a chemical produced within the body which is similar to calcium d-glucarate, a naturally occurring substance found in many fruits and vegetables. As estrogen circulates through the blood, it passes through the liver, where it is bound to glucuronic acid. This binding process inactivates the estrogen, inhibiting it from binding to tissues. It is then secreted into the bile and passed into the intestinal tract, where it is then eliminated from the body via bowel movements.

Unfortunately, certain bacteria in the intestinal tract secrete an enzyme called beta-glucuronidase (B-glucuronidase) which can sabotage the glucuronidation process. B-glucuronidase breaks the newly formed estrogen-glucuronic acid bond apart, which reactivates the estrogen. This free estrogen can then be reabsorbed by the body, thus elevating the level of estrogen circulating through the body.

Luckily, eating a diet rich in glucarate or using glucarate supplements helps to decrease the level of B-glucuronidase by allowing the bond between glucuronic acid and estrogen to be maintained so the body can rid itself of excess estrogen. This helps to prevent your own level of estrogen from rising to toxic levels.

To reduce the total amount of circulating estrogen, I recommend taking 500 to 1,000 mg of glucarate per day with meals. This supplement is very well tolerated with no toxicity or known drug interactions.

GLUCARATE-RICH FOODS

✓ Apples
✓ Apricots
✓ Broccoli

✓ Brussels sprouts
✓ Cherries
✓ Lettuce

Lighten the Load with Limonene

Another ally to help lower your total estrogen load is limonene, a compound usually found in citrus fruits, especially lemons and oranges. In addition to supporting glucuronidation, limonene also promotes healthy detoxification. Specifically, it has been shown to help prevent the development of estrogen-dependent breast cancer by stimulating detoxification enzymes in the liver.

A study published in *Cancer Research* tested to see if limonene could reduce or regress breast cancer in rats. Researchers fed a limonene-rich diet to rats that had developed breast tumors. They found that the rats that were given this diet had significant tumor shrinkage as compared to the control group. However, when the limonene was discontinued, the tumors reappeared. Additionally, researchers found that limonene inhibited the spread or metastasis of the cancer.

To help reduce free-floating estrogen in your body, **I recommend taking 500–1,000 mg of limonene per day or every other day.** *Note:* Women who are allergic to citrus should not take limonene. Additionally, while it appears to be safe and without toxicity, pregnant or nursing should not take limonene since no research has been performed that specifically examines its effect on fetal development.

Flush Out Estrogen With Fiber

Dietary fiber is a key component to eliminating excess estrogen from your body. Once estrogen is broken down and neutralized by your liver, it is secreted into your bile. From there, it enters your small intestines. In your intestinal tract, fiber works by binding to estrogen and removing it through bowel movements. According to a study from Tufts University Medical School, vegetarian women excrete two to three times more estrogen in their bowel movements than do other women who eat a diet lower in fiber and higher in fat. This is great news for estrogen dominant women who are trying to reduce the estrogen load in their body.

In addition to regulating estrogen levels, fiber also binds to cholesterol. This helps to keep your bad cholesterol levels in a healthy range.

Plus, fiber is key for preventing constipation, colon cancer, and many other intestinal disorders. (More than 85,000 cases of colon cancer are diagnosed each year.) Once ingested, fiber undergoes bacterial fermentation in the colon. This process produces butyrate, the main energy source for colonic epithelial cells, which are needed for a healthy, cancer-free colon. This effect was verified in a study published in the *Scandinavian Journal of Gastroenterology*. Researchers followed the health of 20 patients who had undergone surgical treatment for colon cancer. The volunteers were given fiber in the form of psyllium seeds. After one month of supplementation, fecal concentration of butyrate increased by 47 percent.

There are two types of fiber: soluble and insoluble. Soluble fibers (dissolvable in water) are found in fruits, vegetables, nuts, and beans. Insoluble fibers (not dissolvable in water) are found in oatmeal, oat bran, sesame seeds, and dried beans. Sadly, the refining process has removed most of the natural fiber from our foods, creating a nation of people grossly lacking in fiber.

To ensure that you are getting adequate amounts of both kinds of fiber (and therefore ensuring the effective elimination of excess estrogen), be sure to eat whole-grain cereals and flours; brown rice; all kinds of bran; fruits such as apricots, prunes, and apples; nuts and seeds; beans, lentils, and peas; and a wide variety of vegetables. Several of these foods should be included in every meal. Moreover, when you eat apples and potatoes, enjoy them with their skins.

You can further supplement your diet with fibers like oat bran and/or psyllium (1–2 tablespoons per day, mixed with 8–12 ounces of water and swallowed immediately after stirring). You may also try guar gum (which is helpful in regulating your blood sugar level) and pectin (which is derived from apples and grapefruit and can lower the amount of fat that you absorb from your diet). Simply combine ½ teaspoon guar gum and 500 mg of pectin with 8–12 ounces of water. Stir and drink immediately. Use one to three times a day.

Powerful Probiotics

Many women with estrogen dominance tend to eat a high-fat, low-fiber diet. High intake of saturated fats, commonly found in foods such as dairy, butter, and red meat stimulate the growth of unhealthy, anaerobic bacteria in the intestinal tract. These bacteria chemically change the breakdown products of estrogen into forms that can be reabsorbed back into the body.

These bacteria split estrogen from the binding substances that inactivate it in your liver. This splitting process causes free estrogen to be reformed within your intestinal tract. As this free estrogen is reabsorbed into the circulation, it increases free estrogen levels within the blood.

To suppress the growth of these unhealthy bacteria, I suggest that you not only reduce your intake of saturated fat (which can lead to the problem in the first place), but that you also use probiotic supplements. Probiotics help to recolonize your intestinal tract with healthy bacteria such as L. acidolphilus and B. longum. **I recommend taking probiotics that contain at least 1–3 billion live, healthy organisms per day.**

* * *

In addition to decreasing the amount of estrogen in your system by reducing its production and increasing its elimination, you can help to offset the hormone by increasing your progesterone levels. To accomplish this, you need to stimulate ovulation at both the central nervous system and ovarian levels.

Balance Excess Estrogen with Progesterone

The best way I know to increase progesterone production is to stimulate ovulation. This can be done on two levels—through the central nervous system or via the ovaries.

Most women are surprised to learn that you can increase progesterone production through the brain or central nervous system. What many people don't realize is that all hormone production begins in the brain.

We've been traditionally taught that human beings have one brain that is divided into many different parts. But more and more research is putting the "one brain" idea to the test. In fact, it's starting to be widely accepted that the human skull actually houses not one brain, but three—the reptilian brain, the limbic brain, and the neocortical brain.

The reptilian brain is the oldest part of the brain. It controls basic bodily functions like heart rate, breathing, body temperature, hunger, and fight-or-flight responses. Basic drives and instincts, such as defending territory and keeping safe from harm, are other functions of the reptilian brain. The structures in the brain that perform these functions are the brain stem (which controls breathing, heart rate, and blood pressure) and the cerebellum (which controls movement, balance, and posture).

The limbic, or mammalian, brain developed once mammals started roaming the earth. It includes the hippocampus, which controls memories and learning; the amygdala, which controls memory and emotions; and the hypothalamus, which controls emotions (among many other things). Therefore, the limbic brain allows mammals to learn, retain memories, and show emotions.

The neocortical brain, or neocortex, is the complex maze of grey matter that surrounds the reptilian and limbic brains, and accounts for about 85 percent of brain mass. It is found in the brains of primates and humans, and is responsible for sensory perception, abstract thought, imagination, and consciousness. It also controls language, social interactions, and higher communication.

The Chemistry of the Brain

Like the three parts of the brain, there are also three key types of brain chemicals: neuropeptides, neurohormones, and neurotransmitters.

Neuropeptides are responsible for the cell-to-cell communication system in your body. A peptide is a short chain of amino acids connected together, and a neuropeptide is a peptide found in neural tissue. Neuropeptides are widespread in the central and peripheral nervous systems and different neuropeptides have different excitatory or inhibitory actions.

Neuropeptides control such a diverse array of functions in the body. When they work together properly, the wonderful results in your body include elevated mood and other positive behaviors and emotions, stronger bones, better resistance to disease, glowing skin, and boosted metabolism. Conversely, if your neuropeptides function abnormally, the result can be an increased tendency towards neurological and mental disorders such as Alzheimer's disease, epilepsy, and schizophrenia.

There are several types of neuropeptides. Some of the most common include endorphins and beta-endorphins. Endorphins are opiod peptides, meaning they have morphine-like effects within the body. They produce feelings of well-being and euphoria, and a rush of endorphins can lead to feelings of exhilaration brought on by pain, danger, or stress. Endorphins also may also play a role in memory, sexual activity, and body temperature. Beta-endorphins are another form of opiod peptides, but they are stronger than endorphins. They are composed of 31 amino acids and work in the body by numbing pain, increasing relaxation, and promoting a general feeling of well-being.

While there are many, many hormones and hormonal interactions that occur in the brain and body, the most widely known neurohormone is melatonin. (I will discuss melatonin in more detail on page 125.)

Neurotransmitters are naturally occurring chemicals that relay electrical messages between nerve cells throughout your body. While all three types of neurochemicals are important for hormone and overall health, neurotransmitters are particularly important for the production of sex hormones.

In the aggregate, all three types of neurochemicals help to regulate the brain's endocrine glands, specifically the hypothalamus and pituitary gland. The hypothalamus is the master endocrine gland contained within your brain that regulates your production of sex hormones. This gland produces a precursor hormone called gonadotropin releasing hormone (GnRH). When it is released, it travels to your anterior pituitary gland, where it stimulates the secretion of the follicle stimulating (FSH) and luteinizing hormones (LH).

As you now know, these hormones then travel to the adrenals and ovaries, where they stimulate the production of estrogen, progesterone, and testosterone. In women with estrogen dominance, the production of LH needed to trigger ovulation may not proceed in a healthy fashion. This causes menstrual cycles to be estrogen-predominant during the second half of the cycle when progesterone should prevail.

In order to keep this whole process working smoothly, LH and FSH need to be triggered by a balanced mixture of the key neurotransmitters necessary to produce these hormones. As previously mentioned, neurotransmitters are naturally occurring chemicals that relay electrical messages between nerve cells throughout your body. The production of these vital chemicals is synthesized from certain amino acids, vitamins, and minerals that must be obtained through your diet or from supplementation.

First and foremost, the neurotransmitters norepinephrine, epinephrine, dopamine, and serotonin regulate the hypothalamus' release of GnRH. Without proper production and balance of these neurotransmitters, you cannot have proper balance of the sex hormones, including progesterone. This process is supported by precursor amino acids such as tyrosine, phenylalanine, and 5-HTP.

To understand this more fully, let's take a more detailed look at neurotransmitters in action.

Neurotransmitters: The Hormone Messengers

There are two crucial neurotransmitter pathways that help to support your overall health and well-being. The first leads to the production of inhibitory neurotransmitters such as serotonin and GABA, while the second leads to the production of excitatory neurotransmitters like dopamine, norepinephrine, and epinephrine.

Generally speaking, the inhibitor neurotransmitters quiet down the processes of your body, while the excitatory neurotransmitters stimulate them, speeding them up. Thus, the brain chemicals produced through these two pathways oppose and complement one another. Within your brain, serotonin often inhibits the firing of neurons, which dampens many of your behaviors. In fact, serotonin acts as a kind of chemical restraint system.

Of all your body's chemicals, serotonin has one of the most widespread effects on the brain and physiology. It plays a key role in regulating temperature, blood pressure, blood clotting, immunity, pain, digestion, sleep, and biorhythms. Along with another inhibitory neurotransmitter—GABA (gamma-aminobutyric acid)—serotonin also produces a relaxing effect on your mood. Taurine, a type of amino acid, is often used in a similar fashion as these two neurotransmitters because it also has therapeutic, inhibitory effects on your body.

Dopamine, norepinephrine, and epinephrine make up the excitatory neurotransmitter pathway. (Glutamate is another import excitatory neurotransmitter, though not part of the pathway.) Unlike serotonin, which has a relaxing effect on your energy and behavior, excitatory neurotransmitters energize and elevate your mood. In addition to their powerful antidepressant effects, they support alertness, optimism, motivation, zest for life, and sex drive. Plus, the excitatory neurotransmitters are particularly important for the production of progesterone and testosterone.

ARE YOU BALANCED?

If you experience any of the following symptoms on an ongoing, consistent basis, you may have a neurotransmitter imbalance:

Low Inhibitory Neurotransmitters
- ✓ PMS
- ✓ Migraine headaches
- ✓ Chronic pain
- ✓ Irritable bowel syndrome
- ✓ Mood swings, irritability
- ✓ Anxiety
- ✓ Food cravings, binge eating
- ✓ Sleep apnea
- ✓ Fibromyalgia
- ✓ Increased infections
- ✓ Insomnia, poor sleep quality

Low Excitatory Neurotransmitters
- ✓ Depression
- ✓ Fatigue
- ✓ Low thyroid function
- ✓ High stress levels
- ✓ Weight gain, difficulty losing weight
- ✓ Cold hands and feet
- ✓ Mental sluggishness
- ✓ Low libido
- ✓ Irregular menstruation, heavy bleeding

In order to ensure you have adequate neurotransmitter levels needed for healthy hormone production, you need to supplement with key amino acids, vitamins, and minerals. As I indicated earlier, all neurotransmitters are derived from nutrients that you take in through your diet. They are produced from amino acids found in the protein that you eat. The essential amino acid tryptophan is initially converted into an intermediary substance called 5-hydroxytryptophan (5-HTP), which is then converted into serotonin.

While tryptophan is available as a supplement and is abundant in turkey, pumpkin seeds, and almonds, I've found that 5-HTP is a more effective and reliable option for boosting your neurotransmitter production. Numerous double-blind studies have shown that 5-HTP is as effective as many of the more common antidepressant drugs and is associated with fewer and much milder side effects. In addition to increasing serotonin levels, 5-HTP triggers an increase in endorphins and other neurotransmitters that are often low in cases of depression.

The excitatory neurotransmitters are derived from tyrosine, an amino acid produced from phenylalanine, another amino acid. A variety of vitamins and minerals, such as vitamin C, vitamin B_6, and magnesium, act as co-factors and are necessary for the conversion of these amino acids into neurotransmitters.

To maintain proper serotonin levels, it is helpful to take 50–100 mg of 5-HTP once or twice a day, with one of the dosages taken at bedtime. Be sure to start at 50 mg and increase as necessary. If needed during the day, use carefully, as too much serotonin can interfere with your ability to drive or concentrate.

To maintain optimum dopamine levels, take 500–1,000 mg of tyrosine per day. Be sure to take in divided doses, half in the morning and half in the afternoon. Do not take in the evening, as it may interfere with sleep.

As I recommend with all nutritional supplements, you should start at the lower to more moderate dosage, such as 500 mg a day of tyrosine and 50 mg a day of 5-HTP. Stay on this dosage for two weeks. If you don't notice a reduction in your symptoms, gradually increase the dosage by 500 mg for tyrosine and 50 mg for 5-HTP every two weeks until you have either noticed a reduction in your symptoms or have reached the maximum dosages. I generally don't recommend going over 1,000 mg a day of tyrosine, although you may find that you need as much as 100–200 mg of 5-HTP once or even several times a day.

Additionally, be sure to use a high potency multivitamin/mineral nutritional supplement so that you are taking in all of the co-factors needed to produce neurotransmitters. These include vitamin C, vitamin B_6, folic acid, niacin, magnesium, and copper.

Note: I strongly advise that you undertake a program to restore and properly balance your neurotransmitter levels under the care of a complementary physician, naturopath, or nutritionist. You should also have your neurotransmitter levels tested regularly, as dosage needs for the amino acids I've described often vary from woman to woman (see next page).

In addition to creating proper neurotransmitter balance through the use of amino acids derived from your diet, with the help of key vitamins and minerals, there are several other types of nutrients that can help to keep your endocrine glands and precursor hormones functioning properly. My particular favorites include vitex (chaste tree berry), maca, and glandulars.

Vital Vitex

Vitex is an herb native to the Mediterranean area. Also known as chaste tree berry, due to its ability to decrease libido, vitex has been used for centuries to ease heavy menstrual bleeding, promote ovulation, and even restore menstruation in women who suffer from amenorrhea.

Vitex works at the hypothalamic and pituitary levels. Specifically, it inhibits the release of FSH, thereby lowering estrogen production, while also aiding in the production of LH to trigger ovulation, thereby promoting progesterone production.

One study found that vitex helps restore menstruation by increasing progesterone levels. Researchers gave vitex extract to 20 women who had either abnormal or non-existent menstruation. After six months, 15 of the women were available for evaluation. Lab tests revealed that 10 of the 15 women had a return of their menstrual cycles, as well as increased levels of both progesterone and LH. Their FSH levels either remained consistent or decreased slightly.

A similar study found that eight women with abnormally low progesterone levels who were given vitex every day for three months also enjoyed increased progesterone levels. In fact, two of the women became pregnant!

Vitex has also been shown to hinder the release of prolactin, a hormone closely related to human growth hormone, which plays a critical role in lactation. If there is too much prolactin in your system, secretion of LH is disturbed, which in turn can disrupt ovulation, and therefore progesterone production.

Several studies have proven vitex's ability to reduce prolactin levels. One double-blind, placebo-controlled study examined 52 women with luteal phase problems due to increased prolactin levels. They were given 20 mg of vitex a day for three months. At the end of the treatment period, prolactin levels had been significantly reduced.

Similarly, a German study looked at 13 women between the ages of 15 and 48 years, all of whom suffered from menstrual dysfunction. Lab tests showed that all the women had abnormally high prolactin levels. After taking vitex for three months, all the women had "continuous and significant" decreases in their prolactin levels.

A study from *Experimental and Clinical Endocrinology* suggests that vitex works to decrease prolactin by binding to dopamine receptors, which in turn thwart the secretion of prolactin. Interestingly, the researchers found that while prolactin secretion was inhibited, gonadotropin secretion (which leads to FSH and LH secretion) remained unaffected.

Research from several German peer-reviewed publications confirms this finding. For example, the *International Journal of Gynecology & Obstetrics*, and *Hormone and Metabolic Research* have both found that vitex appears to block prolactin secretion by binding to dopamine receptors. However, much research still needs to be done in this area.

To increase progesterone levels and decrease prolactin, I suggest taking 140–275 mg of a standardized extract of vitex (chaste tree berry) every day. Chaste tree berry works slowly, so it may take three or four months before you start to see its full benefit.

Exotic Maca

Maca—referred to as either *Lepidium peruvianum* or *Lepidium meyenii*—is one of the most traditionally used and valued Peruvian herbs, due in large part to its rich nutrient concentration. This malty, butterscotch-flavored root contains a number of minerals, vitamins, fatty acids, plant sterols, amino acids, and alkaloids, among other phytonutrients. In terms of minerals, calcium makes up 10 percent of maca's mineral content. Magnesium, phosphorus, and potassium are also present in significant amounts. Maca also contains a number of vitamins and amino acids, including B_1, B_2, B_{12}, vitamin C, vitamin E, and quercetin, as well as arginine, lysine, tryptophan, tyrosine, and phenylalanine.

German and American researchers begin studying Peruvian botanicals in the 1960's and 1980's. They quickly discovered that maca has many health benefits, including relieving menopausal symptoms; stimulating and regulating the endocrine system (adrenals, thyroid, ovaries, and testes); increasing energy, stamina, and endurance; regulating and normalizing menstrual cycles; and balancing hormone levels.

Maca appears to act as a central nervous system stimulant, at the level of the hypothalamus and pituitary gland. It works to stimulate hormone production, which is a critical part of regulating a woman's physiology. It also operates as an adaptogenic herb to help regulate hormones produced by the endocrine glands. It does this by stimulating your ovaries and adrenals to produce the hormones you need, in the levels you need them.

This was shown in a study published in the *Journal of Veterinary Medical Science*. Researchers tested the effects of maca on mouse sex hormones. They found that while progesterone and testosterone levels increased significantly in the mice that received the maca, their estradiol levels were not increased. In other words, the maca helped to raise the levels of progesterone and testosterone to offset the blood levels of estradiol in the mice. This is exciting news for women suffering from estrogen dominance.

A traditional dosage of maca is 2–10 grams a day. However, dosages are unique to each woman, so you will need to determine which dosage works for you. There have been no acute toxic effects of maca, even at very high doses. In fact, many Peruvians eat it every day! *Note:* If you are sensitive or allergic to herbs, you may want to use maca cautiously. In any event, I suggest starting with the low end of the recommended dosage, as too much can cause increased hot flashes, breast tenderness, or headaches. It is also recommended that you avoid maca if you have a hormone-related cancer (due to lack of formal studies), liver disease, if you are pregnant or nursing, or if you are currently taking conventional HRT.

Transforming Glandulars

Glandular therapy involves the use of purified extracts from the secretory endocrine glands of animals. Most commonly, extracts are drawn from the thyroid and adrenal glands, as well as the thymus, pituitary, pancreas, and ovaries. Most extracts come from cows, with the exception of pancreatic glandular preparations usually drawn from sheep.

There are four common ways to extract glandulars. The first involves quick-freezing the material, washing it with a potent solvent to remove fatty tissues, distilling the solvent out, drying it, and then grinding it into a fine powder that is then encapsulated or pressed into tablets.

The second mixes freshly crushed material with salt and water that also removes fatty tissues. It is then dried and ground into a fine powder to be placed in capsules or made into tablets.

In the third method, the glandular material is freeze-dried, then placed into a vacuum chamber to remove the water. It is then encapsulated. However, with this method, fatty tissues remain.

The final method uses plant and animal enzymes to partially "digest" the material. It is then passed through a filter that separates out the fat-soluble molecules. The remaining material is then freeze-dried. This method seems to be quite effective. Due to the "pre-digestion," all biologically active substances remain intact and can be used therapeutically to support and restore your body's endocrine glands. Healthier endocrine glands are more likely to have healthier hormone production and to be more balanced.

In the past, most experts believed that glandulars could not be effective because the intestinal lining of a healthy person was impenetrable, and that proteins and large peptides could not breach its barrier. However, recent evidence has shown that large macromolecules can and do pass completely intact from the intestinal tract into the bloodstream. In fact, there's further evidence to suggest that your body is able to determine which molecules it needs to absorb whole, and which can be broken down.

Both animal and human studies have proven this theory. In some cases, several whole proteins taken orally, including critical enzymes, have been absorbed intact into the bloodstream. Additionally, many smaller proteins and numerous hormones have also been absorbed intact into the bloodstream, including thyroid, cortisone, and even insulin.

In essence, this means that the active properties of the glandulars stay active and intact, and are not destroyed in the digestive process. This is key to the success of glandular therapy, and explains why they clearly help to restore hormone function by supporting the health of your endocrine glands themselves.

There are multi- and single-glandular systems available from companies like Standard Process—a leader in the field. However, they do require a prescription from a health care practitioner. Other good products are also available in health food stores and should be used as part of a nutritional program to support healthy menstruation.

Examples of widely used and accepted glandulars involve the thyroid and adrenals. Natural thyroid medications such as Armour Thyroid, Naturthyroid, and Bio-Thyroid have been the preference of complementary physicians for decades. Unlike many of the commonly prescribed brands of thyroid therapy that only replace a synthetic form of one of your thyroid hormones (T4), these natural thyroid replacements contain the whole animal-derived thyroid gland, including T3 *and* T4 hormones. This is a significant difference. T3 is more physiologically active than T4, and is critical in regulating normal growth and energy metabolism. Without the use of glandulars, this type of natural thyroid replacement wouldn't be possible. However, the thyroid glandulars sold in the health food stores have the hormone removed and are used to support the function of your own gland.

Adrenal glandular preparations are even more common. With the stress epidemic in this country, the majority of Americans are walking around with depressed adrenal function. Fortunately, whole adrenal extracts have been found to help restore the health and function of compromised adrenal glands. In one research study, eight women suffering from morning sickness (nausea and vomiting) who took oral adrenal cortex extract found relief within four days. A similar study gave both injected and oral adrenal cortex extract to 202 women also suffering from morning sickness. More than 85 percent of the women completely overcame their nausea and vomiting or showed significant improvement.

Another study looked at the use of adrenal glandulars to treat patients with chronic fatigue and immune dysfunction syndrome (CFIDS), as well as fibromyalgia. Researchers found that 5–13 mg of an adrenal glandular preparation significantly reduced pain and discomfort.

Moreover, after six to 18 months, many of the patients were able to reduce and eventually discontinue treatment, while still enjoying relief.

Clearly, glandulars work. **To help support healthy progesterone levels, I suggest taking a good multi-glandular or single glandular product from a company like Standard Process. These could include glandulars such as hypothalamus, pituitary, ovary, adrenal, and thyroid, depending on the specific needs of each individual woman. I also highly recommend that you consider taking a whole brain glandular, if appropriate. To further support your adrenal function, I recommend taking 1,000–3,000 mg of a mineral-buffered vitamin C each day with a meal, 25–100 mg of a vitamin B complex a day, and an additional 250 mg of B$_5$ (pantothenic acid) twice a day.**

While stimulating progesterone production originates in your central nervous system, you also need to support your ovaries and adrenals, which also support progesterone production. Here's a look at the three key nutrients that support its production in the ovaries.

Ovarian Progesterone Production

Progesterone (as well as estrogen and testosterone) are produced by your ovaries, while your adrenal glands produce a precursor to estrogen called androsteredione, which is then converted into estrogen in your fatty tissues. Therefore, it's important to keep your ovaries functioning at their optimal level. To do this, I highly recommend using the following key nutrients: lutein, beta-carotene, and essential fatty acids.

Life-Giving Lutein

Lutein is a carotenoid with powerful antioxidant properties. As you can likely determine from its name, lutein plays a major role in the luteal phase, the time from ovulation to menstruation when the luteinizing hormone (LH) is produced.

While estrogen levels are rising from menstruation through ovulation, LH, which is produced by the pituitary gland, is needed to trigger ovulation. After ovulation, the follicle that contained the egg that was expelled from the ovary during ovulation is then converted into a new structure called the corpus luteum. Lutein is abundant in the corpus luteum and provides it with its distinctive yellow color.

The purpose of the corpus luteum is to switch from the estrogen production, which predominates during the first half of the menstrual cycle (days one to 14) to the production of progesterone and estrogen during the second half of your cycle (days 15 to 28). This is called the luteinizing process. During this time, lutein begins to accumulate on these key cells, and the effectiveness of the luteinizing process may be due, in part, to the amount of lutein found there. **To ensure that you have adequate lutein levels to support normal development of the corpus luteum, I suggest supplementing with 6–12 mg of lutein a day.**

Beneficial Beta-Carotene

Beta-carotene is the plant-based, water-soluble precursor to vitamin A. Like lutein, beta-carotene is abundant in the ovaries, and is found in very high concentrations in the corpus luteum and the adrenal glands—both of which produce progesterone. Some research even suggests that a proper balance between carotene and the retinal form of vitamin A is necessary for proper luteal function.

Researchers have been aware of the reproductive benefits of beta-carotene for more than a century. For example, cows whose diets were deficient in beta-carotene experienced delayed ovulation, decreased progesterone levels, and an increased prevalence of ovarian cysts, as well as cystic mastitis (breast cysts). Both conditions are typically found in women who are progesterone deficient.

Research studies have also found carotenoids such as beta carotene, as well as vitamin A, to be useful in treating conditions related to estrogen dominance, including ovarian cancer, heavy menstrual bleeding, and benign breast disease. A study from the *International Journal of Cancer* found that high carotenoid intake decreased a woman's risk for ovarian cancer. In fact, beta-carotene rich carrots were among the foods most strongly associated with decreased risk.

Studies have also determined that vitamin A helps prevent heavy menstrual bleeding. Researchers tested the blood levels of 71 women suffering with excessive bleeding. They found that all the women had lower than normal levels of vitamin A. After taking vitamin A supplements for just two weeks, 90 percent of them returned to normal menstruation levels.

Finally, a study from *Preventative Medicine* found that high doses of vitamin A can help reverse one form of benign breast disease. Researchers gave 150,000 IU of vitamin A to 12 women with fibrocystic breasts. After three months, more than half the women reported complete or partial remission of the cysts. While I would never suggest that women take this high a dose of vitamin A for fear of toxicity, I believe that beta-carotene would have a similar effect.

To ensure that you have adequate amounts of beta-carotene in your system, I suggest taking 25,000–50,000 IU a day.

Exciting EFAs

Essential fatty acids (EFAs) are health-promoting nutrients that your body needs to perform a whole range of functions. There are two main groups of EFAs: omega-3s and omega-6s. The most common are linoleic acid (omega-6), linolenic acid (omega-3), and the omega-3 fatty acids eicosapentaenoic acid (EPA) and docosahexaenoic acid (DHA).

Your body converts EFAs into series 1 and 3 prostaglandins, potent hormone-like substances with a wide range of benefits that are essential for good reproductive health. Among other things, these prostaglandins help to promote more frequent ovulation at midcycle.

Since prostaglandins are necessary for the rupture of the follicle, which allows the egg to be extruded from the ovary at mid-cycle, this is a critical step for progesterone production to occur during the second half of the cycle.

EFAs are effective for a wide variety of estrogen dominant-related conditions, but they are most commonly heralded for their effectiveness in easing menstrual cramps. Specifically, a study from the *American Journal of Obstetrics and Gynecology* looked at 42 girls between the ages of 15 and 18 years, all of whom had experienced significant menstrual pain during their periods. Those girls who took 1,080 mg of EPA and 720 mg of DHA every day for two months enjoyed a significant decrease in their pain due to menstrual cramps. No change was observed in the placebo group. Additionally, the amount of painkillers the girls took during their menstrual periods decreased by more than 50 percent during the fish oil treatment as compared to the placebo treatment.

The two best sources of EFAs are flaxseed and fish oil. In the case of flaxseed, both the oil and the ground meal are rich in EFAs. Plus, flax has been proven to support progesterone production. Researchers at the University of Minnesota tested 18 women with normal menstrual cycles. During three cycles, the women ate as they normally would. They then added 10 grams of ground flaxseed per day to their diet for an additional three cycles. The women who ate flaxseed had more ovulatory cycles than the women who did not. In addition, ground flaxseed was found to improve the estrogen-to-progesterone ratio, favoring the levels of progesterone within the body. The researchers felt that this was due to the lignans contained in the flaxseed, although I feel strongly that the flaxseed oil was also very beneficial in this regard, as it is also converted into prostaglandins, which are necessary for ovulation to occur. **To promote progesterone production, I suggest taking 1–2 tablespoons of flaxseed oil or 4–6 tablespoons of ground flaxseed per day.**

JUST THE FLAX
When it comes to overcoming estrogen dominance, you cannot forgo the flax. Flaxseed does triple duty, helping combat excess estrogen on three levels:

1. The lignans are weak phytoestrogens that help to modulate estrogen production.
2. The fiber assists the intestines in the excretion of excess estrogen, once it has been inactivated by the liver.
3. The omega-3 and omega-6 fatty acids are converted into series 1 and 3 prostaglandins to help with progesterone production.

If you do not like flaxseed or cannot tolerate it, you may prefer to get your EFAs through fish oil. In addition to also promoting progesterone production and helping to regulate the menstrual cycle, fish oil is extremely beneficial for easing menstrual cramps, endometriosis, and breast cysts due to its anti-inflammatory benefits. **If fish oil is your preference, I suggest taking 3–6 capsules that contain at least 300 mg DHA and 200 mg EPA every day.**

* * *

Clearly, estrogen dominance is a complex condition. And it's one I know first-hand. When I was in my 20's, I too suffered from estrogen dominance. By following the program I've outlined in this chapter, I can happily report that my hormone levels have been balanced for several decades now.

You can enjoy this same balance by reducing estrogen in the five different avenues I've described:

1. Decreasing estrogen production with hormone mimics such as soy, bioflavonoids, and flaxseed.
2. Assisting the breakdown of estrogen in the liver, gallbladder, and intestines with B vitamins, DIM, glucarate, and limonene.
3. Enhancing the elimination of excess estrogen with fiber.
4. Stimulating ovulation (and therefore progesterone) at both the central nervous system level and ovarian level with neurotransmitter precursors, vitex, maca, glandulars, lutein, beta-carotene, and EFAs.
5. Using biochemically identical natural progesterone.

Next, let's take a look at the flip side of the estrogen coin—estrogen deficiency. I'll not only include quizzes and lab tests to help you determine your current levels, but also discuss the use of natural estrogen, as well as plant-based substitutes. Plus, you'll discover how to restore your own levels of this vital hormone with little-known nutrients.

menopause & estrogen deficiency

12

If you are or have been estrogen dominant during the menopause transition, you need to do everything you can to reduce, metabolize, and eliminate as much estrogen as possible from your bodies. However, as you enter menopause, you experience the other side of the coin—estrogen deficiency—and need to do everything you can to increase and maintain your levels of estrogen for your health and physical and emotional well-being. Healthy levels of estrogen are necessary to support so many of your physiological functions, as well as the organs and tissues of your body. But, a healthy balance of this hormone is the key to good health—not too much and not too little.

What is Menopause?

Somewhere between the ages of 43 and 59 years old, most women will usually begin to experience fewer and fewer monthly menstrual periods, and bleeding becomes scanter and scanter. You may also experience hot flashes and other menopause-like symptoms. This is considered the perimenopause phase. Eventually, you will cease menstruation altogether, with the cessation of a menstrual period for 12 straight months signaling the official start of menopause.

Once your periods have stopped completely, you are considered postmenopausal. At this point, estrogen production will have dropped 75 to 90 percent. This life change is due to normal aging of ovaries and egg follicles. Your ovaries and adrenal glands continue to produce a small amount of estradiol (the most potent form of estrogen) and estrone (a middle potency estrogen), and the liver produces some estriol (the weakest form of estrogen). While the action of estrone and estriol is not nearly as strong as the estrogen produced before menopause, these hormones do continue to provide some support for the bones, breasts, brain, heart, vagina, and other tissues.

Menopause by Any Other Name…

There are two different types of menopause. The first type is experienced by most women. It is natural and typically occurs between the ages of 43 and 59. Though the average age for the onset of menopause is 51 years, some women can begin the change in their mid- to late-40's (early-onset) or not until their early-60's (late-onset). About 12.5 percent of women experience early-onset menopause, and this pattern often runs in a woman's family.

Menopause is considered to be late-onset if it occurs after age 55. In fact, less than one percent of women continue menstruating after age 59. The fact that I menstruated into my early 60's is quite rare and is likely due to the fact that I have been supporting and balancing my hormones with my own natural program since I first entered the field of medicine over 30 years ago. As a result, I have had a remarkable level of hormonal health. This is particularly impressive, given the terrible menstrual cramps, PMS, benign breast disease, and irregular menstrual periods that I suffered from during my teenage years and into my 20's.

The second type of menopause is "artificial," meaning that something outside of a woman's natural physiology triggered menopause. Many women who experience menopause in their 30's and 40's fall into this category.

The two most common causes of artificial menopause are chemotherapy and hysterectomy. The chemicals used in chemotherapy can, and often do, interfere with your ovaries' ability to produce estrogen. In the case of hysterectomy, you will always have cessation of periods, but you may or may not still produce your normal levels of hormones. This depends on whether or not you still have your ovaries. If you had only your uterus removed but still have your ovaries, then the surgery will probably not trigger the actual symptoms of hormone deficiency commonly seen with menopause, although hormone levels often fluctuate or even diminish due to the stress of the surgery.

If you've had a hysterectomy that involved the removal of your ovaries as well as your uterus, then your ability to produce hormones has been greatly compromised. Since your ovaries have been removed, your entire hormone production has been drastically reduced, and all of your hormone production is now dependent upon your adrenals. Plus, the shock of the surgery itself may further reduce your adrenals' ability to produce hormones. As a result, menopause symptoms such as hot flashes and vaginal dryness are often experienced almost immediately following this type of surgery.

Now that you understand what menopause is and how it can occur, let's address why it occurs.

The Physiology of Menopause

Your ovaries and adrenal glands produce substantial amounts of estrogen during your active, reproductive years and continue to produce small amounts after menopause. While we are accustomed to using the term *estrogen*, this term actually refers to several different types of estrogens made within the body. At least six types of estrogen have been identified and are classified according to their potency. The term *potency* refers to the time that estrogen is bound to the estrogen receptor within a specific tissue. The higher the estrogen potency, the more time it remains bound to the receptor and, therefore, the more pronounced are the physiological effects that estrogen promotes within that tissue. For example, estrogen is a growth-stimulating hormone, causing tissues to grow and thicken; it also causes water and salt to be retained within the tissues of the body. The more potent and powerful forms of estrogen cause these effects to occur in a more pronounced fashion.

In this book, I focus on the three main types of estrogen produced within the body—estradiol, estrone, and estriol. As I indicated in chapter two, estradiol is the most potent form of estrogen, and the primary type of estrogen produced by the ovaries during a woman's reproductive years. Estrone is an intermediate-potency form of estrogen, 12 times weaker than estradiol. It is mainly produced within the fatty tissue of the body from precursor hormones made by the adrenal glands. Estrone is also produced by the ovaries, and small amounts continue to be produced by the ovaries after menopause, when production of estradiol ceases. Estriol, the liver metabolite of the other two estrogens, is the weakest form of estrogen produced by the body. It is 80 times weaker than estradiol.

In a normal menstrual cycle, you produce primarily estrogen during the first half of your cycle, which lasts approximately 14 days. This is called the follicular phase. At mid-cycle, the egg (or ovum) is extruded from the follicle (the structure that contains each egg), which then undergoes a change in composition, and becomes the corpus luteum (or yellow body). The corpus luteum secretes both estrogen and progesterone during the second half of your cycle.

This entire system is regulated in the brain, which releases hormones secreted by the hypothalamus, and by stimulating hormones made by the pituitary gland. The hormones released by the hypothalamus and pituitary activate and trigger the production of your female hormones by the ovaries and adrenal glands. This primarily works as a negative feedback system.

During this time, your follicle-stimulating hormone (FSH) concentrations become significantly elevated to stimulate estrogen production by the follicles. As estrogen levels begin to rise, your FSH levels begin to fall. In contrast, during the mid and end of your cycle, when estrogen levels are low, your FSH levels rise in an effort to again stimulate estrogen production.

When you enter the menopause transition, your ovaries and their eggs are starting to age and are less responsive to stimulation by FSH in the pituitary. In turn, your pituitary is also starting to show the negative effects of aging, so the whole system starts to unravel and work less efficiently. In fact, a study from the *Journal of the American Medical Association* found that as women age, their hypothalamus and pituitary glands become increasingly insensitive to estrogen.

Due to this decrease in estrogen production, your menstrual period typically becomes significantly shorter. Your FSH levels increase in an attempt to stimulate your follicle to develop more quickly and make more estrogen. Eventually, your estrogen levels drop so low that menstruation ceases altogether. However, FSH levels remain elevated, and soon your levels of luteinizing hormone (LH)—also produced by the pituitary—rise as well, stimulating the supportive tissues of your ovaries to produce more progesterone, testosterone, and androstenedione. This latter hormone is then converted into the second most potent form of estrogen (estrone) by your fatty tissues.

After menopause has begun, your ovaries secrete only small amounts of estradiol. Instead, your adrenal glands become the major source of this potent estrogen. Similarly, the adrenals become your primary source of estrone as well. In other words, while estrogen production does decrease after menopause, it doesn't stop completely. Your ovaries and adrenal glands continue making some estrogen throughout your life. However, the ratios of the types of estrogen changes. You'll go from making mostly estradiol to now making primarily the weaker, mid-level estrone form. As a result, your body has less overall estrogen—and a weaker form—to work with.

Not all women produce the same amounts and/or types of estrogen after menopause. Because androstenedione is converted into estrone in your fatty tissues, women with more body fat have more circulating estrogen than thin women. Additionally, in my practice and in my own personal experience, I've found that women with better nutrition habits and women who are less stressed and more relaxed have healthier estrogen balance and make more estrogen than women who don't watch their food intake and stress levels.

If you are one of these lucky women—and you can be with my program—then you will experience significantly fewer menopausal symptoms, have more energy, and sail through the transition without ever knowing the dark side of menopause.

The Dark Side of Menopause

Ask any menopausal woman what they dislike most about this change of life, and they'll likely give you a list of complaints. In addition to the commonly known hot flashes and night sweats, menopause can bring a whole host of physical, mental, and emotional changes primarily due to a deficiency of estrogen, as well as the other sex hormones.

Hot Flashes/Night Sweats

As many as 85 percent of all menopausal women in the United States experience some degree of hot flashes. Women with more severe symptoms may have as many as 10, 20, or even 40 episodes a day, while other women may only experience them a few times a week or during times of stress. The episodes are the result of increased blood flow to the brain, organs, and skin, causing a sudden sensation of warmth that may be followed by chills. On average, a hot flash lasts about two to five minutes. Most experts agree that hot flashes are caused by either an abrupt withdrawal of estrogen or a sudden increase in the neurotransmitter norepinephrine.

Hot flashes are physically draining, since your body loses fluids and minerals in the process of perspiring. And if they occur at the workplace or during social functions, they can be embarrassing. When they take the form of night sweats, hot flashes may disrupt sleep and soak sheets, leaving you cranky and exhausted. Hot flashes cause a woman to turn pink and either perspire profusely or simply generate a lot of heat within the body. In any case, women often feel like shedding clothes, which is usually not possible in a professional setting.

Fortunately, hot flashes don't last forever. About 50 percent of women see relief within a year. For another 30 percent, hot flashes can last two or three years. And for an uncomfortable 20 percent of women, hot flashes can linger for 5 to 10 years.

Insomnia

A number of studies have shown that estrogen decreases the frequency of awakenings during the night and increases the amount of restorative rapid eye movement (REM) sleep, the type of sleep that occurs when a person is dreaming, which is necessary for feeling rested the next day.

When estrogen levels are deficient, you are likely to sleep more fitfully and for fewer hours. Lacking adequate sleep, you are more likely to feel tired during the day. If you have had an abrupt decline in your estrogen levels by undergoing gynecological surgery, including the removal of your uterus and/or ovaries, you may suffer most acutely from interrupted sleep.

Loss of Libido

When estrogen decreases, vaginal tissues begin to atrophy and your natural lubricants decrease. Your vagina then becomes gradually thinner and less elastic. This can cause intercourse to be painful, and you may experience soreness after sex. Pain during intercourse can also increase your reluctance to have sex.

Also, after menopause, your production of testosterone and other androgens (male hormones) also decline. These hormones normally stimulate sex drive. While androgens are produced throughout your cycle, during your active reproductive years, their levels increase before mid-cycle, thereby increasing your desire for sex just as an egg is ready to be fertilized.

When everything is working perfectly, you have a healthy desire for sex. But as your body shifts gears during the transition to menopause, desire tends to decrease. And while some testosterone still cycles in your bloodstream, the amount may be insufficient to spark desire.

Osteoporosis

Throughout most of your life, your female hormones work to build bone, even as calcium and other alkaline minerals are drawn out of your bones to prevent over-acidity and support the healthy, slightly alkaline pH of your blood.

After menopause, your body continues to draw on your bones' alkaline mineral reserves, but bone building is greatly diminished, due to the significant decline of your female hormone production. The result is more porous, fragile, and brittle bones. Older women with osteoporosis have lost as much as 40 to 45 percent of their total bone mass. In fact, statistics from the National Osteoporosis Foundation indicate that osteoporosis is responsible for 1.5 million fractures each year, and affects more than 20 million women. Fortunately, bone can be rebuilt with my estrogen support program, the right diet, supplements, and exercise.

Heart Disease and Stroke

The incidence of heart disease escalates as women age and estrogen production declines. Estrogen is known to help keep the arteries clear of plaque. From age 30 to 60, cancer is the main cause of death in women, with heart disease ranking second for women age 40 to 60. However, after age 60, heart disease becomes the leading cause of death in American women, claiming the lives of nearly 500,000 women each year, and affecting another three million.

Current research shows that the relationship between estrogen and heart disease is tied to estrogen's role in maintaining healthy cholesterol levels, namely keeping the "good" high-density lipoprotein (HDL) levels elevated. Other research indicates that estrogen increases nitric oxide (NO) levels. This gas naturally inhibits muscle contraction and helps to relax blood vessels. As a result, it helps to promote blood flow and vascular relaxation, and works to make tissues firmer and more elastic.

Vaginal Infections and Dryness

Estrogen causes the uterus and vagina to increase in size. It stimulates the vagina and urinary tract linings to thicken and become more resistant to trauma and infection, thus preparing a woman to eventually become sexually active and bear children. When estrogen decreases, vaginal tissues begin to atrophy and your natural lubricants decrease. These changes can make you more susceptible to vaginal and bladder infections.

If you experience pain during sex or acquire an infection as a result of intercourse, you may be reluctant to have sex. Your doctor may prescribe drugs for infections, but you must be willing to reveal the full range of your symptoms, including lack of sexual desire, to ensure that you get the best treatment available.

Loss of Skin Tone

Estrogen causes an increase in overall body fat, contributing to the softly rounded female contours that we associate with sexual maturation. Firm, youthful-looking skin is also attributable to estrogen, which stimulates collagen, a protein that makes up 90 percent of the skin. Finally, estrogen causes fluid and sodium retention within the tissue, so your skin is plumper and more hydrated.

To this point, research has found that both the amount of collagen and the thickness of your skin decrease by one to two percent each year following menopause. Fortunately, estrogen substitutes and key herbs and nutrients have been found to prevent collagen atrophy, and even restore decreased thickness.

Mental Confusion

The ability to concentrate and remember details depends, in part, on having adequate amounts of estrogen. As a woman's own estrogen production begins to diminish, cognitive function can decline.

I regularly hear complaints from my menopausal patients of muddled thinking, brain fog, and poor memory. When short-term memory fades, a person may misplace their car keys, forget a friend's name, or even enter a room or office at work with no idea of why they went there.

As estrogen replacement therapy became more popular in the 1960's and 1970's, researchers began to study the effects of hormones on cognitive function in young and middle-aged women. In a review article on estrogen and memory done at McGill University, the researcher found that there is a strong indication that estrogen does help to maintain short- and long-term memory in women. These benefits were noted in verbal recall, but not in visual/spatial memory.

Another study published in *Psychoneuroendocrinology* investigated the effects of estrogen on memory function in women with surgically induced menopause. Nineteen women who were scheduled for hysterectomy and removal of the ovaries were given verbal memory tests before surgery, and again two months after their operation. Postoperatively, the women were treated with either 10 mg of estrogen or a placebo. Memory scores of those women treated with estrogen showed no decline after surgery, whereas the scores of those women who received the placebo declined significantly.

Mood Swings

Your emotions are determined, in part, by your estrogen levels. Because estrogen is a natural stimulant, with a mood-elevating effect, fluctuating estrogen levels can cause emotions to go haywire. When estrogen levels are elevated, a woman may experience anxiety and irritability, while a deficiency of estrogen can lead to depression.

With the decline in estrogen production that occurs during menopause, many women notice that their moods may fluctuate. Some of my patients have complained about mood swings varying between increased anxiety and irritability to depression and fatigue. They have reported being bad tempered toward family, friends, and co-workers and responding to daily-life stresses in a more irritable fashion, similar to the emotional ups and downs of PMS.

Although menopause does not inevitably cause depression, some women do become despondent and gloomy as hormone production declines. Research has shown that supplemental estrogen has a mood-elevating effect. Women on some type of hormone replacement therapy may perceive this effect as an enhanced sense of well-being and overall mental balance, which contributes to the relief of other menopausal symptoms such as hot flashes and vaginal dryness. In a study published in *Clinical Obstetrics and Gynecology*, women were given 1.25 mg daily of either conjugated equine estrogen or a placebo for a period of two months. The women were assessed for their degree of irritability and anxiety. Those who received the estrogen treatment reported feeling calmer and more balanced moods with longer periods of well-being.

ADRIANNE'S STORY

Some years back, my friend "Adrianne" was telling me about her experience with menopause. At 52, she had debilitating hot flashes and a loss of sex drive. She had terrible insomnia and searing heartburn. These symptoms affected her career, home life, and relationships.

She tried many different approaches to deal with her symptoms, starting with Premarin—the most frequently prescribed synthetic hormone replacement therapy. It not only made her hot flashes worse, it also caused nausea and facial swelling. Finally, Adrianne settled on an estrogen-alone patch, combined with natural progesterone cream. At my suggestion, she also began using the herb kava root for sleep and sodium bicarbonate (baking soda) and peppermint tea for her heartburn. She was eventually able to find relief with this program.

Adrianne's difficulty in finding relief underscores for me the problem many women have at midlife. Finding a menopause solution that works for you must be individualized. The bottom line is you don't have to feel miserable or accept the idea that it's all downhill from here. Menopause may be a hormone-deficiency state, but with the right dietary support, nutritional supplements, and lifestyle changes, you can write your own ticket to good health and well-being after midlife.

Is It Menopause?

The following checklist can help you determine if you are estrogen deficient. If you answered yes to four or more of these questions, you are very likely in menopause.

- ✓ My last period was 12 months or longer ago
- ✓ My periods are lighter, less frequent, and of shorter duration (late perimenopause)
- ✓ I'm 46 or older
- ✓ I'm having hot flashes
- ✓ Intercourse is painful
- ✓ My desire for sex has faded
- ✓ I have difficulty achieving orgasm
- ✓ I have frequent vaginal infections
- ✓ I leak urine when I laugh, cough, sneeze, exercise, or wait too long to void
- ✓ I've lost my zest for life
- ✓ I have difficulty sleeping through the night
- ✓ I'm frequently tired
- ✓ I'm anxious and irritable
- ✓ I forget small details
- ✓ My skin is drier, thinner, and more wrinkled
- ✓ My muscles are losing their tone
- ✓ I'm gaining weight
- ✓ My joints and/or muscles ache
- ✓ I have itchy, crawly skin
- ✓ I sometimes feel as if electric shocks were going through my body

If you are concerned that this sounds like you, then the next step is to get your hormone levels tested.

Testing for Menopause

As I indicated with estrogen dominance, the method for checking women's hormone levels had severe limitations until the 1990's. A single blood sample was taken and analyzed, though the results of this one-time check were disgracefully unhelpful. In addition, the stress of having blood drawn was enough to throw off a woman's hormone levels and skew the results.

Fortunately, there are saliva female hormone tests that are non-invasive (no needle sticks!) and highly accurate. These tests can take the guesswork out of making a proper diagnosis and make it possible to design individualized treatment that delivers maximum benefit with minimum risk of side effects.

Best of all, saliva hormone testing is accessible. Even physicians who still don't routinely order saliva hormone testing will usually write an order when a patient requests it. You can even order a limited saliva hormone test kit on your own directly from a laboratory, without a doctor's order.

Saliva Versus Blood

Most women are surprised when I suggest saliva testing over blood testing. Let me explain.

Like blood, saliva closely mirrors hormone levels in your body's tissues. However, saliva is a particularly accurate indicator of free (unbound) hormone levels. This is the key, as only free hormones are active, meaning that they can affect the hormone-sensitive tissues in your breasts, brain, heart, and uterus. Saliva testing therefore provides a superior measure of the levels of hormones that actually affect vital body systems, mood, tissue levels of sodium and fluid, and many other important functions.

Additionally, blood testing only provides a one-time "snapshot" of hormone levels, whereas saliva testing provides a dynamic picture of hormonal ebb and flow over an entire menstrual cycle. In fact, 11 samples are collected during the month, all at the same time of day, then sent to a laboratory. The lab measures and charts your progesterone and estradiol (your most prevalent and potent form of estrogen) levels. These results are then compared to normal patterns.

Finally, saliva testing is easy, stress-free and non-invasive. You can collect your own saliva samples, which means you don't have to go to your doctor's office or a lab. Plus, there's no need to draw blood.

Get Tested

If you think saliva hormone testing is right for you, consider consulting your physician. Having your doctor order the test has two advantages: The profile is more extensive, and your insurance may cover the cost. Several laboratories perform the test; in the event your physician does not have a preference, I recommend Genova Diagnostics—formerly Great Smokies Diagnostic Laboratory—(*www.gdx.net* or 800-522-4762), as well as ZRT Laboratory (*www.zrtlab.com* or 866-600-1636). If your doctor doesn't order the test, or you simply want insight to help you develop your own self-care regimen, you can order a test kit from several sources. Aeron Laboratories has a wonderful Life Cycles saliva test kit (*www.aeron.com* or 800-631-7900).

When you get your test results, you'll want to pay particular attention to your estradiol levels. A reading of one to two pico-grams per milliliter (pg/ml) indicates that you are menopausal.

The Cosmetic Effects of Menopause

I never fail to be amazed at how women of all ages are fascinated with the health and beauty of their skin. Several weeks ago, my husband Jim and I were having lunch at a little French restaurant near our house. We were celebrating a special occasion and having a great time when, about halfway through our meal, a group of women came in and sat at the table behind us. The women appeared to be in their 70's and 80's. Some of them were in extremely good health and looked like they could climb mountains, while others had some serious health challenges.

Based on past experience, I fully expected the women to talk about their illnesses, doctor stories, and the like. But instead, the conversation immediately began with a discussion of an incredible skin cream that one of the women had recently discovered. The others were transfixed. They wanted to know all the details about the product—the name, price, ingredients, etc. (Sadly, I missed the name or I would have ran out and bought it myself.) The conversation then moved away from the specific product and turned to comments about skin care in general and how much beautiful skin meant to them.

Clearly, women of all ages are fascinated—even obsessive—when it comes to their skin. Whether they are concerned with acne, wrinkles, dryness, eczema, or puffy eyes, every woman wants beautiful skin.

In my experience, proper female hormonal support is essential throughout life for healthy, moist, and resilient skin, particularly because of the action of estrogen on the skin. Estrogen is responsible for the deposition of fat under the skin, which gives rise to the soft and fine-textured skin that many women enjoy during their younger years. Estrogen also causes fluid and salt retention in tissues, which additionally helps plump up and fill out the skin.

During a woman's active reproductive years, her body produces enough estrogen to properly support the structure of the skin. But much of this support is lost as women go through menopause, when estrogen levels drop significantly. After menopause, skin gradually thins out and becomes drier, and the underlying muscle and fat tissues that help give skin its support also begin to shrink. As a result, wrinkles and creases become apparent and pronounced.

Fortunately, there are many safe, natural, alternative therapies available that have a pronounced estrogen-like effect on tissues, but at much lower potencies. You'll discover all of these treatment options in Chapter 13.

Treat Yourself Like a Queen

The benefits of these estrogen supporters and mimics can be further enhanced when used in combination with nutritional supplements, which, like estrogen, also have hydrating effects on the skin. The moisturizing properties of many different healing substances have been recognized in the Asian medical model of yin and yang for thousands of years. Yin refers to the fluids and tissues of the body, as well as its structure, including flesh, tendons, and bones.

Women are thought to become "yin deficient" when they reach menopause and their tissues become drier and hotter. Traditional Asian medicine uses healing substances, such as royal jelly—the food of the queen bee—to restore the yin. I recommend using ¼ teaspoon of the liquid form of royal jelly twice a day. Royal jelly can be purchased at most health food stores or ordered from Glory Bee at *www.glorybee.com* or 800-456-7923. **Note:** Women who have allergies to bees or have asthma should not take royal jelly.

A House Plant With Punch

Aloe vera, a succulent house plant, also nurtures the yin with its ability to soothe, heal, and moisturize skin. In fact, there is a large body of research that documents the use of aloe for a variety of dermatologic conditions, including rashes, acne scars, dermatitis, psoriasis, burns, and wound healing. When aloe is applied to the skin, it reduces the scaliness, itchiness, and extent of seborrheic dermatitis; prompts the remission of psoriasis; relieves poison ivy; speeds healing of chronic leg ulcers and after dermabrasion, a technique used to remove acne scars and wrinkles.

Drink 2–4 ounces of aloe vera juice per day, either mixed with water or juice or blended in a smoothie. I am partial to Aloe Life's whole leaf aloe juice concentrate (*www.aloelife.com* or 800-414-ALOE). **Note:** Aloe vera can cause diarrhea. If this happens, reduce your intake until you can tolerate it comfortably.

Squalene—Your Skin's Best Friend

Squalene is another skin ally. This powerful, natural antioxidant is found in olive oil and in all human tissues, with the greatest concentration in the skin. I first learned of this wonderful moisturizing oil more than a decade ago when one of my colleagues in the natural health field came to visit me. I was so impressed by her beautiful, soft skin that I had to ask what she was doing for it. Since then, squalene has been one of my absolute favorite skin care products. Even my mother used it for many years, and her skin was absolutely beautiful well into her mid-80's.

I am particularly fond of BioMarine Topical Deep Water Squalene. It contains 99.5-percent pure squalene from deep-water Centrophorus sharks. It comes in a pump bottle, is absorbed easily, and has a very light lavender fragrance, or can be purchased fragrance-free. It can be purchased by calling 800-260-1620 or online at *www.drlark.com*.

Additional sources of squalene include olives, palm oil and wheat germ oil. Use these oils, as well as olive oil, in your salad dressing recipes and when cooking overall to help keep your skin moist and beautiful.

Erase Age Spots

Another common problem among menopausal women is age spots. Sometimes referred to as liver spots, age spots are flat, brownish marks—usually round or oval in shape with irregular edges—that typically begin to show after menopause. They are often the result of free-radical damage throughout the body, often caused by exposure to the sun's ultraviolet rays, heat, trauma, radiation, or heavy metals. The occurrences also affect the formation of melanin, the dark pigment in skin, which hastens the formation of age spots. So when you look at an age spot, what you're actually seeing is an accumulation of debris in your skin's cells.

Poor eating habits—a diet based on dairy, red meat, and saturated fats—can also contribute to age spots. According to Chinese medicine, these foods congest the liver, blocking the chi (or energy), and preventing the liver from purifying the blood. This can also lead to other skin lesions such as acne, eczema, and boils.

The Usual Treatments

Most physicians recommend a cosmetic bleaching cream for treating age spots, but many of these creams contain either monobenzone, an agent that inhibits melanin, or hydroquinone, a white crystalline substance that is also used in film-developing chemicals. But while these substances may be effective at bleaching the surface of the skin, they actually can damage deeper layers of skin and even cause white spots. There are a few vitamin creams on the market that do change the appearance of the surface of the skin to some degree. However, they have not been shown to have an effect on the deeper layers of skin.

Other medical approaches include laser surgery, burning with electricity, freezing, or Retin A-induced peeling—none of which I advocate.

My Age Spot Treatment Plan

The best way to treat age spots is to start from the inside out. Try these natural remedies:

- **Combat free radical damage by eating a diet high in the antioxidants that scavenge free radicals,** especially foods rich in beta-carotene, such as kale, spinach, squash, sweet potatoes, mangoes, cantaloupe, apricots, carrots, and cabbage.
- Research has shown that high **vitamin A intake** can significantly reduce the appearance of age spots. **I suggest 2–4 heaping teaspoons of spirulina (a greens food) a day.** (One heaping teaspoon provides 10,000 IU of vitamin A.)
- Increase your intake of collagen-building **vitamin C (mineral-buffered)** either with supplements **(500–1,000 mg one to three times a day)**, or by eating foods such as cantaloupe, oranges, mangoes, blackberries, broccoli, and cauliflower.
- Take **400–1,600 IU of vitamin E as d-alpha tocopherol per day**. In addition to helping with hyperpigmentation, vitamin E is useful for a wide variety of dermatological complaints such as warts, herpes, and atopic dermatitis. If you have hypertension or are taking insulin, start at 100 IU.
- **Stop smoking.** It hastens the aging of your skin and contributes to free-radical damage throughout your body.
- **Use sunscreen**, at least SPF 15, whenever you go outside.

Halt Hair Loss

In addition to skin concerns, many of my patients have come to me in a panic because their hair was thinning or even falling out. If you can relate to their alarm, I have good news. You can likely turn your hair loss around.

You Are What You Eat

In order for hair to grow thick and healthy, it needs a constant, nutrient-rich supply of blood to its follicles. I have found that a healthy hair diet includes adequate amounts of essential fatty acids (EFAs), zinc, copper, B vitamins, and selenium.

To ensure that you are getting enough EFAs in your diet, eat foods rich in omega-3 fatty acids, like flaxseeds (4–6 tablespoons per serving) and cold-water fish, such as salmon, trout, or halibut (3 times a week).

The best food sources of zinc are wheat germ, oysters, pumpkin seeds, and high protein foods such as chicken breast, eggs, and fish. **You can also take 15 mg of a zinc supplement each day to ensure that you are getting enough of this mineral.**

Don't forget copper, the often-overlooked mineral that helps form collagen in hair. The best food sources for copper are seafood (especially raw oysters), organ meats (beef liver, kidneys, heart), nuts, legumes, chocolate, bran cereals, fruits and vegetables, and blackstrap molasses. **If you prefer, you can take 2–3 mg of copper in supplement form once a day.**

For rich sources of B-complex vitamins, you can turn to a variety of foods, including chickpeas, bananas, and romaine lettuce. Other good sources include brewer's yeast, beans, peas, kelp, mushrooms, whole grains, nuts, and seeds. **If you are supplementing, be sure you're getting at least 100–200 mcg of B_{12}, and 40–50 mg of each of the other B vitamins every day.**

Finally, increase your intake of selenium by including egg yolks, seafood, whole grains, lean red meats, chicken, and mushrooms in your diet. **If supplementing, take 50–200 mcg of selenium a day.**

Lavender Restores Luscious Locks

One of my favorite—and one of the most widely accepted—natural treatments for promoting hair growth and healthy scalp circulation is lavender. A study in *Archives of Dermatology* indicated that 3 drops of lavender (along with 2 drops each of thyme and cedar wood and 3 drops of rosemary in a carrier-oil blend of 1/2 teaspoon of jojoba oil and 4 teaspoons of grapeseed oil) promoted hair growth and healthy scalp circulation. In fact, 44 percent of the treatment group enjoyed new hair growth, as compared to 15 percent of the control group. And there were none of the adverse side effects that can come with conventional treatments for hair loss.

I've outlined below three simple ways you can use lavender to treat your hair loss in the comfort of your home.

- Use a diffuser to disperse micro-particles of the essential oil in the air.
- Apply through your skin by bath, compresses, massage, or simple topical application.
- Spray infused waters in the air or onto your skin.

Essential oils can be purchased in health food and beauty stores, but keep in mind that the quality of the oil may vary. For the highest quality, look for oils packaged in small dark blue or brown vials. Also, prices within a particular brand line will vary, as some essential oils are far more expensive than others. A product line with similar pricing throughout may be offering oils of inferior quality.

As a side note, essential oils can be taken internally for certain conditions, *with proper medical guidance*. An aromatherapist can make an infusion specifically for you and the condition you are seeking to improve. Again, the oils should be taken internally only under the guidance of a practitioner trained in aromatherapy. Ask your chiropractor, energy worker, naturopath, osteopath, or massage therapist to assist you in including aromatherapy in your own health routine.

Twenty Little Mirrors

Lastly, you can't forget your fingernails and toenails. Many women I know have manicures and pedicures done on a regular basis; others enjoy them as a special gift, a reward for working hard, or when attending a special occasion, such as a wedding or reunion.

Yet, even with all of this attention to nails and grooming, many women I have treated have unsightly, brittle, or discolored nails due to unresolved health issues.

Medically speaking, your fingernails and toenails are like tiny little mirrors. Because they're about as far away from your heart and lungs as they can get (and about as low on your body's priority list), any low-grade, chronic stressor of any kind in your general health—for example, if you need a little more of a certain nutrient—will often show up first in your nails.

As a result, if you're paying attention, your nails can give you a gentle, early heads-up, before little problems turn into big ones. In fact, before medicine went high-tech, healers looked to the fingernails and toenails for valuable—and amazingly accurate—diagnostic clues.

Here is a list of several more common nail complaints and what they could be saying about your health.

1. **Thin, brittle, weak nails:** protein deficiency, iron deficiency, calcium deficiency, biotin deficiency, silicon deficiency, or thyroid disease.
2. **Hangnails:** zinc deficiency or dehydrated cuticles.
3. **Brown areas at the tips of your nails:** diabetes, liver disease, or congestive heart failure.
4. **One vertical brown or black streak near your cuticles:** Hutchinson's disease.
5. **Yellow- or green-colored nails:** lung disease or poor circulation.
6. **Yellowish nails:** lymphodema.
7. **Yellowish nails with slight pink color at the base:** diabetes.

8. **Thickened, yellowish nails:** fungal infection.
9. **Half pink or brown, half white nails:** kidney disease.
10. **Red nail beds:** heart problems.
11. **Pale nail bed:** anemia.
12. **White nails:** liver disease.
13. **Ridged nails:** vertical ridges are often inherited and normal; horizontal ridges indicate past illness or stress.
14. **Horizontal "speed bumps" at the edges of your nails:** vitamin A deficiency.
15. **White spots:** not a cause for concern; they will eventually grow out.

If you recognize any of these nail characteristics, especially those that involve serious health conditions such as cardiovascular disease, diabetes, and kidney disease, I urge you to see your physician.

In the meantime, start my Healthy Nail program. In addition to being highly effective, it's also natural and non-toxic. And I promise, if you are patient and diligent, you'll have brand-new fingernails and toenails in just a few months!

My Healthy Nail Program: Three Steps to Healthier Nails

Step One: Daily Tootsies Treatment

- Get a shower stool so you can sit while you work on your feet in the shower. Gently scrub around and under the tip of each nail with a clean nail brush. Polish yellowish cellular debris and dried sweat residues off the nail face with a mildly abrasive bath mitt or loofah. Make sure you use a clean mitt/loofah and brush each day. (I keep a basket of clean mitts by the tub or shower, and launder after each use. I put used nail brushes in a bucket of non-toxic bleach solution, then rinse and run through the dishwasher.)
- After toweling, apply a drop of tea tree oil to the cuticle of each nail (without touching the dropper to the nail). Tea tree oil has the most research behind it as an antifungal. A good second choice would be oregano and eucalyptus oil. In a 1999 study at the University of California at San Francisco, 80 percent of 40 patients who'd had toenail fungus for six to 60 weeks, in spite of having been treated with conventional treatment, were cured after 16 weeks of treatment with a cream containing tea tree oil.
- Spread the tea tree oil across the length of the cuticle with a clean cotton swab, then into the crevices at the sides and over the nail face. Make sure you use a separate swab for problem nails. Do this every day to ensure healthy, fungus-free toenails.

Step Two: Trim with Care

Make sure you trim toenails straight across to avoid ingrown toenails. To reduce your risk of breakage, keep fingernails an attractive "sport" length (no longer than a millimeter or two past the tip of your finger).

Step Three: Feed Your Nails

Make sure your diet and nutritional supplements give your body the tools it needs to build healthy nails. Although we grew up thinking Knox gelatin would do the trick, it usually doesn't strengthen weak nails because most North Americans aren't protein-deficient, especially in this age of low-fat, low-carbohydrate fad diets. Plus, gelatin doesn't address other healthy-nail nutrients such as biotin, zinc, and calcium.

Instead, make sure you are getting adequate amounts of the following nutrients:

- **Biotin:** A 1993 Swiss study demonstrated 25-percent improvement in fingernail thickness when patients took supplemental biotin. Veterinarians prescribing biotin for horses with weak, brittle hooves report faster growth, improved hardness and resilience, and corrected microscopic hoof structure. **I recommend taking 30–300 mcg a day.**
- **Zinc** is essential for maintenance and normal healing of cuticles. It must be properly balanced with copper—an excess of one can interfere with assimilation of the other. I recommend **taking 10–25 mg of zinc a day**, as well as **2–3 mg of copper a day** to avoid copper depletion.
- **Silicon:** Levels of this nutrient tend to decline with age and can result in weak, thin, brittle nails and sweaty odorous feet. Natural dietary sources are few in the North American diet, so supplementation is often needed. **I recommend 25 mg per day.**
- **Calcium:** Deficiencies are increasingly common in women approaching and beyond the menopausal years. For the average adult woman, **I recommend taking 1,000–1,500 mg a day** in divided doses to ensure proper absorption. If you consume a lot of protein, caffeine, sugar, and/or alcohol, and if you have osteoporosis, you'll need 1,500–2,000 mg a day.
- **Since you need to balance calcium and magnesium intake for the proper 2:1 ratio, you'll also want to take 500–1,000 mg of magnesium.** If you have chronic stress or low stomach acidity, take calcium before bed.
- **Iron:** Iron deficiency is uncommon in postmenopausal women, and supplementation can be dangerous when there is no deficiency, as too much iron can lead to heart disease. That's why I recommend a range of dosages of iron for women at different stages of the life cycle. **If you are still menstruating, 18 mg a day is ideal. Women with anemia or heavy menstrual bleeding may**

need as much as 30–70 mg a day. For women who are no longer losing blood through menstruation, 10 mg a day is plenty. To be absorbed properly, iron must be taken with at least 75 mg of vitamin C.

The Lure of Fools' Gold

With all the uncomfortable and downright scary symptoms and medical conditions associated with estrogen deficiency, it's no surprise that women began taking conventional HRT in droves. Moreover, the medical establishment "proved" its benefit, citing study after study that showed HRT lowered postmenopausal women's risk of cardiovascular disease (CVD) by 35 to 50 percent. The risk reduction was even higher among women known to have heart disease before starting HRT.

A few critics pointed to flaws in the studies, but they were largely ignored. The numbers were good and the medical profession believed it had struck gold in the fight against postmenopausal heart disease. A prescription for HRT was considered the equivalent of "heart disease insurance policy."

But now we know better. As I indicated in Chapter 8, the latest research shows that synthetic HRT is not only ineffective in protecting women against postmenopausal heart disease, it actually increases cardiac risk! The studies leave no room for doubt about HRT and its effects on the cardiac health of postmenopausal women:

- It does not reduce women's risk of heart disease, rather it increases risks of heart attack, stroke, and blood clots.
- It does not reverse pre-existing heart disease.
- It places healthy women and women with a history of cardiac disease at increased risk of heart attack within the first year or two of usage.
- It raises levels of C-reactive protein, an indicator of inflammation that is a strong predictor of a future heart attack.

Even worse, conventional HRT has also been shown to increase your risk of breast cancer. According to a study from the *Lancet*, conventional HRT increased the risk of breast cancer with each year of use. Women using HRT for five or more years were at 35 percent greater risk.

Interestingly, according to a study reported at the San Antonio Breast Cancer Symposium, U.S. breast cancer rates plunged 7.2 percent in 2003. With 200,000 cases of the disease projected for 2003, this means that 14,000 fewer women were diagnosed with breast cancer. This drop in cancer rates comes just one year after millions of women stopped taking conventional HRT, thanks in large part to the abovementioned findings that HRT is conclusively associated with an increased risk of breast cancer and heart disease. Researchers found that the largest decline was among women aged 50–69, the exact age group most likely to use HRT. In fact, the drop was three times greater than that of any other age group.

This is great news! It means that more and more women are saying "no" to the dangers of conventional HRT. However, many of them may continue to suffer from menopausal symptoms.

Fortunately, there's a safe and effective solution that will not only ease and even prevent menopausal symptoms, but can also protect you from heart disease and breast cancer.

A Better Option

After all this, you are likely asking yourself, "Now what?" Many women fear that giving up HRT means a return of dreaded menopausal symptoms such as hot flashes, night sweats, and anxiety. Fortunately, the answer is quite simple—my program helps to safely increase your own estrogen levels to help you restore healthy hormone balance. You receive the benefit of your own estrogen to reduce and eliminate menopausal symptoms, and to restore the estrogenic support needed for your tissues and organs.

Best of all, my program is safe, gentle, natural, and highly effective. Plus, it works even if you are on conventional HRT! Let's take an in-depth look at each element of the program and the key nutrients I use to help you begin feeling better than ever.

treating estrogen deficiency

13

Finding safe and truly effective therapies to treat the symptoms and health concerns related to menopause is one of the top concerns among my female patients. Over the past three decades, I've researched and fine-tuned my incredibly successful menopause program, helping thousands upon thousands of women sail through perimenopause and menopause with nary a symptom. My powerful approach works to restore and support your own hormones by using natural substances that don't cause the risky side effects of conventional HRT.

Not only is my program safe, gentle, and incredibly effective, it helps to give you even better hormonal balance than you had during your pre-menopausal years. You achieve this balance by restoring and supporting your entire hormone system, including estrogen. By increasing and balancing all your hormone levels, as well as those substances that support hormone production, you can relieve menopausal symptoms, improve and support your health, and start feeling more like yourself again. The program also slows down the detoxification, breakdown, and elimination of estrogen, and safeguards you against postmenopausal conditions, such as osteoporosis and heart disease.

This program consists of three parts: (1) nutrients that can help you actually produce more of your own estrogen and help to slow down your metabolism and excretion of the estrogen you do produce, thereby increasing your own estrogen to a higher and healthier level that can eliminate menopause symptoms and support your tissues and organs; (2) nutrients that have estrogen-like activity and can help relieve symptoms of estrogen deficiency typically seen in perimenopause and menopause; and (3) biochemically identical estrogen replacement therapy, if you feel that you truly need direct hormone support.

Best of all, my program is very flexible. These approaches can be used separately or in combination, depending upon your own unique needs. Simply take all of the information you'll find here and customize it to what feels best for your body. For example, some women love herbs, others don't. Some women like soy, others have trouble digesting it. By overlapping treatments from all the different options, you will be sure to find the blend that works best for you.

Hysterectomy—Surgical Menopause

While most women enter menopause as part of the natural aging process, some women are "forced" into menopause surgically after undergoing a complete hysterectomy, which involves the removal of your ovaries as well as your uterus. If you have had a complete hysterectomy, you have been placed in a very compromised situation with respect to your ability to produce hormones.

That's why I always encourage women to do everything they can to avoid having their ovaries removed. I have found that some physicians will do this, even if it's not truly warranted. Get second and third opinions to see if you can keep your ovaries intact, at least partially. They are a precious resource and will continue to produce hormones to support your health and well-being. They are especially important after hysterectomy to maintain and sustain the tissues of your body.

As I indicated earlier, estrogen, progesterone, and testosterone are produced by your ovaries and adrenal glands. If your ovaries have been removed, your entire hormone production has been drastically reduced, and all of your hormone production is now dependent upon your adrenals. Plus, the shock of the surgery itself may reduce your adrenals' ability to produce hormones even more. As a result, menopause symptoms are often experienced almost immediately following this type of surgery.

Luckily, my nutritional support program can help to restore your strength and energy after the surgery, and help to promote more rapid healing. The truth is there are also a variety of natural hormone-supportive therapies available to you, as you'll discover throughout this chapter. Under these circumstances, I suggest you start using my natural hormone restoration program, as well as natural hormone replacement therapy (HRT), immediately (see page 145). This will help alleviate some of the severe symptoms, such as hot flashes, insomnia, and mood swings while you are trying to heal from the procedure. Like other post-menopausal women, you will also need to address long-term health issues, including bone health, heart protection, libido concerns, mood health, and the appearance of your skin—all of which depend upon appropriate hormone levels and proper dietary and nutritional support.

It is also crucial that you support your adrenal glands, as they are currently your sole source of hormone production. Plus, they will help you feel more energized. Similarly, your neurotransmitters promote alertness and zest for life, as well as your libido and mood, so it's important for you to sustain the health of your brain and entire endocrine system.

When "Marla" came to see me, she was 37-years-old and had already had a total hysterectomy as a result of endometriosis. Her case of endometriosis had been quite severe, with years of ever-worsening menstrual cramps, which began 10 to 12 days before each menstrual cycle. She also experienced pain during the middle of her cycle, around the time of ovulation.

Marla also had endometrial implants in her colon, which caused painful bowel movements and intestinal irritability, as well as an irritable bladder. Unfortunately, the hysterectomy only swapped her problems for a set of new ones. Thanks to her "surgical menopause," she now had severe hot flashes, vaginal dryness, and sleeplessness, as well as extreme fatigue.

Her physician prescribed conventional hormone replacement therapy, which she could not tolerate due to the fact that it reactivated her endometriosis! Marla was very depressed and upset when she finally came to see me. She said that she literally felt trapped with no place to turn.

Luckily, my hormonal support and balancing program proved to be very helpful, and her symptoms started to resolve.

The Hysterectomy Decision

If your doctor has suggested a hysterectomy but you have not yet had the surgery, I strongly suggest getting a second and third opinion. This is extremely crucial in making a decision of this magnitude.

If you do decide to have the surgery, find the best surgeon for you. Again, be sure to find one who will do their best to allow you to keep your ovaries, if at all possible, as that will greatly boost your ability to continue producing your own hormones, even after a hysterectomy. Get referrals from your physician or a friend who has had a hysterectomy. Be sure to interview all surgeons. In addition to the obvious requirement—surgical skill—you want to trust this individual and feel that your questions and concerns are addressed with care and attention.

Pre-Op Prep

A few weeks before surgery, you'll want to get your body get into the best possible condition to handle the stress of anesthesia and surgery. Here are some recommendations to get you as prepared as possible for surgery.

Two to four weeks pre-op, start taking:

- A top quality multinutrient daily.
- 50–100 mg of vitamin B_5 and 25–100 mg of vitamin B_1 daily to accelerate healing and support collagen synthesis.
- 500–3,000 mg of mineral-buffered vitamin C two to three times daily to counteract surgical stress and enhance healing. Reduce your dosage if you begin to experience loose bowel movements, which can occur with high-dose vitamin C.
- 10–25 mg zinc daily to facilitate wound healing.
- 300–600 mg daily of quercetin and 1,000–2,000 mg daily of citrus bioflavonoids to prevent excessive inflammation and protect against infection.
- 25,000 IU a day of beta carotene to boost the strength and resilience of the scar.

Two weeks pre-op, **stop** *taking:*
Any supplements that can affect blood clotting and alter the effects of anesthesia and other drugs, such as:

- Vitamin E
- *Ginkgo biloba*
- Fish oil
- Ginger
- Feverfew
- St. John's wort
- Flax oil

If you're taking other herbs such as chamomile, valerian, or echinacea, ask your doctor about possible drug interactions. (Doctors rarely ask about the supplements their patients take.) When in doubt, stop taking the herb.

Two Weeks Pre-Op:

Intensify your stress-reduction program. Include meditation and deep breathing in your daily routine to reduce your level of stress hormones and help oxygenate your blood. If you are having difficulty coping with the emotional ramifications of your upcoming hysterectomy, seek help from a good counselor to work through it preoperatively.

Continue taking the other pre-op supplements, and two days before surgery and for at least four weeks afterward take:

- 300–500 mg of bromelain four times daily, between meals, to minimize swelling, bruising, and pain from surgery.

- 50 mg of grapeseed extract per day to reduce postoperative swelling.
- Colostrum, the first pre-milk from cows, which improves immune function and reduces postoperative diarrhea and intestinal inflammation. Colostrum is available as capsules or in liquid form at health food stores. Take as directed on the package.

Post-Op Planning

After recovering from anesthesia and for two weeks afterward, use an alkalinizing supplement that contains two parts sodium bicarbonate and one part potassium bicarbonate, such as my Daily Balance Alkalinizer (available by calling 888-314-5275 or by visiting *www.drlark. com*). Or, you can simply take sodium bicarbonate (baking soda)—one-half to one teaspoon dissolved in a glass of spring water in the morning and at night.

Swelling, hemorrhage, and physical changes in the injured tissues impair oxygenation and blood flow, leading to an accumulation of wastes and acidity. By maintaining a slightly alkaline body pH, you can help prevent inflammation and tissue acidosis from surgery and hasten your recovery.

From the first day to 12 weeks after surgery:
Resume taking vitamin E—800–1,000 IU daily. It speeds skin healing and reduces pain. In addition, I recommend that you:

- Apply arnica gel or ointment three times daily around (but not directly on) the incision site to reduce bruising, pain, and swelling.
- Take showers, not baths, for the first two to six weeks, depending on how your incision heals. A solid, flexible, watertight scar is needed to keep bath water from seeping in and causing infection.
- Don't lift anything heavier than a gallon of milk for the first two weeks, and do nothing that requires tension in your abdominal muscles. Straining can cause little rips in the tissues. If they bleed and ooze, your body reacts with inflammation, which prolongs recovery and increases the risk of adhesions. And, it could be disastrous if you pop any stitches. You only get one chance to heal right!
- Do Kegel exercises. Hysterectomies can weaken pelvic muscles, which may contribute to urinary incontinence. To make sure you're doing Kegels correctly, ask your physician or find physical therapy services that offer guidance in Kegel exercises.
- Be extra good to yourself. You're likely to have many internal stitches that can take up to a year for your body to dissolve and absorb. This takes energy and time. Minimize stress, say "no" to projects that deplete your energy, and eat less quantity but great quality food, so you'll get the nutrients you need without packing on extra pounds.

With good preparation and a commitment to healing, you can emerge from this experience with optimal physical, emotional, and sexual health. In addition to my recommendations here, you can also find some excellent tips at www.hystersisters.com, a hysterectomy recovery support site. I highly recommend connecting with other women who've had a hysterectomy—they may have some excellent advice to share, as well!

KAY'S STORY

At age 42, "Kay" had the terrifying situation of being diagnosed with breast cancer. She was treated with aggressive chemotherapy, which stopped her menstrual periods entirely.

She came to me because her physician told her he could not treat her with conventional HRT, due to the risk of further stimulating the growth of the cancer. She asked me if I could help her deal with her uncomfortable hot flashes and other symptoms of menopause that she never dreamed she'd be dealing with in her early 40's.

Fortunately, she found my all-natural program—including the use of breast-safe nutrients like bioflavonoids, vitamin E, black cohosh, soy, and melatonin—to be extremely effective in **providing symptom relief**.

Restore Your Own Hormones

Whether you enter menopause naturally or due to hysterectomy or even chemotherapy for cancer treatment, I am certain that my powerful and effective program will work wonders for you. My program supports all of the components necessary for healthy and balanced estrogen levels within your body. It will help you support the stimulation of hormone production by the central nervous system, estrogen production in the ovaries and adrenal glands, and reduce the breakdown and elimination of estrogen safely and gently. My goal is to nudge your estrogen levels back into a healthier, more functional range to eliminate such uncomfortable and debilitating symptoms like hot flashes, night sweats, insomnia, vaginal dryness, low libido, forgetfulness, increased dryness and wrinkling of the skin, as well as promote healthier bones, heart, and joints.

Hormone Production Begins in the Brain

As I described earlier in the book, the stimulation of all hormone production begins in the brain. Thus, you can begin to increase estrogen production by supporting the health of your brain and the endocrine glands contained within the brain.

Traditionally, we've always been told that humans have one brain that is divided into many different parts. But more and more research is putting the "one brain" idea to the test. In fact, it's starting to be widely accepted that the human skull actually houses not one brain, but three—the reptilian brain, the limbic brain, and the neocortical brain.

The reptilian brain is the oldest part of the brain. It controls basic bodily functions like heart rate, breathing, body temperature, hunger, and fight-or-flight responses. Basic drives and instincts, such as defending territory and keeping safe from harm, are other functions of the reptilian brain. The structures in the brain that perform these functions are the brain stem (which controls breathing, heart rate, and blood pressure) and the cerebellum (which controls movement, balance, and posture).

The limbic, or mammalian, brain developed once mammals started roaming the earth. It includes the hippocampus, which controls memories and learning; the amygdala, which controls memory and emotions; and the hypothalamus, which controls emotions (among many other things). Therefore, the limbic brain allows mammals to learn, retain memories, and show emotions.

The neocortical brain, or neocortex, is the complex maze of grey matter that surrounds the reptilian and limbic brains, and accounts for about 85 percent of brain mass. It is found in the brains of primates and humans, and is responsible for sensory perception, abstract thought, imagination, and consciousness. It also controls language, social interactions, and higher communication.

The Chemistry of the Brain

Like the three parts of the brain, there are also three key types of brain chemicals: neuropeptides, neurohormones, and neurotransmitters.

Neuropeptides are responsible for the cell-to-cell communication system in your body. A peptide is a short chain of amino acids connected together, and a neuropeptide is a peptide found in neural tissue. Neuropeptides are widespread in the central and peripheral nervous systems and different neuropeptides have different excitatory or inhibitory actions.

Neuropeptides control such a diverse array of functions in the body. When they work together properly, the wonderful results in your body include elevated mood and other positive behaviors and emotions, stronger bones, better resistance to disease, glowing skin, and boosted metabolism. Conversely, if your neuropeptides function abnormally, the result can be an increased tendency towards neurological and mental disorders such as Alzheimer's disease, epilepsy, and schizophrenia.

There are several types of neuropeptides. Some of the most common include endorphins and beta-endorphins. Endorphins are opiod peptides, meaning they have morphine-like effects within the body. They produce feelings of well-being and euphoria, and a rush of endorphins can lead to feelings of exhilaration brought on by pain, danger, or stress. Endorphins also may also play a role in memory, sexual activity, and body temperature. Beta-endorphins are another form of opiod peptides, but they are stronger than endorphins. They are composed of 31 amino acids and work in the body by numbing pain, increasing relaxation, and promoting a general feeling of well-being.

While there are many, many hormones and hormonal interactions that occur in the brain and body, the most widely known neurohormone is melatonin. (I will discuss melatonin in more detail on page 125.)

Neurotransmitters are naturally occurring chemicals that relay electrical messages between nerve cells throughout your body. While all three types of neurochemicals are important for hormone and overall health, neurotransmitters are particularly important for the production of sex hormones.

In the aggregate, all three types of neurochemicals help to regulate the brain's endocrine glands, specifically the hypothalamus and pituitary gland. The hypothalamus is the master endocrine gland that regulates your production of sex hormones. This gland produces precursor hormones called gonadotropin releasing hormones (GnRH). When they are released, they travel to your anterior pituitary gland, where they stimulate the secretion of the follicle stimulating (FSH) and luteinizing hormones (LH). As you now know, these hormones then travel to the adrenals and ovaries, where they stimulate the production of estrogen, progesterone, and testosterone.

In order to keep the whole process working smoothly, FSH and LH need to be triggered by a balanced mixture of the key neurotransmitters necessary to produce these hormones. Neurotransmitters are naturally occurring chemicals that relay electrical messages between nerve cells throughout your body. The production of these vital chemicals is synthesized from certain amino acids, vitamins, and minerals that must be obtained through your diet or from supplementation.

For women who are estrogen dominant, it is critical to increase levels of LH to help trigger ovulation and progesterone production. In the case of menopause and estrogen deficiency, just the opposite is true. You want to favor estrogen production. Additionally, if you have an estrogen deficiency-fast processor hormonal profile, you'll want to increase the production of neurotransmitters like serotonin and GABA, which slow down your brain processes, and promote more peace, better sleep, and a more balanced mood, as well as favoring estrogen production. However, if you are an estrogen deficiency-slow processor type, promoting the production of the more stimulating, excitatory neurotransmitters like dopamine and norepinephrine can be quite helpful for more energy, sex drive, and zest for life. Let's look at this in more detail.

Serotonin: The Neurotransmitter to Love

All neurotransmitters stimulate hormone production, but menopausal women are most particularly in need of serotonin. Serotonin is an inhibitory neurotransmitter. This means it quiets down the processes of your body, rather than speeding them up. Within your brain, serotonin often inhibits the firing of neurons, which dampens many of your behaviors. In fact, serotonin acts as a kind of chemical restraint system.

Of all your body's chemicals, serotonin has one of the most widespread effects on the brain and physiology. It plays a key role in regulating temperature, blood pressure, blood clotting, immunity, pain, digestion, sleep, and biorhythms. It also produces a relaxing effect on your mood.

When you are low in serotonin, you are most likely not a lot of fun to be around. Low levels often lead to mood swings, depression, insomnia, chronic pain, food cravings, migraine headaches, and irritable bowel syndrome. It can even increase your likelihood of infection and sleep apnea.

Menopausal women are most at risk of decreased levels of serotonin, thanks to a complementary relationship between this neurotransmitter and estrogen. According to research from both the *American Journal of Psychiatry* and *Behavioral and Cognitive Neuroscience Reviews*, as goes estrogen, so goes serotonin. It appears that estrogen stimulates serotonin production. If you don't have adequate amounts of estrogen, you are not producing adequate amounts of serotonin. Additionally, low estrogen also triggers your brain to release monoamine oxidase (MAO), an enzyme that degrades serotonin. So decreased estrogen levels have a double-whammy effect on serotonin.

This relationship is the key to postmenopausal depression and anxiety. By increasing estrogen, you increase serotonin, and thereby elevate your mood and reduce many of the symptoms related to menopause. This is particularly important for estrogen deficient women who are fast processors and really need to calm and slow down their body chemistry and metabolism.

The essential amino acid tryptophan is initially converted into an intermediary substance called 5-hydroxytryptophan (5-HTP), which is then converted into serotonin. While tryptophan is available as a supplement and is abundant in turkey, pumpkin seeds, and almonds, I've found that 5-HTP is a more effective and reliable option for boosting your neurotransmitter production. Numerous double-blind studies have shown that 5-HTP is as effective as many of the more common antidepressant drugs and is associated with fewer and much milder side effects. In addition to increasing serotonin levels, 5-HTP triggers an increase in endorphins and other neurotransmitters that are often low in cases of depression.

THE SEROTONIN-THYROID CONNECTION

Serotonin is intimately bound with thyroid hormone. Healthy thyroid function plays an important role in supporting healthy serotonin production and concentration, as well as preventing serotonin reuptake. As a result, strong, healthy thyroid levels result in an increased level of serotonin in the brain.

If you exhibit symptoms of low thyroid—cold hands and/or feet, weight gain, constipation, fatigue, dry skin, brittle nails, depression, loss of hair—then you need to have a thyroid test performed. If you are determined to have low or hypothyroid, I strongly suggest bringing your thyroid hormone up to normal levels to ensure that you have adequate, healthy levels of serotonin.

To maintain proper serotonin levels, it is helpful to take 50–100 mg of 5-HTP once or twice a day, with one of the dosages taken at bedtime. If needed during the day, use carefully, as too much 5-HTP can interfere with your ability to drive or concentrate.

Be sure to start at 50 mg. Stay on this dosage for two weeks. If you don't notice a reduction in your symptoms, gradually increase the dosage by 50 mg every two weeks until you have either noticed a reduction in your symptoms or have reached the maximum dosage.

Conversely, if you are an estrogen deficient-slow processor with a more placid, peaceful temperament and a tendency towards lower energy, weight gain, fluid retention, and even depression, stimulating the brain excitatory pathways that help to speed up the processes of your body will be more helpful for you.

The excitatory neurotransmitter pathways are primarily made up of substances like dopamine, norepinephrine, and epinephrine. Unlike serotonin, which has a calming and relaxing effect on your energy and behavior, excitatory neurotransmitters energize and elevate your mood. They act as powerful antidepressants and also support alertness, optimism, motivation, zest for life, and sex drive.

The excitatory neurotransmitters are derived from tyrosine, an amino acid produced from phenylalanine (another amino acid). A variety of vitamins and minerals, such as vitamin C, vitamin B_6, and magnesium, act as co-factors and are necessary for the conversion of these amino acids into neurotransmitters.

To maintain optimum dopamine levels, take 500–1,000 mg of tyrosine per day. Be sure to take in divided doses, half in the morning and half in the afternoon. Do not take in the evening, as it may interfere with sleep.

Note: I strongly advise that you undertake a program to restore and properly balance your neurotransmitter levels under the care of a complementary physician, naturopath, or nutritionist. You should also have your neurotransmitter levels tested regularly, as dosage needs for the amino acids I've described often vary from woman to woman (see next page).

There are three key nutrients that will also help to raise estrogen levels—melatonin, glandulars, and ginseng. Let's take a look at each of them in more detail.

Mighty Melatonin

Melatonin is a hormone produced from serotonin and secreted by the pineal gland. Its secretion takes place at night and is inhibited by light. As such, it sets and regulates the timing of your body's natural circadian rhythms, such as waking and sleeping.

Unfortunately, as you get older, you produce less and less melatonin. This is due, in part, to menopause. Women who have poor sleep patterns, such as night shift workers, are also more likely to have decreased melatonin production.

As I mentioned earlier, melatonin is produced from serotonin, and serotonin production is stimulated by estrogen. Low estrogen equates to low serotonin, which results in low melatonin…which means you can't fall asleep or stay asleep easily.

In fact, a study from the *Annals of the New York Academy of Sciences* found that there is a cause-effect relationship between decreased nighttime levels of melatonin and the onset of menopause. Researchers found that women who took 3 mg of melatonin a day for six months enjoyed decreased FSH levels (with levels returning to those of a younger woman), and nearly a third of the menopausal women experienced a return of normal menstrual cycles. And, as I mentioned earlier, when women enter menopause, their levels of FSH and LH production in the pituitary increase in an effort to trigger greater estrogen production. Additionally, the study showed a significant improvement in thyroid function and relief of menopause-related depression in the women using melatonin.

Another research study published in the *Journal of Clinical Endocrinology and Metabolism* studied men and women over the age of 50 who suffered from insomnia to assess the best melatonin dosage necessary to promote healthy sleep. Researchers looked at three dosages: 0.1 mg; 0.3 mg; and 3.0 mg (the same dosage used in the *Annals of the New York Academy of Sciences* study). Unfortunately, they found that the 3.0 mg dosage had some downsides. It decreased body temperature and caused melatonin levels to stay elevated throughout the day. However, the lower doses—especially the 0.3 mg dosage—restored sleep without these negative side effects.

Research has also shown that melatonin is cancer-protective. One study looked at 250 patients with a wide variety of advanced, metastatic tumors, including lung cancer, breast cancer, gastrointestinal cancer, and head and neck cancer. None of the patients who received chemotherapy alone enjoyed a complete response, while six of the patients who received chemo and 20 mg of intravenous melatonin did, and another 36 patients achieved a partial response. Moreover, the one-year survival rate was significantly higher in the melatonin/chemo group (51 percent) than the chemo-alone group (23 percent). Researchers concluded that melatonin may be a secret weapon in the war on cancer.

To ensure that you have adequate levels of melatonin, I suggest supplementing with 0.3–1 mg at bedtime. Some women may find that they do better with a higher dosage. In this case, I suggest taking 1.5–3 mg. In my own hormone support product, I have erred on the side of caution and included 0.3 mg of melatonin. For melatonin to be effective, your bedroom should be dark, as light suppresses its release.

MELATONIN DEPLETERS

The following drugs deplete melatonin. If you are taking these drugs, be sure to supplement with adequate amounts of melatonin.

- Aspirin
- Beta-blockers
- Sleeping pills
- Ibuprofen
- Calcium channel blockers
- Tranquilizers

CAROL'S STORY

"Carol" was a 68-year-old patient of mine who, for about 15 years after reaching menopause, experienced mild depression and mood swings. When she came to see me, her depression had worsened and sleeplessness had set in. Even more frustrating for her was that she felt sleepy and depressed during the day, but as soon as the sun went down, she became restless and couldn't sleep for more than three hours. This cycle of sleepiness and sleeplessness was beginning to affect her work and even her simple, everyday tasks—but even more upsetting was that her marriage was starting to sour.

Carol's situation is common in women who have neurotransmitter imbalances. Testing showed that Carol did indeed have a neurotransmitter imbalance—in particular, her serotonin levels were too low.

I put Carol on a combination of 5-HTP and melatonin, as well as other nutrients. Soon, she was feeling like her old self again and sleeping better than ever.

HOPE'S STORY

"Hope," a 62-year-old woman, came to see me with worsening urinary incontinence, which was interfering with her ability to take long hikes she used to do at least three times a week in the forested area near her home. She was also distressed by her diminished ability to handle stress.

Hope shared with me that she was reacting to her husband's bad moods and her grown children's family issues with much greater anxiety than she had in the past. She went on to tell me that her sleep was also being affected, and she was waking up much more frequently in the middle of the night. She also mentioned that she continued to have hot flashes on and off, which were definitely more frequent when she felt particularly stressed.

I suggested that she start using my hormonal restoration program immediately, which included among other things 5-HTP, melatonin, and GABA. After several weeks, Hope was much calmer and more relaxed. She was sleeping better and was even able to reduce her urinary incontinence.

Transforming Glandulars

I am a big fan of glandular therapy, which involves the use of purified extracts from the secretory endocrine glands of animals. The most common extracts are drawn from the thyroid and adrenal glands, as well as the thymus, pituitary, pancreas, and ovaries. Most extracts come from cows, with the exception of pancreatic glandular preparations, which are usually drawn from sheep.

There are four common ways to extract glandulars. The first involves quick-freezing the material, washing it with a potent solvent to remove fatty tissues, distilling the solvent out, drying it, and then grinding it into a fine powder that is then encapsulated or pressed into tablets.

The second mixes freshly crushed material with salt and water that also removes fatty tissues. It is then dried and ground into a fine powder to be placed in capsules or made into tablets.

In the third method, the glandular material is freeze-dried, then placed into a vacuum chamber to remove the water. It is then encapsulated. However, with this method, fatty tissues remain.

The final method uses plant and animal enzymes to partially "digest" the material. It is then passed through a filter that separates out the fat-soluble molecules. The remaining material is then freeze-dried. This method seems to be quite effective. Due to the "pre-digestion," all biologically active substances remain intact and can be used therapeutically to support and restore your body's endocrine glands. Healthier endocrine glands are more likely to create healthier hormone production.

In the past, most experts believed that glandulars were not effective because the intestinal lining of a healthy person was impenetrable, and that proteins and large peptides could not breach its barrier. However, recent evidence has shown that large macromolecules can and do pass completely intact from the intestinal tract and into the bloodstream. In fact, there's further evidence to suggest that your body is able to determine which molecules it needs to absorb whole, and which can be broken down.

Both animal and human studies alike have proven this theory. In some cases, several whole proteins taken orally, including critical enzymes, have been shown to be absorbed intact into the bloodstream. Additionally, many smaller proteins and numerous hormones have also been found to be absorbed intact into the bloodstream, including thyroid, cortisone, and even insulin.

In essence, this means that the active properties of the glandulars stay active and intact, and are not destroyed in the digestive process. This is key to the success of glandular therapy, and explains why they clearly help to restore hormone function. When the gland is healthy, you will have fewer hormone-related problems because the feedback loop of the central nervous system and the endocrine glands are working properly. In essence, if you optimize the function, you bring *all* your hormones back into balance.

Examples of widely used and accepted glandulars involve the thyroid and adrenals. Natural thyroid medications such as Armour® Thyroid, Naturethroid, and Bio-Thyroid have been the preference of complementary physicians for decades. Unlike many of the commonly prescribed brands of thyroid therapy that only replace a synthetic form of T4 (one of four thyroid hormones), these natural thyroid replacements contains the whole animal-derived thyroid gland, including T3 *and* T4. This is a significant difference. T3 is more physiologically active than T4, and is critical in regulating normal growth and energy metabolism. Without the use of glandulars, this type of natural thyroid replacement wouldn't be possible. However, the thyroid glandulars sold in the health food stores have the hormone removed and are used to support the function of your own gland.

Adrenal glandular preparations are even more common. With the stress epidemic in this country, the majority of Americans are walking around with depressed adrenal function. Fortunately, whole adrenal extracts have been found to help restore the health and function of compromised adrenal glands. In one research study, eight women suffering from morning sickness (nausea and vomiting) who took oral adrenal cortex extract found relief within four days. A similar study gave both injected and oral adrenal cortex extract to 202 women also suffering from morning sickness. More than 85 percent of the women completely overcame their nausea and vomiting or showed significant improvement.

Another study looked at the use of adrenal glandulars to treat patients with chronic fatigue and immune dysfunction syndrome (CFIDS), as well as fibromyalgia. Researchers found that 5–13 mg of an adrenal glandular preparation significantly reduced pain and discomfort. Moreover, after six to 18 months, many of the patients were able to reduce and eventually discontinue treatment, while still enjoying relief.

To support the endocrine glands that make estrogen (and other female hormones), as well as those that regulate estrogen production—including the pineal gland, which secretes melatonin—I suggest taking a good multi-glandular or single glandular product such as pineal or hypothalamus from a company like Standard Process. I also highly recommend that you consider taking a whole brain glandular, if appropriate. Standard Process is a leader in the field; however, they do require a prescription from a health care practitioner. Other good products are also available in health food stores and should be used as part of a nutritional program to support your entire hormone system. I suggest consulting with a complementary health care provider if you are interested in using glandular therapy.

Glorious Ginseng

Panax ginseng is an ivy-like ground cover originating in the wild, damp woodlands of northern China and Korea. Its use in Chinese herbal medicine dates back more than 4,000 years. In colonial North America, ginseng was a major export product. The wild form is now rare, but panax ginseng is a widely cultivated plant.

Ginseng has a legendary status amongst herbs. While extravagant claims have been made about its many uses, scientific research has yielded inconsistent results in verifying its therapeutic properties. However, enough good research does exist to demonstrate ginseng's activity, especially when high-quality extracts, standardized for active components, are used.

Ginseng has a balancing, tonic effect on the systems and organs of the body involved in the stress response. It contains at least 13 different saponins, a class of chemicals found in many plants, especially legumes, which take their name from their ability to form a soaplike froth when shaken with water. These compounds (triterpene glycosides) are the most pharmaceutically active constituents of ginseng. Saponins benefit cardiovascular function, hormone production, immunity, and the central nervous system.

During times of stress, ginseng acts as a general stimulant, delaying the alarm phase in Selye's classic model of stress. (Hans Selye is a distinguished Canadian physiologist whose groundbreaking research led to the modern theories regarding how your body adapts to stress. The alarm phase indicates the first stage of stress, when your have an immediate, acute reaction to an irritant or stressor. Such reactions can take the form of nervousness, restlessness, and agitation.)

The saponins found in ginseng act on the hypothalamus and pituitary glands, increasing the release of adrenocorticotrophin, or ACTH (a hormone produced by the pituitary that promotes the manufacture and secretion of adrenal hormones). As a result, ginseng increases the release of adrenal cortisone and other adrenal hormones, including an estrogen precursor, and prevents their depletion from stress. Other substances associated with the pituitary are also released, such as endorphins.

In a double-blind study published in *Drugs Under Experimental and Clinical Research*, two groups of volunteers suffering from fatigue due to physical or mental stress were given nutritional supplementation over a 12-week period. One hundred sixty-three volunteers were given a multivitamin and multimineral complex, and 338 volunteers received the same product plus a standardized Chinese ginseng extract. Once a month, the volunteers were asked to fill out a questionnaire during a scheduled visit with a physician. This questionnaire contained 11 questions that asked them to describe their current level of perceived physical energy, stamina, sense of well-being, libido, and quality of sleep.

While both groups experienced similar improvement in their quality of life by the second visit, the group using the ginseng extract almost doubled their improvement, based on their questionnaire responses, by the third and fourth visits. Thus, ginseng, when added to a multivitamin and multimineral complex, appears to improve many parameters of well-being in individuals experiencing significant physical and emotional stress, including those commonly associated with menopause, such as loss of libido, poor sleep, and mood imbalances.

Ginseng also enhances mental capacity, as demonstrated in both animal studies and clinical trials in humans. Improvements in logical deduction, reaction time, mental arithmetic, alertness, and accuracy have been observed. ACTH (the hormone that stimulates the adrenal cortex) and adrenal hormones, which ginseng stimulates, are known to bind to brain tissue, increasing mental activity and acuity during stress.

Many of my patients have used ginseng and have found it to have energizing effects. When trying to replenish yin, I suggest using the more cooling Chinese and American forms of ginseng, and avoid Korean red ginseng, which is considered to be "hotter" and more yang. This type of ginseng can have the reverse effect, causing a decrease in normal menstrual flow and dryness of the skin and mucous membranes.

To further support hormone function at the central nervous system level, I suggest taking 100 mg of American or Chinese ginseng in capsule form twice a day. For maximum benefit, be sure to take a high-quality preparation, standardized for ginsenoside content and ratio. If this is too stimulating, especially before bedtime, take the second dose mid-afternoon, or take only the morning dose.

In addition to stimulating hormone production at the endocrine and nervous system levels, you can also use nutrients such as wheat germ oil and boron to increase estrogen production.

Wonderful Wheat Germ

Wheat germ oil is rich in vitamin E, which we already know has mildly estrogenic properties. In fact, wheat germ oil contains the same fatty acids and other nutrients like vitamin E that your body needs to support and produce hormones such as estrogen.

Wheat germ oil is so effective, it has even been shown to increase estrogen production and reestablish healthy menstrual cycles in young women. Living under the stress of war is often associated with widespread disruption of menstrual cycles. This was true of women living in an internment camp in Manila during World War II. Doctors who treated these women observed that menstruation had stopped abruptly after the first bombing of Manila, before a nutritional deficiency would have been experienced. These physicians conducted a small study, published in the *Journal of the American Medical Association* (*JAMA*), in which 10 women with amenorrhea (a lack of menstruation) were given 20 drops of wheat germ oil as a source of vitamin E. The doses were taken orally, three times a day, for a period of 10 days, preceding the onset of each woman's expected menstrual flow. Of the 10 women, eight began to menstruate or had uterine bleeding.

Another study found that wheat germ oil was beneficial in treating vaginitis in menopausal women. One particular patient had such an extreme case of the condition that the physician couldn't even examine her. After 10 days on wheat germ oil, the burning eased and 17 days later, she reported to be "better than in months."

I suggest taking 2,000–2,400 mg of wheat germ oil in capsule form a day, in divided doses. I am particularly fond of the Standard Process and Viobin brands (*www.standardprocess.com* and *www.viobinusa.com*). I've found wheat germ oil to be a very effective part of my menopause treatment program, although not all women can tolerate it.

Bountiful Boron

Boron is a trace mineral found in such foods as apples, grapes, almonds, legumes, honey, and dark green leafy vegetables like kale and beet greens. Unfortunately, the foods most commonly consumed—meat, dairy products, and refined flour—are *not* good sources of boron, so many Americans are deficient in this vital mineral.

According to a study conducted by the U.S. Department of Agriculture, there is some evidence that boron enhances estrogenic activity. When women on estrogen therapy supplemented their normally low-boron diet with 3 mg of boron, their blood levels of estrogen, specifically beta-estradiol, were significantly elevated. It appears that boron boosts estrogen production and mimics some effects of estrogen. There is also anecdotal evidence that boron may reduce hot flashes.

Moreover, boron is critical in the fight against osteoporosis. One study published in *Nutrition Today* found that boron reduced urinary excretion of calcium by 44 percent and significantly reduced excretion of magnesium as well. It also found that it increased levels of both beta-estradiol and testosterone.

To help boost estrogen levels and prevent osteoporosis, I suggest taking 3 mg of boron a day.

Fend Off a Breakdown

While plant-based nutrients, vitamins, and minerals all work to support estrogen production, you can also decrease the metabolism and elimination of estrogen to help maintain higher levels of the hormone. This will also help to relieve symptoms of estrogen deficiency. Let's take a look at the best ways to accomplish this.

Women with estrogen dominance need to be sure they are breaking down, metabolizing, and eliminating excess estrogen effectively. However, women in estrogen deficiency need to do everything they can to slow down this breakdown and excretion cycle.

During estrogen metabolism in the liver, the most potent estrogen (estradiol) is converted into the mid-level potency form of estrone. They are both then metabolized to the weakest and least potent form—estriol.

Estrogen is also inactivated as it passes through the liver, where it is bound to sulfuric and glucuronic acid. This binding process inactivates the estrogen, inhibiting it from binding to tissues. It is then secreted into the bile and passed into the intestinal tract, where it is then eliminated from the body via bowel movements.

To slow this process down, you need hormone potentiators, nutrients that help to slow down your body's normal breakdown of hormones, thereby causing a gentle, yet helpful, elevation of the levels of estrogen circulating through the body. That's where PABA and cobalt chloride (or cobalt derived from vitamin B_{12}) come in.

Powerful PABA

PABA (para-aminobenzoic acid) is a fat-soluble B vitamin necessary for the production of folic acid. It helps to break down protein in the body, supports red blood cell production, and maintains the health of the intestines. PABA also works to absorb ultraviolet light, and may be useful in alleviating some skin conditions, such as the over-pigmentation or under-pigmentation of skin.

More importantly, studies indicate that PABA helps to safely and effectively impede the breakdown of estrogen and other hormones in the liver. Research has shown that higher levels of PABA are associated with better mood and outlook, less thinning hair, better vaginal lubrication, and increased libido—all of which are also indicative of higher estrogen levels. In fact, PABA is the only substance (other than testosterone) that has been proven to increase libido!

In addition to increasing estrogen levels, PABA has also been found to increase adrenal and thyroid hormone levels, as well as enhance the effects of cortisone. Because of its cortisone-like effects, PABA was used to treat rheumatoid arthritis in the 1940's. Specifically, PABA has been shown to be beneficial in helping to relieve the stiffness and pain associated with arthritis. In fact, high doses of PABA have been found to prevent and even reverse the accumulation of fibrous tissue.

One study from the *American Journal of Medical Sciences* found that rheumatoid arthritis sufferers who took low doses of cortisone and high doses of PABA enjoyed considerable pain relief. Specifically, they found that patients who took 12 grams of PABA, along with low amounts of cortisone, enjoyed significantly more relief than those people taking cortisone alone.

Moreover, PABA has also been found to be effective in overcoming infertility. Researchers gave 16 infertile women 100 mg of PABA four times a day for three to seven months. Twelve of the 16 become pregnant.

If you are tired, depressed, irritable, or show signs of anxiety, you may be deficient in PABA. **I recommend taking 400–500 mg a day, which may be taken in divided dosages as a hormone potentiator.**

> ### LINDA'S STORY
> "Linda" was 71 years old when she first came to see me. She had been taking conventional HRT for nearly 20 years. When she read the study results from the July 2002 issue of the *Journal of the American Medical Association* on the connection between synthetic HRT and heart disease and breast cancer, she quit taking her medications cold turkey.
>
> Within days, she began experiencing terrible hot flashes, worse than she remembered from her early 50's. She also had insomnia, which kept her up most nights. She started using PABA, glandulars, and a few other nutrients to help ease her symptoms. She was delighted to find that her symptoms decreased in a very short period of time.

Control Estrogen With Cobalt

One of the most exciting, and little known, nutrients for menopausal women is cobalt. Research has shown that cobalt slows down the excretion of estrogen, thus allowing you to better maintain your own production of estrogen, as well as that of supplemental estrogen.

Cobalt is able to retain estrogen and other hormones by stimulating production of heme oxidase. This, in turn, promotes the breakdown of cytochrome p450, a substance that normally metabolizes and detoxifies estrogen. By breaking down this substance, cobalt helps to prevent estrogen metabolism and excretion.

Physicians who have used cobalt have found that it has significant therapeutic benefits for their patients, helping to reduce night sweats, insomnia, hot flashes, depression, mood swings, and memory loss. It has even improved the therapeutic effects of women using conventional HRT who were not experiencing symptom relief due to their hyperexcretion of the hormones.

To impede the breakdown and excretion of estrogen, **I suggest taking 400–500 mcg of cobalt a day. To further improve your cobalt status, you can also take 100–500 mcg of B_{12} a day.** Research has shown that cobalt is supplied in your body by B_{12}. If you have adequate amounts of B_{12}, you are likely to have adequate amounts of cobalt as well.

Protect Your Health With Hormone Safeguards

As you've seen, specific herbs, plants, vitamins, minerals, and even neurotransmitters all work to help you produce and maintain vital, healthy levels of estrogen. My entire program has been formulated to help promote healthy hormonal balance, which, in itself, is protective against the negative side effects that can occur from either too many or too few hormones in your cells and tissues.

I have also added additional safeguards to my program, so that any estrogen, whether it's your own or estrogen derived from HRT, is handled by your body in the safest, least toxic way. This will greatly reduce your risk of diseases that can accompany menopause, including breast cancer, heart disease, and arthritis, as well as help to significantly improve your overall health and well being.

Beat Breast Cancer

Researchers have found that diindolylmethane (DIM), an interesting little compound found in *Brassica* vegetables such as broccoli, bok choy, cauliflower, cabbage, and Brussels sprouts, is quite beneficial in promoting estrogen metabolism. Specifically, DIM helps to metabolize estrogen into its safer form.

As I indicated earlier, estrogen is converted from the potent estradiol into estrone. Estrone then becomes either 2-hydroxyestrone—a "good" estrogen metabolite—or 16-alpha-hydroxyestrone—a "bad" estrogen metabolite. The good metabolite (2-hydroxyestrone) is then converted into 2-methoxyestrone and 2-methoxyestradiol. These two estrogen metabolites have been shown to inhibit the growth of malignant tumors; however, 16-alpha-hydroxyestrone has been strongly associated with cancer growth.

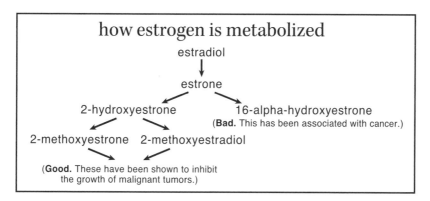

This is where DIM comes in. Research has shown that when DIM is ingested, it not only encourages its own metabolism, but that of estrogen. While it is not an estrogen or even an estrogen-mimic, its metabolic pathway exactly coincides with the metabolic pathway of estrogen. When these pathways intersect, DIM favorably adjusts the estrogen metabolic pathways by simultaneously increasing the good estrogen metabolites and decreasing the bad 16-alpha-hydroxyestrone.

Since higher levels of bad estrogen circulating in the bloodstream have been associated with higher breast cancer rates, scientists theorized that by increasing the good to bad estrogen ratio, you could protect against estrogen-fed cancer. Here's what they found:

In a study released in 1998, researchers in England looked at estrogen pathways to determine if in fact the ratio of the good 2-hydroxyestrone to the bad 16-alpha-hydroxyestrone actually affected breast cancer risk. They took urine samples from more than 5,000 women ages 35 and older. These samples were then frozen and stored for up to 19 years. Researchers found that those women with the highest good estrogen metabolite to bad estrogen metabolite ratio had a 30 percent decreased risk for breast cancer.

Here in the United States, researchers collected and tested the urine of nearly 11,000 women aged 35 to 69. At the time of testing, all women were cancer-free and not on HRT. After an average storage time of 5.5 years, the samples were tested for 2-hydroxyestrone and 16-alpha-hydroxyestrone levels and compared to those women who had developed breast cancer in that time. Researchers found that the women who had higher ratio of 2-hydroxyestrone to 16-alpha-hydroxyestrone at the start of the study were at less risk for breast cancer.

Once researchers became more confident that the 2-hydroxyestrone to 16-alpha-hydroxyestrone ratio was a good predictor of breast cancer risk, they set out to determine if consumption of *Brassica* vegetables such as broccoli and cabbage could influence this ratio. In a study from *Epidemiology*, American researchers took urine samples from 34 healthy postmenopausal women. They then added 10 grams of broccoli a day to the women's diets. After taking another urine sample, researchers found that this dietary change significantly increased the 2-hydroxyestrone to 16-alpha-hydroxyestrone ratio.

A similar study looked at the dietary habits of postmenopausal Swedish women aged 50 to 74. When asked how often, on average, they consumed a wide variety of foods, including 19 different commonly eaten fruits and vegetables, researchers found that those women who ate 1 to 2 servings of *Brassica* foods a day had a 20 to 40 percent lower risk of breast cancer than those women who ate virtually none.

Finally, a study from *Biochemical Pharmacology* found that DIM may have another intriguing benefit. Researchers at the University of California at Berkeley found that DIM not only blocked DNA synthesis in human breast cancer cells, but also stopped the cells from spreading. They discovered that DIM also caused the cancerous cells to die. I am very excited about this early in vitro research and will keep you apprised of further findings.

I am a huge advocate of DIM and personally take it every day. I strongly suggest you do the same. In addition to eating more *Brassica* vegetables like broccoli and cauliflower, I recommend taking 30 mg of DIM a day with meals.

B Vitamins Protect Against Estrogen Toxicity

The vitamin B complex—a group of 11 separate, water-soluble nutrients, including B_1 (thiamine), B_2 (riboflavin), B_3 (niacin), B_5 (pantothenic acid), B_6 (pyridoxine), B_{12} (cobalamin/cyanocobalamin), biotin, folic acid, PABA, choline and inositol—have been shown to help your liver break down your more potent estrogens into the weaker, but effective, estriol. Estriol is the least potent and safest form of estrogen, yet when present in sufficient levels, it is very effective in ameliorating and eliminating many symptoms of estrogen deficiency, such as hot flashes, vaginal dryness, and urinary tract conditions. (For more on the benefits of estriol, see page 147.)

According to a study conducted by Guy Abraham, M.D., at UCLA Medical School, 500 mg of a particular B vitamin (vitamin B_6) helped to change the blood levels of both estrogen and progesterone and bring them into balance.

PABA, which I discussed earlier, also has a protective benefit, as it slows down the metabolism of many hormones, including estrogen. This helps to promote a healthier overall hormone balance.

To help promote the healthy breakdown of estrogen into estriol, I suggest taking 50–100 mg of a vitamin B-complex a day. Be sure it includes 50–100 mg of vitamin B_6 and 400–500 mg of PABA.

Benefit From Estrogen-Like Hormone Substitutes

The second part of my program involves the use of many herbs and nutrients that replicate estrogen's role in your body. In my practice, I have used a combination of plant-based foods and nutrients, yin herbs, and key vitamins. These hormone substitutes provide a safe, estrogen-like effect, and using all or a combination of these daily, in sufficient amounts, can improve your hormone status.

Feel Better With Phyto Foods

Weak estrogenic activity is found in a variety of plant foods and herbs. However, for therapeutic purposes, only soybeans contain sufficient active compounds to approximate the effects of estrogen produced by the body. Soy contains two main phytoestrogens—genistein and daidzein, which belong to the class of chemicals called isoflavones.

Soy isoflavones were first discovered during the 1930's, but their potency was not assayed until the 1950's. At that time, genistein was found to be 50,000 times weaker than a powerful synthetic estrogen. Asian women eat much more soy products in their traditional diet than American women, whose isoflavone intake is virtually zero. This was confirmed in a study published in the *Lancet*, which found that Japanese women who regularly eat a range of soy products had 100 to 1,000 times more isoflavone breakdown products in their urine than Western women. Additionally, menopausal women in Japan are rarely troubled by symptoms such as hot flashes.

I've been recommending soy foods to my patients since the 1970's. Like all legumes, soybeans are superb sources of fiber, essential fatty acids, and other key nutrients. They contain high quality, low-fat protein, provide relief from menopausal symptoms, help conserve bone mass, and reduce your risk of heart disease. And, according to a study from the *British Medical Journal*, soy is useful in reducing vaginal atrophy.

MAKING SENSE OF SOY

It seems that we are bombarded on a daily basis with new information about soy—in some cases praising its benefits, and in other cases making it the scapegoat for everything from Alzheimer's to early maturation of teenage girls. While a handful of the critical studies have some merit, many are based on questionable research or test tube science. These studies really lose their impact when compared to the hundreds of clinical, animal, and epidemiological studies that attest to soy's health-protective benefits.

Still, I receive questions almost weekly about the dangers of soy and breast cancer and/or thyroid function. In my experience, I believe that it is fine for women with breast cancer to eat soy foods in moderation, with one caveat. In a study published in *Cancer Research*, researchers investigated the interactions between dietary genistein and the prescription drug tamoxifen and breast cancer by implanting estrogen-dependent breast cancer cells in mice who had had their ovaries and thymus removed. They found that genistein negated or overwhelmed the inhibitory effect of tamoxifen. Based on these findings, they urged postmenopausal women to exercise caution when consuming dietary genistein while taking tamoxifen. To date, I have not seen anything in the literature to negate this conclusion. Therefore, if you have breast cancer and are taking tamoxifen, I suggest that you use caution and avoid using pure soy isoflavones unless further, more conclusive studies contradict these findings.

In the case of hypothyroidism, I believe that the concern over soy's impact on thyroid function is unwarranted. First, no well-controlled, statistically significant human studies have shown that soy interferes with thyroid function. In fact, several studies conducted on humans have found no difference in thyroid function between those women who ate soy and those who did not. Second, the lack of evidence regarding this topic has led the FDA to reverse its earlier position that soy adversely affected the thyroid. Even more compelling is the fact that the American Foundation of Thyroid Patients has reviewed the current medical literature on soy and thyroid health and now recommends soy for all its members.

Based on the research as well as my experience, I see no reason for you to avoid soy or soy products if you have a thyroid condition. The only exception I have is if you have inflammatory bowel disease and autoimmune thyroiditis, combined with a known allergy or sensitivity to soy. In this small, specific instance, I recommend avoiding soy, as it may aggravate your condition.

Eating soy-based foods also has several other long-term health benefits. Unlike prescription estrogen, soy does not appear to have a carcinogenic effect on uterine cells or breast tissue. In fact, it appears to be cancer-protective for several reasons. Not only does soy reduce the production of estrogen within the body, but it also directly inhibits the growth of breast cancer cells. A review article appearing in the *Journal of the American Dietetics Association* confirmed that two compounds in soy—protease inhibitors and phytic acid—both have anticarcinogenic activity. The writers noted that soybean intake is associated with reduced rates of prostate, colon, and breast cancer. Once again, we see this benefit in Japanese women, who have an incidence of breast cancer four to six times lower than that of women who do not include soy in their diet.

Other studies currently in progress suggest that soy can have a beneficial effect on both blood fats and bone metabolism. While estrogen is often prescribed to prevent heart disease and osteoporosis, soy offers a food-based approach to the same health issues.

To enjoy a symptom-free menopause while protecting against cancer and heart disease, I recommend consuming whole soy foods. There is often a synergistic effect among the active elements that make the whole food more than the sum of its parts. And, in the case of soy, there are so many healthful components that it would be a shame to miss any of them.

If you are allergic to soy, then obviously you need to avoid consuming it entirely. If you find that soy foods cause digestive upset such as gas, bloating, or intestinal discomfort, I suggest taking a high-potency digestive enzyme such as bromelain or papain whenever you consume soy foods, or simply opt for supplemental soy isoflavones capsules. **I recommend that you take in 50–100 mg of soy isoflavones each day, either through soy foods or isoflavone capsules, or a combination of both.**

ISOFLAVONES IN SOY FOODS

Whole soybeans (½ cup)—150 mg	Tempeh (½ cup)—35 mg
Soy milk (one cup)—35–40 mg	Tofu (½ cup)—35 mg

KATHLEEN'S STORY

When "Kathleen" first consulted with me, she was a busy 60-year-old woman, lived on unhealthy but convenient fast food meals, was 25 pounds overweight, and often felt nervous and over-stressed. She was postmenopausal, with high blood pressure and cholesterol. Moreover, she had lost considerable bone mass.

continued on next page

The Healing Power of Plants

Many herbs are estrogen-like in their activity, including common culinary herbs such as fennel and anise, as well as licorice. Other herbs, such as black cohosh and red clover, have been used medicinally as part of healing traditions for thousands of years. While their estrogenic activity is a small fraction of the activity of the estrogen a woman produces (at least 400 times less active), their benefit is that these herbs usually do not cause unwanted side effects for most women.

One of the most effective estrogenic herbs is black cohosh. Native to America, black cohosh was well known and accepted in Native American herbal medicine and was widely prescribed in colonial times as a treatment for menstrual cramps and menopausal symptoms.

The effectiveness and safety of black cohosh are well documented. Clinical studies have shown that black cohosh relieves hot flashes, night sweats, heart palpitations, headaches, and vaginal dryness and atrophy. It is also effective in relieving other symptoms such as depression, anxiety, sleep disturbances, and a decline in libido.

Currently, in Germany, a special extract of black cohosh is the most thoroughly studied and widely used natural alternative to hormone replacement therapy. This research has prompted at least six well-publicized studies on the standardized extract of black cohosh and its ability to treat menopausal symptoms. According to a review of five key studies on black cohosh from the *American Journal of Medicine*, black cohosh is most effective at easing hot flashes.

In one of the largest studies on black cohosh, women with menopausal complaints received 40 drops of liquid black cohosh extract twice a day for six to eight weeks. Within four weeks of treatment, a distinct improvement was seen in nearly 80 percent of the women. After six to eight weeks, all symptoms had completely disappeared in half of the women.

Another study found similar results. Scientists gave women with menopausal symptoms either high- or low-dose black cohosh for a 12-week period. At the conclusion of the study, approximately 80 percent of both patients and physicians rated the treatment as "good to very good." The investigators reported no differences in either effectiveness or adverse reactions between the two groups.

Other studies have focused on black cohosh and its relationship to breast cancer. One in particular concluded that black cohosh actually inhibits the growth rate of breast cancer cells due to the fact that the herb does not trigger estrogen-like effects in certain breast cancer cell linings whose growth is dependent upon estrogen. Laboratory experiments have shown that black cohosh inhibits the effects of estrogen-induced stimulation and actually binds to those receptors. By doing so, it does not increase production of endometrial cells, nor does it change the makeup of vaginal cells. Also, it does not exert estrogen-like effects on the endometrium or breast, nor does it exhibit any toxic, mutagenic, or carcinogenic properties.

Given its apparent safety, I consider black cohosh a safe therapy for women who suffer from the acute symptoms of menopause, such as hot flashes, night sweats, sleeplessness, vaginal dryness and mood swings. I am particularly fond of Klimadynon® from Bionorica. Compelling research from several different journals, including *Maturitas: The European Menopause Journal and Menopause: The Journal of the North American Menopause Society*, has shown that Klimadynon® (CR BNO 1055) safely and effectively eases hot flashes and night sweats, promotes plumping of the vaginal wall, decreases vaginal dryness, and even promotes bone growth. Moreover, Klimadynon® does not cause proliferation of the uterine lining or of breast cells. This means that it, very likely, does not increase your risk of uterine or breast cancer.

Note: A recent study from the *Australian Adverse Drug Reactions Bulletin* found that, in rare instances, black cohosh can cause liver toxicity. More common and minor effects include occasional gastrointestinal disturbances, headaches, heaviness in the legs, and possible weight problems. There are no known drug interactions and the only contraindication is during pregnancy, with the possibility of premature birth due to overdose.

Additionally, an article in the *Journal of Agricultural & Food Chemistry* found that three of 11 black cohosh supplements tested didn't even contain the herb! Instead, they contained less expensive extracts of a similar Chinese herb. To be sure this doesn't happen to you, I suggest buying black cohosh from a reputable retailer or look for Bionorica's Klimadynon® brand.

To treat your menopausal symptoms safely and effectively, I suggest taking 40–80 mg of a standardized extract of black cohosh such as Klimadynon® twice a day. This dose should contain 2 to 4 mg of the active components (triterpenes, calculated as 27-deoxyacteine). You should see results within four weeks. In my practice, I have seen women experience relief from hot flashes and mood swings in as little as two to seven days.

Relief with Red Clover

I'm also a big fan of red clover for easing hot flashes and improving cardiovascular health. Red clover contains four phytoestrogens (estrogen-like plant compounds thought to have an effect on menopause-related symptoms such as hot flashes) called genistein, daidzein, biochanin A, and formononetin, and has become increasingly popular among menopausal women here in the United States.

And for good reason. While some studies have questioned the efficacy of red clover, comparing it to that of a placebo, it does appear to help reduce hot flashes. According to a review of five studies published in *The American Journal of Medicine*, red clover helps to significantly reduce the frequency of hot flashes. Other research has shown that the herb is also beneficial for cardiovascular health. Both the aging process and menopause itself reduce the elasticity of major arteries (called arterial compliance). This tends to make blood vessels more rigid and less flexible. Over time, these changes can lead to high blood pressure, or hypertension, and increase the workload on the heart. In one placebo-controlled study reported in the *Journal of Clinical Endocrinology and Metabolism*, red clover improved arterial compliance. Other known potential cardiovascular benefits of red clover isoflavones include the inhibition of platelet clumping or aggregation, which can clog arteries, and the herb's action as a potent antioxidant, which also helps reduce buildup of "bad" low-density lipoprotein (LDL) cholesterol in arteries.

If you would like to try red clover, I recommend taking a standardized extract that contains 40 mg of total isoflavones.

Yin is In

Traditional Asian medicine maintains that health and well-being are believed to be a balance of two equally important, but opposing, principles—yin and yang. Yin is associated with attributes such as femininity, receptivity, calmness, coolness, and moisture. Yin also regulates the fluids, blood, and tissues of your body, as well as its structural components, including flesh, tendons, and bones. It is protective and nurturing. Yang, on the other hand, is more associated with growth, masculinity, aggression, heat, and dryness. It also regulates your body's energy, which acts as the spark plug to your structural elements.

Balance between yin and yang is essential if you are to achieve and maintain optimal health and well-being. In younger, healthy women, the balance between this duality seems to be maintained almost effortlessly. Young women can become either very yin or very yang in response to the demands and stresses in their lives. They can study hard, work overtime, eat anything they want, and still have the ability to return to the balanced middle point, where yin and yang co-exist as a unified reality.

Maintaining an optimal yin-yang balance becomes much more difficult once you reach middle age and menopause, when it's common to experience symptoms such as hot flashes, night sweats, tissue dryness, insomnia, mood swings, and thinning of skin, hair, bones, and connective tissue. In the traditional Asian medical model, these symptoms occur, in part, because yin becomes deficient. To help bring your body back into balance, I suggest using a variety of yin-supportive herbs that work on the kidneys, which contain the reserve energy of the body and support your hormonal production. These herbs also improve blood and fluid circulation, ovarian health, and your sleep-wake cycle. In particular, I'd like to focus on royal jelly, dong quai, and saffron.

Royal jelly—the food of the queen bee—has been used for centuries to promote reproductive health and longevity and ease menopausal symptoms. Doctors from France have reported that women who ate royal jelly during menopause had a complete remission of symptoms, and some were even able to conceive again! Other doctors have found that royal jelly had a libido-increasing effect and helped promote vaginal secretions. Additionally, royal jelly has been found to be a natural antibiotic, fat metabolizer, immune booster, and metabolic catalyst, and even supports adrenal health.

I recommend using ¼ teaspoon of the liquid form of organic royal jelly twice a day. Royal jelly can be purchased at most health food stores. Just be sure to avoid royal jelly from China. Recent reports have shown that royal jelly imported from China was found to contain trace amounts of a dangerous (and possibly carcinogenic) antibiotic called chloramphenicol. To avoid this concern, be sure to purchase royal jelly that is produced by bees from the United States under healthy, organic conditions. Additionally, women who are allergic to bees or have asthma should not take royal jelly.

Dong quai (also called dang gui) has been used for thousands of years as a female health tonic to prevent or treat symptoms of PMS and menopause. Traditionally, dong quai has been used to treat abnormal menstruation and menopausal hot flashes. Many naturopathic physicians and herbalists today regularly prescribe this herb for their female patients.

In China, most women consume dong quai as a food, cooking the root in soup or other liquid mixture to soften it. **I recommend that you take dong quai in powdered form in a 500 mg capsule. Take two capsules two to three times a day.** Do not take dong quai if you are on a blood-thinner, as it may reinforce the effect of the anticoagulants and could increase your risk for bleeding.

Lastly, saffron is a bright yellow Indian spice that has also been used traditionally to reduce menopausal symptoms, enhance calmness, and reduce irritability. To preserve its medicinal properties, stir saffron into hot, cooked food. **Use ¹⁄₁₀ of a teaspoon or less per day, as higher amounts can be toxic**, causing stomach and intestinal maladies, and even death. Additionally, too much saffron can have a narcotic effect, causing sedation and sleepiness.

I also want to tell you about an amazing multi-herb blend called Formula D-34. This impressive blend of 10 herbs works to restore kidney yin. In fact, a study of 20 menopausal women found that Formula D-34 significantly increased blood levels of estradiol, the most potent and chemically active estrogen produced by your body. Additionally, the women reported a considerable reduction in menopausal symptoms, including hot flashes, depression, and anxiety. Formula D-34 is made by Draco Natural Products. I have included this amazing formula as one of the components in my own hormonal restoration product that I formulated for women with estrogen deficiency (see "Resources" for more information).

Vital Vitamins

Like phytoestrogens found in plants and herbs, certain vitamins have also been found to offer a natural way to reduce the symptoms of menopause—such as hot flashes, night sweats, insomnia, headaches, nervousness, and irritability—with little risk of side effects. The two vitamins with the most research in the area of menopause are vitamin E and bioflavonoids.

The original research on vitamin E's usefulness as an estrogen substitute was done between the 1930's and the early 1950's. Some of this research was done on breast and uterine cancer patients who were in menopause and were known to be poor candidates for estrogen replacement therapy, since it was understood as far back as the 1930's and 40's that estrogen could stimulate the growth of any remaining tumor cells. Vitamin E was found to be both effective and safe in alleviating menopausal symptoms in these patients, and it could be safely used by breast cancer patients. Between 67 and 95 percent of the women followed in various studies had relief of such common menopausal symptoms as hot flashes, fatigue, mood swings, and muscle aches and pains. Vitamin E was less successful for the treatment of vaginal atrophy, being helpful in only 50 percent of the cases.

One such study from the *British Medical Journal* found that vitamin E not only helped reduce hot flashes in 64 percent of women tested, but also helped reduce symptoms of vaginal aging. Fifty percent of the women reported healing of vaginal atrophy, as well as a decrease in pain during sex.

A similar study published in the *Journal of the American Medical Association* found that of the 25 menopausal women treated with 10 mg of vitamin E (about 15 IU), all found either complete relief or significant improvement in frequency and severity of hot flashes, as well as an improved mood and outlook on life. In another study of 66 women with menopause-related depression and irritability, 91 percent of the women found relief from their symptoms with vitamin E.

To relieve menopause-related symptoms, I suggest you take 400–2,000 IU of natural vitamin E daily, as d-alpha in a base of mixed tocopherols. Start with a lower dose and increase this by 400 IU every two weeks until the desired effect is achieved. ***Note:*** Oil-based capsules can also be used topically to treat irritation caused by the thinning of the vaginal walls that can occur at menopause. Simply open the capsule and apply the vitamin oil directly to vaginal tissues. Just be sure to test the vitamin first to make sure that there is no adverse skin reaction. A tiny amount of vitamin E can be applied over a few days before using larger doses topically.

Bioflavonoids have also been found to be mildly estrogenic. The potency of bioflavonoids is so low that they have no side effects for most women, yet they can relieve hot flashes as well as vaginal dryness. A study of 94 women at Loyola University Medical School showed the effectiveness of a bioflavonoids–vitamin C combination in controlling hot flashes for most of the women tested. In addition, bioflavonoids were suggested in this particular study as an estrogen substitute for cancer patients who cannot use traditional replacement therapy because their tumors are estrogen-sensitive.

I suggest taking 750–2,000 mg of bioflavonoids per day. Bioflavonoids are considered to be very safe and have virtually no side effects.

Estriol: Your Body's Natural Estrogen

If you feel the need for direct hormonal support, the final step of my program involves the use of biochemically identical hormones—namely estriol. Estriol can be used very safely in combination with many of the natural therapies I've already discussed. It is produced in the laboratory from active steroid molecules found in soy and wild yam. The resulting molecules are structurally the same as those produced in your body.

Of the three estrogens, estriol is the weakest, and more importantly, it is probably the safest type of natural estrogen. Based on various animal and human studies, it appears that estriol is less likely to promote excessive tissue growth, and even helps prevent breast and endometrial cancers. Several human studies indicate that it may be the ratio of estriol to estradiol and estrone that is protective. Women with higher amounts of estriol in relation to the other hormones were less likely to develop cancer, perhaps because estriol attaches to estrogen receptors that might otherwise bind to much more potent forms of estrogen that more readily promote cell proliferation. And, unlike conventional HRT that may cause fluid retention, headaches, nausea, and the build up of uterine tissue, estriol has few, if any, side effects.

One study published in the *Journal of the American Medical Association* found that estriol was particularly effective in treating vaginal atrophy, mood swings, and hot flashes. Researchers selected 52 symptomatic, postmenopausal women and separated them into four groups, giving each group either 2 mg, 4 mg, 6 mg, or 8 mg of estriol per day for six months. On average, women in every group experienced a decrease in their menopausal symptoms after one month of treatment. Furthermore, in the three higher-dosage groups, women who had ranked their symptoms as severe now felt that their symptoms were very mild.

Another study from Alternative Medicine Review found that estriol provides the protection of conventional HRT without the risks. Additionally, estriol was shown to ease menopausal symptoms, including hot flashes, insomnia, vaginal dryness, and urinary tract infections.

A study from Taiwan showed similar results. Researchers gave 20 menopausal patients, aged 44–62 years, 2 mg of estriol a day for two years. They found that estriol was significantly effective in easing menopausal symptoms (especially hot flashes and insomnia) in 86 percent of patients. Additionally, estriol did not cause proliferation of cells in the uterine lining. This is great news for women at high risk for endometrial cancer, such as those who are significantly overweight.

Other studies have supported estriol benefit in treating recurrent urinary tract infections. In a study from the *New England Journal of Medicine*, researchers looked at 93 postmenopausal women with a history of recurrent urinary tract infections. After four months of treatment, the patients using estriol needed to use significantly fewer antibiotics for their bladder infections during the course of the study. Additionally, 95 percent of those who received the estriol remained disease-free. The only side effects noted with the use of estriol have been occasional mild itching and irritation.

Early research also suggests estriol may offer some protection to your bones. One study in particular found that estriol significantly improved bone mineral density. Researchers divided 24 elderly women into two groups. The first group received 2 mg of estriol a day for six months, while the other received a placebo; both groups were given 1,000 mg of calcium chloride per day. They found the group who took estriol enjoyed an increase in bone mineral density, while the control group actually saw a decrease in bone density.

A similar study published in the *Journal of Obstetrics and Gynecology Research* found that menopausal women who received 2 mg of estriol a day for 50 weeks enjoyed a significantly slower breakdown of bone. This was most noticeable in women who had been in menopause for at least five years. Patients also reported an improvement in menopausal symptoms.

More importantly, researchers found that estriol did not stimulate the uterine lining, which translates to a reduced risk for uterine cancer. Plus, the fact that it attaches to estrogen receptors in breast tissue means estriol may help to block the more potent, and therefore carcinogenic, estrogens like estradiol from attaching to these receptors.

Lastly, an exciting study from the *Annals of Neurology* has reported that 8 mg of oral estriol (considered to be a "pregnancy dose") appears to have a protective immune response in non-pregnant women with relapsing-remitting multiple sclerosis. Estriol also decreased the number and volume of a certain type of lesion associated with the disorder. In fact, the average total enhancing lesion volumes decreased by 79 percent and number of lesions by 82 percent within the first three months. Over the next three months, lesion volumes decreased by 82 percent and numbers by 82 percent. This is very exciting news for women who suffer from multiple sclerosis.

CINDY'S STORY

"Cindy" was 57 years old and had been in menopause for several years. She began suffering from severe vaginal dryness and irritation that made sex with her husband very uncomfortable. She was also experiencing recurrent bladder infections, with as many as three in one year. This was particularly surprising to her, as she hadn't had a bladder infection since she was in her early 20's.

Her physician treated her infection with antibiotics, and even suggested that she use antibiotics prophylacticly. However, whenever she went off the medication, her bladder infection returned.

I suggested she use a regimen that included biochemically identical HRT (including estriol) and estriol cream. Within weeks, her problem had totally resolved. She was able to resume an enjoyable sex life with her husband, and the bladder infections completely disappeared.

Using Biochemically Identical Estrogen

Estriol can be taken orally or used topically. **If taken orally, I recommend using 2–4 mg daily, in capsule form. When used topically, I suggest applying one gram of the cream to your vagina every night for two to four weeks, then use twice a week for maintenance.** Many women with vaginal or bladder symptoms may choose just to use the vaginal cream locally, limiting their total body exposure to estrogen. However, I recommend covering the urethral and outer genital area with a thin layer of the cream as well as applying it intra-vaginally during the first few weeks of use.

In addition to estrogen alone, some researchers advocate the use of estriol in combination with estradiol (bi-estrogen or bivalent) or with estradiol and estrone (tri-estrogen or trivalent). In these combinations, the amount of estriol is far greater than the other forms of estrogen. In the case of trivalent estrogen, the ratios are usually 80 percent estriol and just 10 percent each estradiol and estrone. These combinations are also highly effective, and have also been shown to reduce menopausal symptoms, improve bone density, and increase "good" high-density lipoprotein (HDL) cholesterol.

Estriol and all biochemically identical estrogen have to be prescribed by your physician. I have found that physicians in my area will often prescribe estriol when asked to by their patients. Estriol is available at most compounding pharmacies, as well as a few mainstream pharmacies. I am particularly fond of the Women's International Pharmacy in Madison, Wisconsin, which sends estriol formulations to physicians throughout the U.S. You can find them online at *www.womensinternational.com* or by calling 800-279-5708.

TAPERING OFF CONVENTIONAL HRT

If you are currently taking conventional HRT and would like to start a natural therapy program instead, slowly taper down your HRT over a period of a few months. This tapering down method will help to ease any menopausal symptoms you may experience as you make the transition.

Tapering Off Estrogen Only or Separate Estrogen/Progestin Prescriptions

If you are on estrogen only or are taking two separate prescriptions (one for estrogen, one for progestin), cut your estrogen prescription in half each month for one or two months. Then cut back to every other day for a month. Then cut back to twice a week for one month, and finally to once a week for a month before you stop. As you decrease your estrogen, begin to increase your intake of natural estrogen substitutes like soy isoflavones, black cohosh, and vitamin E or potentiators such as PABA and cobalt to help cushion the estrogen withdrawal that will occur when you stop using prescription HRT. If you simply stop cold turkey, you might experience a recurrence of symptoms like hot flashes and night sweats.

If you are taking a separate prescription for synthetic progestin and are on a two- or three-week cycle with a rest period, you should finish your cycle, and then switch to the natural progesterone. If you're on a continuous program where you are taking progestin every day of the month, you can immediately substitute natural progesterone for the progestin.

continued on next page

TAPERING OFF CONVENTIONAL HRT   *continued*

Tapering Off a Combination Prescription

If your HRT prescription is a single pill combination of estrogen/progestin, cut your prescription dosage in half each month for one to two months. Then cut back to every other day for a month. Then cut back to twice a week for one month, and finally to once a week for a month before you stop. As you decrease your prescription, begin to increase your intake of natural estrogen substitutes like soy isoflavones, black cohosh, or vitamin E or potentiators such as PABA and cobalt to help cushion the estrogen withdrawal that will occur when you stop using prescription HRT.

Once you are completely weaned off your prescription and onto the natural estrogen substitutes and potentiators, you may want to add natural progesterone to your regimen to support your bone health, enjoy better sleep quality, and improve your mood.

* * *

Clearly, estrogen deficiency is a complex issue. Fortunately, there is much you can do to preserve your body's estrogen levels. I know this first-hand, as I've personally used this program to maintain my own hormone health well in to my 60's.

You can enjoy a healthier hormonal balance and combat symptoms of estrogen deficiency by using the therapies I've discussed in this chapter. These include:

1. Stimulate estrogen at the central nervous system level with glandulars and ginseng.
2. Decrease FSH and LH levels with melatonin.
3. Increase estrogen production with wheat germ oil and boron.
4. Impede the breakdown of estrogen in the liver with PABA and cobalt.
5. Protect your body from estrogen toxicity and side effects by taking DIM, and B vitamins (including PABA).
6. Use estrogen substitutes, such as soy, black cohosh, red clover, vitamin E, and bioflavonoids.
7. Replenish your yin with royal jelly, dong quai, and saffron.
8. Increase estradiol levels with the herbal mixture Formula D34.
9. Use biochemically identical estrogen, especially estriol.

Next, we'll take a look at estrogen's complement—progesterone. You'll find quizzes and lab tests to help you determine your current levels, as well as techniques to stimulate your own progesterone production. Plus, you'll discover the secret of biochemically identical progesterone, and what frauds to watch out for.

14 health-promoting progesterone

Whatever your age—whether you are in active reproduction, premenopause, peri-menopause, or menopause—maintaining healthy progesterone levels is crucial to your female health and overall well-being. Deficiency of this important hormone can produce uncomfortable and deleterious symptoms, and relate to many female health issues at all stages of life.

Fortunately, I have developed a program more than 30 years ago to help women restore and boost their own progesterone production. Over the years, my program has helped thousands of female patients, often with dramatic results.

I first started to use it with my PMS and premenopause patients. The results were so positive—and often occurred so rapidly, *usually* within one or two menstrual cycles—that I began to expand the program to many of the women I worked with, no matter what their age, including many postmenopausal women. I also pioneered the use of biochemically identical hormones, and was one of the very first physicians to introduce this very beneficial hormonal therapy to patients, again with great benefit.

In this chapter, I'll discuss why progesterone is so critical to female health, then in Chapter 15, I give you the details of my "restore and boost" program.

What is Progesterone?

As I've indicated earlier, progesterone is one of your primary female hormones, derived directly from pregnenolone, the "mother" hormone from which all the other sex hormones are produced. Progesterone is primarily produced by the corpus luteum of your ovary, the "yellow body" that is created during the second half of your menstrual cycle. If pregnancy occurs, progesterone is also secreted by the placenta.

While estrogen causes tissues to grow and thicken, progesterone has more of a maturing and limiting effect on tissue. It also stimulates secretions throughout your body. For example, when progesterone production is stimulated during the second half of your menstrual cycle, the lining of your uterus secretes nutrients critical to the development of an embryo. Similarly, progesterone also causes secretion of those cells in your breasts that are necessary to produce breast milk.

Progesterone has a balancing effect on estrogen in many other ways. It is calming and sedating, while estrogen is stimulating. Estrogen lowers blood sugar levels while progesterone increases them. Additionally, estrogen tends to cause salt and fluid retention, while progesterone acts as a natural diuretic. This is why it is so critical to ensure that all of your hormone levels are in proper balance.

Progesterone's Role in Your Body

Progesterone is similar in structure to the other sex hormones. And like the other sex hormones, it too is produced by conversion from the precursor hormone pregnenolone.

Progesterone plays a key role in menstruation and pregnancy. The entire process of menstruation depends on the balanced interaction of several hormones, especially estrogen and progesterone. Working together, they prepare the lining of the uterus (the endometrium) to receive a fertilized egg, should pregnancy occur. The surge of progesterone after an egg is released from the ovarian follicle greatly stimulates the libido, which increases the likelihood that a sperm will enter the female and unite with the egg.

The increase in production of progesterone at mid-cycle causes a rise in body temperature, which many women monitor to identify when ovulation is most likely to occur and, therefore, the days when they are fertile. If the egg does not unite with a sperm, progesterone output declines. This stimulates the cells of the uterine lining to slough off and be excreted, which is experienced as menstruation. A rapid decline in progesterone triggers your monthly menstrual bleeding.

During your monthly cycle, the level of progesterone rises and falls dramatically, from 2–3 mg per day in the first half of the month, to 22 mg per day in the second half of the month. For some women, this number can be as high as 30 mg per day.

Should pregnancy occur, the placenta also begins to produce progesterone, greatly adding to the amount of hormone in circulation. By the fourth month of gestation, a woman produces 10 times her normal amount. During the last months of pregnancy, daily production can be as high as 300–400 mg a day. To appreciate the significance of this quantity, consider that the various hormones produced within the body are usually measured in micrograms (a thousand-fold less).

Besides its role in the menstrual cycle, progesterone participates in several other vital functions. These other metabolic actions are especially important because they help women to maintain general good health and help prevent disease. For instance, progesterone helps keep blood sugar levels normal, aids the activity of the thyroid, and functions as a natural diuretic. It also normalizes zinc and copper levels, promotes the metabolic conversion of fat into energy, and normalizes blood clotting.

Having sufficient levels of progesterone also helps to prevent the development of a variety of diseases. For example, progesterone prevents the uterine lining from becoming too thick during the second half of the menstrual cycle and even, over time, from becoming cancerous. Progesterone also prevents menstrual bleeding from becoming too profuse or long lasting.

How Progesterone Deficiency Occurs

Unfortunately, the balance between estrogen and progesterone does not remain intact as a woman ages. By the time you are in your 30's, progesterone production begins to decline. Having an irregular menstrual cycle can also affect your progesterone production.

This decline continues in perimenopause, when changes occur in both the length of the menstrual cycle and the amount of blood lost. Often, this occurs during your mid- to late-40's, although the age can vary greatly. Women can begin this process as young as their 30's and well into their late 50's, and it can last as briefly as one year or as long as five or six years.

In the early stages of menopause, the ovarian follicles begin to atrophy, reducing your ability to produce estrogen. You ovulate less frequently, thereby producing less progesterone or no progesterone at all during certain months. In an attempt to force the ovaries to manufacture more hormones, the levels of the pituitary hormone FSH (follicle-stimulating hormone) become elevated. (As I indicated before, FSH is the hormone that triggers follicular function in the ovaries.) Paradoxically, your ovaries may go into overdrive in response to the pituitary stimulation. In fact, for a time, your ovaries may produce high levels of estrogen until they are finally exhausted. When this occurs, estrogen levels may drop permanently, and menstruation ceases. As a result, hormonal levels may fluctuate during this time, and the balance between estrogen and progesterone is disrupted.

Although both estrogen and progesterone stimulation are needed for healthy menstruation, the overabundance of estrogen and lack of progesterone can cause changes in the menstrual cycle. Too much estrogen causes the uterine lining to grow and thicken excessively. Without the addition of progesterone during the second half of the cycle, the lining continues to thicken and proliferate until it finally outgrows its blood supply and begins to shed. Heavy, irregular bleeding can be the unfortunate result for many women.

At menopause, the production of progesterone declines more than that of estrogen. While estrogen production can fall 75–90 percent, progesterone production becomes almost negligible in postmenopausal women. Fortunately, there are ways to determine if you have decreased levels of this vital hormone.

Symptoms of Progesterone Deficiency

Unlike too much estrogen (which tends to affect premenopausal women) or too little estrogen (which is often the issue for perimenopausal or menopausal women), progesterone deficiency can affect a woman at any stage of life. If you are in premenopause, there are a wide variety of negative health issues that can often result from decreased levels of progesterone. In addition to the discomfort of premenstrual syndrome, you may experience more severe conditions such as uterine fibroids tumors, endometriosis, ovarian cysts, or even endometrial cancer.

If you are in perimenopause or menopause, your progesterone deficiency concerns will likely include typical menopausal symptoms like hot flashes and insomnia, as well as increased risk for osteoporosis.

Let's take a more in-depth look at the issues surrounding decreased levels of progesterone during both phases of life.

Progesterone Deficiency During Premenopause

As one of the major female sex hormones, progesterone affects many body systems and tissues. Decreased levels of this crucial hormone can trigger a wide variety of negative health conditions, ranging from the discomfort of PMS to more life-threatening conditions, such as uterine cancer.

PMS

Premenstrual syndrome (PMS) is thought to be a result of hormonal changes, diet, and lifestyle. Studies have shown that women with PMS tend to have relatively high levels of estrogen and relatively low levels of progesterone.

Low progesterone levels play a particularly large role in the emotional symptoms associated with PMS, including anxiety, irritability, and depression. In fact, progesterone has a significant effect on mood. For example, pregnant women, who produce abundant quantities of progesterone, tend to have an exceptional sense of well-being. Conversely, after childbirth, when progesterone production suddenly plummets, women may develop postpartum depression.

The association of progesterone with mood swings is evident when considering the years in a woman's life in which they most commonly occur. About 60 percent of women have mild to moderate PMS in their late 30's and 40's. For many women, this is a time when their hormone production begins to go out of balance. An additional 15–20 percent of women will have symptoms severe enough to disrupt their ability to function both at home and at work.

Fortunately, increasing progesterone through proper diet, exercise, and the right combination of nutrients (and in severe cases, the use of natural progesterone) can ease most, if not all, PMS-related symptoms.

Ovarian Cysts

During normal ovulation, a follicle (the fluid-filled structure that houses an egg before it's released into the fallopian tube) grows to a certain size and then ruptures, releasing the egg. The follicle is then converted into a larger structure, the *corpus luteum*—which produces both estrogen and progesterone needed to promote proper growth and maturation of your uterine lining during the second half of your menstrual cycle.

An ovarian cyst forms when the follicle continues to grow, instead of releasing the egg and dissolving like it's supposed to. In other words, the cyst is a failed ovulation, and as such, is a clear indicator that you aren't producing the proper levels of progesterone.

Ovarian cysts are so common that conventional medicine considers them normal. In fact, most cysts do go away on their own within a couple of months. In the event they don't go away, your treatment options aren't so positive—surgically draining, cauterizing, or removing the cyst (along with a section of the ovary); removing the ovary; and/or taking synthetic hormones—all of which only treat the symptoms, not the cause.

Fortunately, increasing your progesterone levels will likely help to reduce or even eliminate symptoms and help cause the cysts to shrink.

Benign Breast Disease

Benign breast disease is a catch-all term for changes in the breast that *aren't cancer*. According to the American Cancer Society, nine out of 10 women have some type of benign breast disease at some point in their lives. Often, it manifests as breast swelling, pain, and engorgement that can last several days to two weeks during each cycle. In many cases, women complain that their breasts are so tender they can't bear to have them touched. Some women even have to stop running during this period because of the pain.

JANE'S STORY

"Jane" was a 38-year-old woman who suffered from cystic changes in her breast, as well as breast swelling and pain for one week prior to the start of her menstrual periods. Her breast swelling and engorgement were so pronounced that she had to buy a larger bra just for this time of the month.

She loved to jog and would run four miles each day as her preferred exercise, except during the time just before her period, when her breast tenderness made running too difficult. She also noticed abdominal bloating, some swelling in her fingers (which made it more difficult for her to take her rings on and off her fingers), and a tendency toward mood swings and crankiness with her husband. Luckily, her symptoms subsided dramatically with the use of my dieting and nutritional recommendations.

Hyperplasia and Endometrial (Uterine) Cancer

Endometrial hyperplasia usually affects women between the ages of 50 and 70. In some women, this can be a pre-cancerous condition, in which there is an overgrowth of the cells of the uterine lining, or endometrium (a precursor to endometrial or uterine cancer). In the early stages, there may not be any symptoms, but as the condition progresses, more common symptoms like abnormal vaginal bleeding may occur.

Prevention of endometrial cancer is the primary reason physicians prescribe progesterone. This became evident several decades ago when the incidence of uterine cancer increased in American women who were prescribed unopposed estrogen. Estrogen use fell into decline among the menopausal female population until studies showed that combined estrogen therapy could protect women from the development of this cancer. Without the addition of progesterone to an estrogen treatment regimen, the incidence of endometrial (uterine) cancer increases four- to eight-fold in women with an intact uterus.

SUSAN'S STORY

I first saw "Susan" when she was 40 years old. At that time, she was suffering from mood swings, irritability, bloating, and sugar cravings due to the PMS that had occurred after the birth of her second child. Her PMS symptoms resolved relatively quickly on my nutritional and supplement program and she was able to handle her day-to-day routine without suffering from PMS.

At age 48, Susan consulted me again. She explained that she had felt extremely well and her menstrual cycles had been normal until the past year when she began to transition into a new phase of her life—premenopause. At that time, her menstrual periods, which had been regular (4–5 days in length, with a moderate amount of bleeding) had now become much heavier, lasted longer, and were more irregular.

She sought help from her gynecologist, who did an endometrial biopsy and told her that she had endometrial hyperplasia, which needed to be watched carefully and treated so that it did not progress to endometrial cancer. He also told her that the condition was caused by her estrogen levels being too high without sufficient production of progesterone.

Susan asked me if she could resolve this problem using natural healing methods, as she had done with her PMS. I explained to her that with the use of diet and a nutritional supplement program—including natural, biochemically identical progesterone—we could absolutely bring her hormones back into a healthy balance.

Some six months later, I received a very excited phone call from Susan, telling me that upon retesting, her endometrial hyperplasia had totally resolved, and her uterine lining was now normal.

Progesterone Deficiency During Perimenopause and Menopause

During the perimenopause and menopause years, the side effects of decreased progesterone levels continue to plague many women. Not only does progesterone deficiency intensify the symptoms of menopause, but it is also a risk factor for heart disease, osteoporosis, and even certain nerve diseases.

Menopausal Symptoms

Between 15–20 percent of women who are making the transition into menopause experience hot flashes, even while they're still having fairly regular menstrual periods. They may also experience heavy bleeding and premenstrual tension.

Fortunately, progesterone used alone can relieve hot flashes and other vasomotor symptoms in about 60–80 percent of women. Because of its sedative and calming effects, progesterone is also useful in treating menopausal mood swings.

Insomnia

Women deficient in progesterone often have trouble falling or staying asleep. Fortunately, increasing your levels of this hormone can help to restore normal sleep patterns. In fact, progesterone therapy during perimenopause and the postmenopausal years can potentially reduce fatigue and increase energy by improving sleep quality.

Another reason for progesterone's sleep benefits is that it helps to boost and support the effects of GABA (gamma-aminobutyric acid), a calming, inhibitory neurotransmitter, a chemical that relays information from one part of your brain to another.

Decreased Sex Drive

Progesterone levels are an important component of your ability to maintain your libido, or sex drive. This is thought to occur through progesterone's effect on the brain, as libido is primarily a brain function.

For most women, continuing to have fulfilling sexual activity is an essential part of life. Restoring progesterone levels offer one way to restore this ability in those women who have experienced a decline in this function. Animal studies have demonstrated that while estrogen readies the brain cells involved with libido, progesterone is the hormone that activates them.

Brain Fog

Mental acuity and the ability to concentrate depend on adequate progesterone levels within the body. After menopause, when ovarian progesterone production has ceased, many women experience brain fog, periods of forgetfulness, and difficulty remembering names, phone numbers, etc.

Progesterone has also been effective in elderly people who have become senile, helping them to regain some degree of mental alertness. This effect of progesterone may be due to several factors involving brain function. Relatively large amounts of progesterone are present in brain cells, 20 times greater than in the blood. It is thought that progesterone enhances the amount of oxygen in the cells of the brain, thereby increasing mental acuity.

Mood Swings

According to recent research, changes in levels of progesterone have been shown to influence the production and breakdown of brain chemicals that modulate mood. These include the neurotransmitters dopamine, norepinephrine, acetylcholine, and serotonin. Both the peripheral and the central nervous systems have hormone receptors and react to changes in the level of progesterone. Therefore, low progesterone levels will have a direct impact on your ability to maintain a level and balanced mood. It is thought that the ability of progesterone to generate a sense of well-being depends on its brain-related activity.

Stress and Anxiety

As progesterone helps promote a natural calm, a deficiency in this vital hormone can lead to stress and anxiety. In fact, progesterone is sometimes referred to as a natural tranquilizer, as it has a calming and even mildly sedating effect. Taken in high dosages, it has been used as an anesthetic.

It is thought that this calming effect is due to the conversion of progesterone into substances that slow activity at GABA (gamma-aminobutyric acid) receptors. GABA is an amino acid that inhibits neurotransmitters (chemicals that relay information from one part of the brain to another) and has a calming effect. While progesterone has a sedating effect on its own, having a balance between estrogen and progesterone levels is crucial for remaining even-tempered under pressure.

Heart Disease

There has been quite a bit of controversy surrounding the connection between progesterone and heart disease. Some experts believe that progesterone has no positive effects on the heart, while others claim that it actually increases the "bad" low-density lipoprotein (LDL) cholesterol and decreases the "good" high-density lipoprotein (HDL) cholesterol.

While the experts still debate these issues, what is clear is that the answer lies in the use of natural progesterone versus synthetic progestins. There is strong evidence that natural progesterone causes less fluid retention than progestins, and that the oral, micronized type of natural progesterone may lower blood pressure.

Other research indicates that while synthetic progestins may cause constriction and/or spasms of the blood vessels, natural progesterone has the opposite effect, and actually promotes a widening of the blood vessels—a critical aspect of heart health.

Osteoporosis

Although there has recently been a great deal of media attention on the role of estrogen in bone health, the benefits of progesterone have received far less attention. Nevertheless, research has shown that progesterone plays an important role in bone metabolism.

While estrogen does help to prevent osteoporosis by inhibiting calcium loss from the bone and facilitating calcium absorption from the intestinal tract, the addition of progesterone to a treatment regimen may provide even greater benefits. Medical studies have shown that progesterone therapy increases bone mass by promoting new bone formation. Recent research has led to the conclusion that progesterone acts directly to stimulate new bone by attaching to the osteoblast cell receptors—the cells from which new bone tissue is created.

HELGA'S STORY

I have worked with patients with decreased bone density, but who have refused conventional estrogen/progestin therapy. One such woman, "Helga," chose instead to use natural progesterone cream, along with a variety of dietary and plant-based estrogens, as well as a high-potency nutritional supplement that contained critical vitamins and minerals for bone health. She also adopted a vegetarian-based diet and started performing resistance exercises with weights.

Although she had a higher than normal risk of osteoporosis, given a 25 percent loss of bone mass by age 50, she showed a steady improvement in her bone density in the years after initiating my program.

Nerve Disease

Decreased progesterone levels can mean decreased health of your nervous system. Nerves extend throughout your body and are coated with a protective covering called a myelin sheath. These sheaths help protect your nerves from injury caused by trauma and chemical damage, and prevent the electrical impulses from being short-circuited. Myelin is produced by specialized cells called Schwann cells. These cells also produce progesterone, which makes the manufacture of myelin possible.

Besides helping to maintain healthy nerves, progesterone may also be of use in repairing nerve damage. Animal studies have shown that progesterone levels near the site of a nerve injury are far more concentrated than they normally are in the blood, and when the animals receive additional progesterone, the myelin sheaths surrounding the nerves thicken. This association suggests the possibility that progesterone may one day be useful in the treatment of diseases involving nerve damage, such as multiple sclerosis, which involves a loss of myelin and a resulting impairment of communication functions of the nerves.

Are You Progesterone Deficient?

The following checklists can help you determine if you are deficient in progesterone. If you are still menstruating, refer to the first list. If you are in perimenopause or menopause, then the second list is for you.

Women in Premenopause

If you answer yes to four or more of these questions, you very likely need to increase your progesterone levels.

- ✓ Are you over age 35?
- ✓ Have you gained more than 10 pounds?
- ✓ Do you have heavy periods?
- ✓ Do you have irregular periods or spotting?
- ✓ Do you suffer from premenstrual syndrome (PMS), including premenstrual anxiety, irritability and mood swings?
- ✓ Do you experience premenstrual edema or swollen breasts?
- ✓ Do you get menstrual migraine headaches?
- ✓ Are you retaining fluids?
- ✓ Have you been diagnosed with ovarian cysts?
- ✓ Have you been told you have fibroid tumors?
- ✓ Do you have symptoms of endometriosis?
- ✓ Do you have a decreased interest in sex?
- ✓ Are you experiencing sleep difficulties?
- ✓ Do you have bouts of brain fog—forgetting your friend's first name, where you put your car keys, or the point of a text you recently studied?
- ✓ Have you recently discovered cysts in your breasts?
- ✓ Have you been diagnosed with either hyperplasia or endometrial cancer?

Women in Perimenopause or Menopause

If you answer yes to four or more of these questions, you very likely need to increase your progesterone levels.

- ✓ Are you age 45 or older?
- ✓ Are you in perimenopause?
- ✓ Are you in menopause?
- ✓ Are you having hot flashes?
- ✓ Has your desire for sex faded?

- ✓ Do you have difficulty achieving orgasm?
- ✓ Is your sleep quality poor?
- ✓ Are you often unable to concentrate?
- ✓ Are you unable to remain calm under stress?
- ✓ Are you frequently tired?
- ✓ Are you anxious and irritable?
- ✓ Do you forget small details?
- ✓ Do your joints and/or muscles ache?
- ✓ Do you have osteoporosis?
- ✓ Do you have a history of nerve damage?

If you are concerned that either of these checklists sounds like you, you may want to get your hormone levels tested.

Testing for Progesterone Deficiency

In addition to blood testing, there are also saliva tests for female hormones. Unlike blood tests, saliva tests are non-invasive (no needle sticks!) and highly accurate. These tests can take the guesswork out of making a proper diagnosis and make it possible to design individualized treatment that delivers maximum benefits with minimum risk of side effects.

Best of all, saliva hormone testing is accessible. Even physicians who still don't routinely order saliva hormone testing will usually write an order when a patient requests it. You can even order a limited saliva hormone test kit on your own directly from a laboratory, without a doctor's order. (See below for specific recommendations.)

Like blood, saliva closely mirrors hormone levels in your body's tissues. However, saliva is a particularly accurate indicator of free (unbound) hormone levels. This is the key, as only free hormones are active, meaning that they can affect the hormone-sensitive tissues in your breasts, brain, heart, and uterus. Saliva testing therefore provides a superior measure of the levels of hormones that actually affect vital body systems, mood, tissue levels of sodium and fluid, and many other important functions.

Additionally, blood testing only provides a one-time "snapshot" of hormone levels, whereas saliva testing provides a dynamic picture of hormonal ebb and flow over an entire menstrual cycle. In fact, 11 samples are collected during the month, all at the same time of day, then sent to a laboratory. The lab then measures and charts your progesterone levels. These results are compared to normal patterns.

Get Tested

If you think saliva hormone testing is right for you, consider consulting your physician. Having your doctor order the test has two advantages: The profile is more extensive, and your insurance may cover the cost. Several laboratories perform the test; in the event your physician does not have a preference, I recommend Genova Diagnostics—formerly Great Smokies Diagnostic Laboratory—(*www.gdx.net* or 800-522-4762), as well as ZRT Laboratory (*www.zrtlab.com* or 866-600-1636). If your doctor doesn't order the test, or you simply want insight to help you develop your own self-care regimen, you can order a test kit from several sources. Aeron Laboratories has a wonderful Life Cycles saliva test kit (*www.aeron. com* or 800-631-7900).

Progesterone levels are also commonly assessed through blood testing. If you opt for saliva testing, keep in mind that the level of progesterone measured in your saliva represents about one percent of the total blood concentration.

This test is thought to be representative of the free versus the bound progesterone within your body. Peak levels with supplemental progesterone use, whether taken orally or as a cream, occur about three hours after use. The lowest levels occur just prior to the next scheduled dose. Readings of progesterone levels help detect luteal insufficiency in the early stages of pregnancy. Progesterone levels are also monitored in women on replacement therapy.

Ranges of salivary progesterone without supplementation:
Follicular phase:	< 0.1 ng/ml*
Luteal phase:	0.1 to 0.5 ng/ml*

Ranges in saliva with progesterone supplementation:
Transdermal cream users:	1.0 to 10 ng/ml)*
Oral micronized progesterone users	0.1 to 0.5 ng/ml*
Ranges of blood progesterone:	
Menstruating women, luteal phase (midcycle):	5 to 20 ng/ml**
Normal, untreated, postmenopausal women:	< 1.0 ng/ml**

If your results indicate that you are deficient in progesterone (or if you scored high on the questionnaire), you are far from alone. I have treated thousands of women with decreased levels of this hormone. Let's take a look at how you can replenish your progesterone levels safely and effectively.

* figures from Aeron Biotechnology
** figures from MedlinePlus (a service of the US National Library of Medicine and the National Institutes of Health)

15 restoring progesterone

Throughout my many, many years in the field of women's health, I've worked with a number of substances that have been very useful in helping women increase their own progesterone production. I have had wonderful success over the years using these safe, gentle, effective nutritional and other lifestyle-related therapies to accomplish this goal.

My program is a better, safer way to help you navigate through the progesterone deficiency often related to premenopause, as well as perimenopause and menopause, with greatly diminished symptoms. In the case of premenopause-related conditions, my program has helped women avoid surgical procedures like hysterectomies, as well as reduce or eliminate the need to use medications that can cause very severe side effects, and treat conditions such as uterine fibroids, endometriosis, and severe PMS.

With my program, you'll use nutrients to help you stimulate progesterone production at the nervous system level as well as in the ovaries. You'll also learn how supplemental, natural, biochemically identical progesterone can help increase levels of this vital hormone.

Let's get started!

Stimulate Progesterone Production

To increase progesterone production, it is necessary to stimulate and support ovulation. This can be done on two levels—through the central nervous system or via the ovaries.

While women are surprised to learn that you can increase progesterone production through the brain or central nervous system, the truth is that all hormone production begins in the brain.

We've been traditionally taught that human beings have one brain that is divided into many different parts. But more and more research is putting the "one brain" idea to the test. In fact, it's starting to be widely accepted that the human skull actually houses not one brain, but three—the reptilian brain, the limbic brain, and the neocortical brain.

The reptilian brain is the oldest part of the brain. It controls basic bodily functions like heart rate, breathing, body temperature, hunger, and fight-or-flight responses. Basic drives and instincts, such as defending territory and keeping safe from harm, are other functions of the reptilian brain. The structures in the brain that perform these functions are the brain stem (which controls breathing, heart rate, and blood pressure) and the cerebellum (which controls movement, balance, and posture).

The limbic, or mammalian, brain developed once mammals started roaming the earth. It includes the hippocampus, which controls memories and learning; the amygdala, which controls memory and emotions; and the hypothalamus, which controls emotions (among many other things). Therefore, the limbic brain allows mammals to learn, retain memories, and show emotions.

The neocortical brain, or neocortex, is the complex maze of grey matter that surrounds the reptilian and limbic brains, and accounts for about 85 percent of brain mass. It is found in the brains of primates and humans, and is responsible for sensory perception, abstract thought, imagination, and consciousness. It also controls language, social interactions, and higher communication.

The Chemistry of the Brain

Like the three parts of the brain, there are also three key types of brain chemicals: neuropeptides, neurohormones, and neurotransmitters.

Neuropeptides are responsible for the cell-to-cell communication system in your body. A peptide is a short chain of amino acids connected together, and a neuropeptide is a peptide found in neural tissue. Neuropeptides are widespread in the central and peripheral nervous systems and different neuropeptides have different excitatory or inhibitory actions.

Neuropeptides control such a diverse array of functions in the body. When they work together properly, the wonderful results in your body include elevated mood and other positive behaviors and emotions, stronger bones, better resistance to disease, glowing skin, and boosted metabolism. Conversely, if your neuropeptides function abnormally, the result can be an increased tendency towards neurological and mental disorders such as Alzheimer's disease, epilepsy, and schizophrenia.

There are several types of neuropeptides. Some of the most common include endorphins and beta-endorphins. Endorphins are opiod peptides, meaning they have morphine-like effects within the body. They produce feelings of well-being and euphoria, and a rush of endorphins can lead to feelings of exhilaration brought on by pain, danger, or stress. Endorphins also may also play a role in memory, sexual activity, and body temperature. Beta-endorphins are another form of opiod peptides, but they are stronger than endorphins. They are composed of 31 amino acids and work in the body by numbing pain, increasing relaxation, and promoting a general feeling of well-being.

While there are many, many hormones and hormonal interactions that occur in the brain and body, the most widely known neurohormone is melatonin. (I discussed melatonin in more detail on page 125.)

Neurotransmitters are naturally occurring chemicals that relay electrical messages between nerve cells throughout your body. While all three types of neurochemicals are important for hormone and overall health, neurotransmitters are particularly important for the production of sex hormones.

In the aggregate, all three types of neurochemicals help to regulate the brain's endocrine glands, specifically the hypothalamus and pituitary gland. The hypothalamus is the master endocrine gland contained within your brain that regulates your production of sex hormones. This gland produces a precursor hormone called gonadotropin releasing hormone (GnRH). When it is released, it travels to your anterior pituitary gland, where it stimulates the secretion of the follicle stimulating (FSH) and luteinizing hormones (LH).

These hormones then travel to the adrenals and ovaries, where they stimulate the production of estrogen, progesterone, and testosterone. In women with decreased levels of progesterone, the production of LH needed to trigger ovulation may not proceed in a healthy fashion.

In order to keep this whole process working smoothly, LH and FSH need to be triggered by a balanced mixture of the key neurotransmitters necessary to produce these hormones. The production of these vital chemicals is synthesized from certain amino acids, vitamins, and minerals that must be obtained through your diet or from supplementation.

First and foremost, the neurotransmitters norepinephrine, epinephrine, dopamine, and serotonin regulate the hypothalamus' release of GnRH. Without proper production and balance of these neurotransmitters, you cannot have proper balance of the sex hormones, including progesterone. This process is supported by precursor amino acids such as tyrosine, phenylalanine, and 5-HTP.

To understand this more fully, let's take a more detailed look at neurotransmitters in action.

Neurotransmitters: The Hormone Messengers

There are two crucial neurotransmitter pathways that help to support your overall health and well-being. The first leads to the production of the inhibitory neurotransmitter serotonin, while the second leads to the production of the excitatory neurotransmitters dopamine, norepinephrine, and epinephrine.

Generally speaking, the inhibitory neurotransmitters quiet down the processes of your body, while the excitatory neurotransmitters speed them up. Thus, the brain chemicals produced through these two pathways oppose and complement one another. Within your brain, serotonin often inhibits the firing of neurons, which dampens many of your behaviors. In fact, serotonin acts as a kind of chemical restraint system.

Of all your body's chemicals, serotonin has one of the most widespread effects on the brain and physiology. It plays a key role in regulating temperature, blood pressure, blood clotting, immunity, pain, digestion, sleep, and biorhythms. Along with another inhibitory neurotransmitters GABA (gamma-aminobutyric acid) and taurine, serotonin also produces a relaxing effect on your mood. Glutamate is another important excitatory neurotransmitter, though it is not part of the pathway.

Dopamine, norepinephrine, and epinephrine make up the excitatory neurotransmitter pathway. Unlike serotonin, which has a relaxing effect on your energy and behavior, excitatory neurotransmitters energize and elevate your mood. In addition to their powerful anti-depressant effects, they support alertness, optimism, motivation, zest for life, and sex drive. Plus, the excitatory neurotransmitters are particularly important for the production of progesterone.

ARE YOU BALANCED?

If you experience any of the following symptoms on an ongoing, consistent basis, you may have a neurotransmitter imbalance.

Low Inhibitory Neurotransmitters
- ✓ PMS
- ✓ Migraine headaches
- ✓ Chronic pain
- ✓ Irritable bowel syndrome
- ✓ Mood swings, irritability
- ✓ Anxiety
- ✓ Food cravings, binge eating
- ✓ Sleep apnea
- ✓ Fibromyalgia
- ✓ Increased infections
- ✓ Insomnia, poor sleep quality

Low Excitatory Neurotransmitters
- ✓ Depression
- ✓ Fatigue
- ✓ Low thyroid function
- ✓ High stress levels
- ✓ Weight gain, difficulty losing weight
- ✓ Cold hands and feet
- ✓ Mental sluggishness
- ✓ Low libido
- ✓ Irregular menstruation, heavy bleeding

In order to ensure that you have adequate neurotransmitter levels for healthy hormone production, you need to supplement with key amino acids, vitamins, and minerals. All neurotransmitters are produced from amino acids found in the protein that you eat. The essential amino acid tryptophan is initially converted into an intermediary substance called 5-hydroxytryptophan (5-HTP), which is then converted into serotonin.

While tryptophan is available as a supplement and is abundant in turkey, pumpkin seeds, and almonds, I've found that 5-HTP is a more effective and reliable option for boosting your neurotransmitter production. Numerous double-blind studies have shown that 5-HTP is as effective as many of the more common anti-depressant drugs and is associated with fewer and much milder side effects. In addition to increasing serotonin levels, 5-HTP triggers an increase in endorphins and other neurotransmitters that are often low in cases of depression.

The excitatory neurotransmitters are derived from tyrosine, an amino acid produced from phenylalanine, another amino acid. A variety of vitamins and minerals, such as vitamin C, vitamin B₆, and magnesium, act as co-factors and are necessary for the conversion of these amino acids into neurotransmitters.

To maintain proper serotonin levels, it is helpful to take 50–100 mg of 5-HTP per day, preferably at bedtime. You may want to start as low as 50 mg and increase as necessary. If needed during the day, use carefully, as too much serotonin can interfere with your ability to drive or concentrate.

To maintain optimum dopamine levels, take 500–1,000 mg of tyrosine per day. Be sure to take in divided doses, half in the morning and half in the afternoon. Do not take in the evening, as it may interfere with sleep.

As I recommend with all nutritional supplements, you should start at the lower to more moderate dosage, such as 500 mg a day of tyrosine and 50 mg a day of 5-HTP. Stay on this dosage for two weeks. If you don't notice a reduction in your symptoms, gradually increase the dosage by 500 mg for tyrosine and 50 mg for 5-HTP every two weeks until you have either noticed a reduction in your symptoms or have reached the maximum dosages. I generally don't recommend going over 1,000 mg a day of tyrosine, although you may find that you need as much as 100–200 mg of 5-HTP once or even several times a day.

Additionally, be sure to use a high potency multivitamin/mineral nutritional supplement so that you are taking in all of the co-factors needed to produce neurotransmitters. These include vitamin C, vitamin B₆, folic acid, niacin, magnesium, and copper.

Note: I strongly advise that you undertake a program to restore and properly balance your neurotransmitter levels under the care of a complementary physician, naturopath, or nutritionist. You should also have your neurotransmitter levels tested regularly, as dosage needs vary from woman to woman (see below).

TEST YOUR NEUROTRANSMITTER LEVELS

State-of-the-art neurotransmitter testing is currently available and can accurately pinpoint your exact levels of these essential brain chemicals. NeuroScience, Inc., (888-342-7272 or *www.neurorelief.com*) is a leader in the development of neurotransmitter testing. They have developed sensitive testing for these neurochemicals that can be done through your urine. The test is simple to do, non-invasive, and can be done in the privacy of your own home. In addition to NeuroScience, there are many other similar laboratories that offer neurotransmitter testing.

I would strongly recommend that you consider such testing if you suspect that you suffer from a moderate to severe neurotransmitter deficiency. Your health care provider will need to order these tests for you.

In addition to creating proper neurotransmitter balance through the use of amino acids derived from your diet, with the help of key vitamins and minerals, there are several other types of nutrients that can help to keep your endocrine glands and precursor hormones functioning properly. My particular favorites include vitex (chaste tree berry), maca, and glandulars.

Vital Vitex

Vitex is an herb native to the Mediterranean area. It works at the hypothalamic and pituitary levels. Specifically, it aids in the production of LH to trigger ovulation, thereby promoting progesterone production.

One study found that vitex helps restore menstruation by increasing progesterone levels. Researchers gave vitex extract to 20 women who had either abnormal or non-existent menstruation. After six months, 15 of the women were available for evaluation. Lab tests revealed that 10 of the 15 women had a return of their menstrual cycles, as well as increased levels of both progesterone and LH.

A similar study found that eight women with abnormally low progesterone levels who were given vitex every day for three months also enjoyed increased progesterone levels. In fact, two of the women became pregnant!

Vitex has also been shown to hinder the release of prolactin, a hormone closely related to human growth hormone, which plays a critical role in lactation. If there is too much prolactin in your system, secretion of LH is disturbed, which in turn can disrupt ovulation, and therefore progesterone production.

Several studies have proven vitex's ability to reduce prolactin levels. One double-blind, placebo-controlled study examined 52 women with luteal phase problems due to increased prolactin levels. They were given 20 mg of vitex a day for three months. At the end of the treatment period, prolactin levels had been significantly reduced.

A study from *Experimental and Clinical Endocrinology* suggests that vitex works to decrease prolactin by binding to dopamine receptors, which in turn thwart the secretion of prolactin. Interestingly, the researchers found that while prolactin secretion was inhibited, gonadotropin secretion (which leads to FSH and LH secretion) remained unaffected.

Research from several German peer-reviewed publications confirms this finding. For example, the *International Journal of Gynecology & Obstetrics*, and *Hormone and Metabolic Research* have both found that vitex appears to block prolactin secretion by binding to dopamine receptors. However, much research still needs to be done in this area.

To increase progesterone levels and decrease prolactin, I suggest taking 140–275 mg of a standardized extract of vitex (chaste tree berry) every day. Chaste tree berry works slowly, so it may take three or four months before you start to see its full benefit.

Exotic Maca

Maca—referred to as either *Lepidium peruvianum* or *Lepidium meyenii*—is one of the most traditionally used and valued Peruvian herbs, due in large part to its rich nutrient concentration. This malty, butterscotch-flavored root contains a number of minerals, vitamins, fatty acids, plant sterols, amino acids, and alkaloids, among other phytonutrients. In terms of minerals, calcium makes up 10 percent of maca's mineral content. Magnesium, phosphorus, and potassium are also present in significant amounts. Maca also contains a number of vitamins and amino acids, including B_1, B_2, B_{12}, vitamin C, vitamin E, and quercetin, as well as arginine, lysine, tryptophan, tyrosine, and phenylalanine.

German and American researchers begin studying Peruvian botanicals in the 1960's and 1980's. They quickly discovered that maca has many health benefits, including relieving menopausal symptoms; stimulating and regulating the endocrine system (adrenals, thyroid, ovaries, and testes); increasing energy, stamina, and endurance; regulating and normalizing menstrual cycles; and balancing hormone levels.

Maca appears to act as a central nervous system stimulant, at the level of the hypothalamus and pituitary gland. It works to stimulate hormone production, which is critical to regulate so much of a woman's physiology. It also operates as an adaptogenic herb to help regulate hormones produced by the endocrine glands. It does this by stimulating your ovaries and adrenals to produce the hormones you need, in the levels that you need them.

This was shown in a study published in the *Journal of Veterinary Medical Science*. Researchers tested the effects of maca on mouse sex hormones. They found that progesterone and testosterone levels increased significantly in the mice that received the maca.

A traditional dosage of maca is 2–10 grams a day. However, dosages are unique to each woman, so you will need to determine which dosage works for you. There have been no acute toxic effects of maca, even at very high doses. In fact, many Peruvians eat it every day! *Note:* If you are sensitive or allergic to herbs, you may want to use maca cautiously. In any event, I suggest starting with the low end of the recommended dosage, as *too* much can cause increased hot flashes, breast tenderness, or headache. It is also recommended that you avoid maca if you have a hormone-related cancer (due to lack of formal studies), liver disease, if you are pregnant or nursing, or if you are currently taking conventional HRT.

Glorious Glandulars

Glandular therapy involves the use of purified extracts from the secretory endocrine glands of animals. Most commonly, extracts are drawn from the thyroid and adrenal glands, as well as the thymus, pituitary, pancreas, and ovaries. Most extracts come from cows (bovine glandulars), with the exception of pancreatic glandular preparations usually drawn from sheep (ovine glandulars).

There are four common ways to extract glandulars. The first involves quick-freezing the material, washing it with a potent solvent to remove fatty tissues, distilling the solvent out, drying it, and then grinding it into a fine powder that is then encapsulated or pressed into tablets.

The second mixes freshly crushed material with salt and water that also removes fatty tissues. It is then dried and ground into a fine powder to be placed in capsules or made into tablets.

In the third method, the glandular material is freeze-dried, then placed into a vacuum chamber to remove the water. It is then encapsulated. However, with this method, fatty tissues remain.

The final method uses plant and animal enzymes to partially "digest" the material. It is then passed through a filter that separates out the fat-soluble molecules. The remaining material is then freeze-dried. This method seems to be quite effective. Due to the "pre-digestion," all biologically active substances remain intact and can be used therapeutically to support and restore your body's endocrine glands. Healthier endocrine glands are more likely to have healthier hormone production and to be more balanced.

In the past, most experts believed that glandulars could not be effective because the intestinal lining of a healthy person was impenetrable, and that proteins and large peptides could not breach its barrier. However, recent evidence has shown that large macromolecules can and do pass completely intact from the intestinal tract into the bloodstream. In fact, there's further evidence to suggest that your body is able to determine which molecules it needs to absorb whole, and which can be broken down.

Both animal and human studies alike have proven this theory. In some cases, several whole proteins taken orally, including critical enzymes, have been shown to be absorbed intact into the bloodstream. Additionally, many smaller proteins and numerous hormones have also been found to be absorbed intact into the bloodstream, including thyroid, cortisone, and even insulin.

In essence, it means that the active properties of the glandulars stay active and intact, and are not destroyed in the digestive process. This is key to the success of glandular therapy, and explains why they clearly help to restore hormone function by supporting the health of your endocrine glands themselves.

There are multi- and single-glandular systems available from companies like Standard Process—a leader in the field. However, they do require a prescription from a health care practitioner. Other good products are also available in health food stores and should be used as part of a nutritional program to support healthy menstruation.

Examples of widely used and accepted glandulars involve the thyroid and the adrenals. Natural thyroid medications such as Armour Thyroid, Naturthyroid, and Bio-Thyroid have been the preference of complementary physicians for decades. Unlike many of the commonly prescribed brands of thyroid therapy that only replace a synthetic form of T4, these natural thyroid replacements contains the whole animal-derived thyroid gland, including T3 *and* T4. This is a significant difference. T3 is more physiologically active than T4, and is critical in regulating normal growth and energy metabolism. Without the use of glandulars, this type of natural thyroid replacement wouldn't be possible. However, the thyroid glandulars sold in the health food stores have the hormone removed and are used to support the function of your own gland.

Adrenal glandular preparations are even more common. With the stress epidemic in this country, the majority of Americans are walking around with depressed adrenal function. This can also manifest as fatigue, susceptibility to infection, allergies, and infection.

Fortunately, whole adrenal extracts have been shown to possess cortisone-like properties that help treat asthma, eczema, rheumatoid arthritis, and even psoriasis. They have also been found to help restore the health and function of comprised adrenal glands. In one research study, eight women suffering from morning sickness (nausea and vomiting) who took oral adrenal cortex extract found relief within four days. A similar study gave both injected and oral adrenal cortex extract to 202 women also suffering from morning sickness. More than 85 percent of the women completely overcame their nausea and vomiting or showed significant improvement.

Another study looked at the use of adrenal glandulars to treat patients with chronic fatigue and immune dysfunction syndrome (CFIDS), as well as fibromyalgia. Researchers found that 5–13 mg of an adrenal glandular preparation significantly reduced pain and discomfort. Moreover, after six to 18 months, many of the patients were able to reduce and eventually discontinue treatment, while still enjoying relief.

Clearly, glandulars work. **To help support healthy progesterone levels, I suggest taking a good multi-glandular or single glandular product from a company like Standard Process. These could include glandulars such as hypothalamus, pituitary, ovary, adrenal, and thyroid, depending on the specific needs of each individual woman. I also highly recommend that you consider taking a whole brain glandular, if appropriate. To further support your adrenal function, I recommend taking 1,000–3,000 mg of a mineral-buffered vitamin C each day with a meal, 25–100 mg of a vitamin B complex a day, and an additional 250 mg of B$_5$ (pantothenic acid) twice a day.**

While stimulating progesterone production originates in your central nervous system, you also need to support progesterone production in your ovaries.

Ovarian Progesterone Production

Like estrogen and testosterone, progesterone is also produced by your ovaries, making it critical that you keep your ovaries functioning at their optimal level. To do this, I highly recommend using the following key nutrients: lutein, beta-carotene, and essential fatty acids.

Life-Giving Lutein

Lutein is a carotenoid with powerful antioxidant properties. As you can likely determine from its name, lutein plays a major role in the luteal phase, the time from ovulation to menstruation when the luteinizing hormone (LH) is produced.

While estrogen levels are rising from menstruation through ovulation, LH, which is produced by the pituitary gland, is needed to trigger ovulation. After ovulation, the follicle that contained the egg that was expelled from the ovary during ovulation is then converted into a new structure called the corpus luteum. Lutein is abundant in the corpus luteum and provides it with its distinctive yellow color.

The purpose of the corpus luteum is to switch from the estrogen production, which predominates during the first half of the menstrual cycle (days one to 14) to the production of progesterone and estrogen during the second half of your cycle (days 15 to 28). This is called the luteinizing process. During this time, lutein begins to accumulate in these key cells, and the effectiveness of the luteinizing process may be due, in part, to the amount of lutein found there. **To ensure that you have adequate lutein levels to support normal development of the corpus luteum, I suggest supplementing with 6–12 mg of lutein a day.**

Beneficial Beta-Carotene

Beta-carotene is the plant-based, water-soluble precursor to vitamin A. Like lutein, beta-carotene is abundant in the ovaries, and is found in very high concentrations in the corpus luteum. Some research even suggests that a proper balance between carotene and the retinal form of vitamin A is necessary for proper luteal function.

Researchers have been aware of the reproductive benefits of beta-carotene for more than a century. For example, cows whose diets were deficient in beta-carotene experienced delayed ovulation, decreased progesterone levels, and an increased prevalence of ovarian cysts, as well as cystic mastitis (breast cysts). Both conditions are typically found in women who are progesterone deficient.

Studies have also determined that high doses of vitamin A can help reverse one form of benign breast disease. In a study from Preventative Medicine, researchers gave 150,000 IU of vitamin A to 12 women with fibrocystic breasts. After three months, more than half the women reported complete or partial remission of the cysts. While I would never suggest that women take this high a dose of vitamin A for fear of toxicity, I believe that beta-carotene would have a similar effect.

To ensure that you have adequate amounts of vitamin A (as beta-carotene) in your system, I suggest taking 25,000–50,000 IU of beta-carotene a day.

Exciting EFAs

Essential fatty acids (EFAs) are health-promoting nutrients that your body needs to perform a whole range of functions. There are two main groups of EFAs: omega-3s and omega-6s. The most common are linoleic acid (omega-6), linolenic acid (omega-3), and the omega-3 fatty acids eicosapentaenoic acid (EPA) and docosahexaenoic acid (DHA).

Your body converts EFAs into series 1 and 3 prostaglandins, potent hormone-like substances with a wide range of benefits that are essential for good reproductive health. Among other things, these prostaglandins help to promote more frequent ovulation at mid-cycle. Since prostaglandins are necessary for the rupture of the follicle, which allows the egg to be extruded from the ovary at mid-cycle, this is a critical step for progesterone production to occur during the second half of the cycle.

The two best sources of EFAs are flaxseed and fish oil. In the case of flaxseed, both the oil and the ground meal are rich in EFAs. Plus, flax has been proven to support progesterone production. Researchers at the University of Minnesota tested 18 women with normal menstrual cycles. During three cycles, the women ate as they normally would. They then added 10 grams of ground flaxseed per day to their diet for an additional three cycles. The women who ate flaxseed had more ovulatory cycles than the women who did not. In addition, ground flaxseed was found to improve the estrogen-to-progesterone ratio, favoring the levels of progesterone within the body. The researchers felt that this was due to the lignans contained in the flaxseed, although I feel strongly that the flaxseed oil was also very beneficial in this regard, as it is also converted into prostaglandins, which is needed to allow ovulation to occur. **To promote progesterone production, I suggest taking 1–2 tablespoons of flaxseed oil or 4–6 tablespoons of ground flaxseed per day.**

If you do not like flaxseed or cannot tolerate it, you may prefer to get your EFAs through fish oil. In addition to also promoting progesterone production and helping to regulate the menstrual cycle, fish oil is extremely beneficial for easing menstrual cramps, endometriosis, and breast cysts due to its anti-inflammatory benefits. **If fish oil is your preference, I suggest taking 3–6 capsules that contain at least 300 mg DHA and 200 mg EPA every day.**

Supplement With Progesterone

Before the 1980's, all progesterone therapy had to be administered by injection in the doctor's office. The development of oral progesterone-like chemicals made this hormone much more readily available. Initially, a synthetic type of progesterone was combined with estrogen in birth control pills for younger women. Then progesterone's important role in preventing endometrial cancer in postmenopausal women on estrogen replacement therapy (ERT) was discovered in the 1970's. In one study, cited in a review article in the *American Family Physician*, 5,563 postmenopausal women were followed for nine years. In women using estrogen alone, the incidence of endometrial cancer was 390.6 cases per 100,000 women per year. In contrast, with combined estrogen and progesterone therapy, the incidence was only 99 cases per 100,000 women per year.

Not only does progesterone confer protection in women using estrogen replacement therapy, but it actually appears to protect against the development of endometrial cancer in all postmenopausal women. In the same study, women using no estrogen therapy at all were at higher risk than those on progesterone because of their own endogenous estrogen. These women developed 245.5 cases of endometrial cancer per 100,000 women per year. Not only has the rate of this cancer declined with the use of progesterone, but those women who develop it tend to do so at a later age. After this and other similar studies, progesterone therapy rapidly became part of the standard hormonal regimen for postmenopausal women who still had their uterus intact.

The progesterone used in replacement therapy today, whether described as synthetic or natural, is all produced by commercial laboratories. The terms *natural* and *synthetic* refer to the actual structure of the progesterone molecule. Progesterone that is natural has the same structure as the hormone the body produces. In contrast, while synthetic progesterone has somewhat the same function as the progesterone produced by the body—but many negative side effects—its structure differs slightly. In the United States, most prescriptions are for the synthetic form, called a progestin. The most common progestin is Provera, or medroxyprogesterone.

Natural, biochemically identical progesterone became available in the early 1980's, but initially only as a rectal or vaginal suppository. I was one of the very first physicians in the U.S. to use natural, biochemically identical progesterone with my patients, who benefited tremendously from this therapy. Although many women found the use of natural progesterone to be helpful, using it as a suppository was messy, since it tended to leak from the rectum or vagina. Progestin remained the preferred form because it was easy to take as a pill and also more absorbable. However, a natural progesterone was subsequently developed in a micronized form (pulverized into tiny particles) that is readily absorbed and is taken orally. The prescription name of this form of oral, natural progesterone is Prometrium, and must be prescribed by your physician.

It's important to thoroughly understand the difference between synthetic and natural progesterone, as they do not have the same chemical structure and do not behave the same biologically. They also differ in their benefits and side effects. Let's take a more in-depth look at the two main progesterone replacements available—progestins and natural progesterone.

Synthetic Progestins

The first chemical (or synthetic) progestin was developed in the early 1950's by Mexican chemist Luis Miramontes. Over the last half century, it has continued to gain acceptance in the conventional medical community and is still commonly prescribed by many mainstream physicians.

Progestins have been traditionally used during the transition into menopause. Perimenopausal women may produce too much estrogen without ovulating, which can cause heavy periods lasting as long as 10 to 12 days, or even longer. Taking progestins alone can help prevent erratic heavy periods. Progestins also help prevent the heavy buildup of endometrial lining by making sure that the lining is completely shed each month. By promoting a regular menstrual period each month, the use of progestins can also help reduce the number of endometrial biopsies a woman's physician needs to perform.

Progestins are used 10 to 13 days per month. The most commonly used brand of progestins is Provera (Upjohn). Norlutate (Parke-Davis) is also frequently prescribed, but it may cause side effects similar to those of androgens, such as oily skin and acne. A third progestin currently on the market is Amen (Carnick).

Physicians have also used progestins for many years as part of a conventional HRT regimen that is prescribed by most doctors. This is most often used by women who are menopausal, or those who have had surgically induced menopause, but still have their ovaries. Progestins can even be used alone by women who cannot take (or cannot tolerate) estrogen. Although it is not as effective as estrogen for reducing the severity of hot flashes, many women can still find some relief with a progestin. In fact, one study found that an injectable progestin (Depo-Provera) relieved hot flashes in nearly 90 percent of women.

However, the use of progestins has many drawbacks. In addition to increased risk of breast cancer and heart disease, some women taking progestins experience debilitating side effects. These often include abnormal bleeding, fatigue, headaches, depression and mood changes, bloating, breast tenderness and enlargement, vaginal dryness, and increased appetite. If any of these occur, physicians will often reduce the dosage.

Progestins can also cause more serious problems, such as an increased risk of heart disease. A study published in the *Journal of the American College of Cardiology* looked at monkeys that were made vulnerable to coronary spasms. The researchers treated the monkeys with estrogen, and this tendency was completely reversed. Then six monkeys were given a combined treatment of estrogen plus progesterone, and six others estrogen plus progestins. The progestin treatment resulted in coronary-artery spasms in all the monkeys, while those receiving natural progesterone had no spasms.

In human trials, progestins (especially when combined with synthetic estrogen) also prove to be problematic. In the Postmenopausal Estrogen/Progestin Intervention (PEPI) trial study, all of the women who took estrogen alone, estrogen and the progestin medroxyprogesterone (Provera), or estrogen with micronized (oral) progesterone experienced increases in their C-reactive protein levels. C-reactive protein, an indicator of inflammation, is now known to be a very strong predictor of future heart attacks, superior to LDL or HDL levels. Similarly, in the Heart and Estrogen/Progestin Replacement Study (HERS) trial, women taking a synthetic estrogen/progestin combination suffered significantly more heart attacks and other heart problems than those receiving a placebo.

Worse yet, progestins also appear to lower the "good" HDL cholesterol associated with a lower risk of heart disease, though the results of some studies do conflict with this. In the PEPI trials, women taking estrogen and progestins had lower HDL levels, while women on estrogen and natural, biochemically identical progesterone maintained higher levels of HDL.

There is also evidence that progestins may have a harmful effect on various systems of the body if taken over a long period, and can increase the risk of birth defects if taken during the first four months of pregnancy.

Natural Progesterone

In my opinion, any woman considering taking progesterone for its performance, as well as health benefits, should consider using natural progesterone rather than the progestins. As I mentioned earlier, I have been recommending natural progesterone since the early 1980's, and was one of the first physicians to have clinical experience in using it. I initially prescribed it for my PMS patients, but also found that it was useful for problems related to estrogen dominance, as well as menopause.

Natural (or biochemically identical) progesterone is produced from dioscorea, the active component of the Mexican wild yam—as are pregnenolone and DHEA. It can also be manufactured from soybeans. In either case, the resultant hormone has the same chemical structure and range of activity as the progesterone made by your body.

Natural progesterone appears to confer an equal amount of protection against uterine cancer and functions as a diuretic and an anti-anxiety treatment. It can also stimulate libido, help prevent and treat fibrocystic breast disease, regulate thyroid hormone activity, stabilize blood sugar levels, and assist in normal blood clotting. Plus, natural progesterone is essential for the production of cortisone in the adrenal cortex, and helps convert fat to energy.

Beyond all these benefits, natural progesterone also plays an important role in the prevention and reversal of osteoporosis. In a study conducted by John Lee, published in *Medical Hypotheses*, 100 postmenopausal women were treated with natural progesterone for a minimum of three years. Without treatment, these women would have had an expected bone loss of 4.5 percent. However, the bone density of the women was found to increase—10 percent in the first year on average, followed by a yearly increase of 3 to 5 percent thereafter.

When natural progesterone is taken in normally prescribed amounts (see next page), there are no known side effects. However, very high doses can cause drowsiness, due to its sedative effect on the brain, and huge doses of the hormone can be an anesthetic or cause a person to feel drunk. During the beginning stages of supplementing with progesterone, a woman may have symptoms of estrogen dominance. This happens because progesterone can increase the sensitivity of estrogen receptor sites. However, this sensitivity will disappear after a few weeks.

Using Natural Progesterone

Women of all ages (from their 30's on up) are currently using natural progesterone cream, which is now available in many health food stores and does not require a doctor's prescription (although the other forms of natural progesterone do require a prescription). Natural progesterone can be taken in oral micronized form or as a skin cream, rectal or vaginal suppository, or sublingual drops. Be sure to check the label of any product that you buy to make sure it truly contains pharmaceutical-grade, natural progesterone in therapeutic doses.

Oral Micronized Progesterone

Initially, natural progesterone could not be taken orally because it was destroyed during digestion and never reached the bloodstream. However, a micronized form of progesterone is now available that is protected from destruction by stomach acid and enzymes and can be absorbed and used by the body.

One study published in the *British Medical Journal* followed 23 women for four months. Each woman received 300 mg of oral progesterone daily for two continuous months. Those women receiving treatment had a clear improvement in concentration. Similar increases in mental acuity and the ability to remain focused on a subject have also been found in premenopausal and postmenopausal women.

Research has shown that oral progesterone can also reduce blood pressure. In a study also published in the *British Medical Journal*, researchers gave postmenopausal women and older men 200, 400, or 600 mg of oral progesterone or a placebo every day for two weeks. Those taking the progesterone enjoyed a significant decrease in their systolic blood pressure (the top number), as compared to the placebo group. In fact, participants who took 600 mg lowered their systolic blood pressure by about 19.7 mm Hg and their diastolic blood pressure (the bottom number) by about 9.6 mm Hg.

In menopausal women, dosages of 100–200 mg of natural, oral progesterone (Prometrium) taken daily can be effective, although the dose can vary in either direction. You need these high doses, as 85–90 percent of the amount consumed will be metabolized by the liver soon after it has been ingested. Like the synthetic progestins, perimenopausal women should use oral micronized progesterone 10–13 days per month. If you are in menopause, most physicians recommend using it every day.

Skin Cream

Progesterone cream is getting rave reviews from women and researchers alike. According to a randomized, double-blind, placebo-controlled study from *Obstetrics & Gynecology*, transdermal progesterone cream relieved menopausal vasomotor symptoms.

Researchers tested 90 postmenopausal women who were within five years of menopause and had not used any hormones for at least 12 months prior to the study. The women were tested for follicle-stimulating hormone levels; bone mineral density of the lumbar spine and hip; cholesterol levels; LDL, HDL, and triglyceride levels, and thyroid-stimulating hormone levels. All of the tests were repeated after one year. During that time, each woman kept a log of the number and severity of hot flashes.

The women were divided into two groups. In the first group, 43 of the women used ¼ teaspoon (20 mg) of progesterone cream a day, regularly rotating the application on their arm, breasts, or thighs. The other 47 women used a placebo. Of the women using the progesterone cream, 83 percent enjoyed fewer hot flashes, as compared to just 19 percent in the placebo group.

This finding was also confirmed by a study reported in *Gynecological Endocrinology*. Researchers found that women using 40 mg of transdermal progesterone cream a day for one year reported a significant reduction in hot flashes.

Other studies have shown that progesterone creams are also just as effective in increasing progesterone levels and easing menopausal symptoms as oral progestins—but significantly safer. According to a study presented at the annual meeting of the American Society for Clinical Pharmacology and Therapeutics, women given either natural progesterone cream or a synthetic oral progestin exhibited the same blood levels of the hormone.

A range of progesterone creams, available without a prescription, contain anywhere from less than 2 mg to more than 400 mg of the hormone per jar. Pro-Gest cream, which contains more than 400 mg in a container, is one of the better-known brands. The cream is applied to the skin and absorbed into the general circulation and reaches more body tissues than oral progesterone, which is first metabolized by the liver and converted into three different compounds.

A typical dosage of natural progesterone is 40 mg a day. A two-ounce jar should last for over one month. If you are perimenopausal, you should apply the cream from day 12 to day 26 of your menstrual cycle. If you are menopausal and not taking estrogen, you may use progesterone for two to three weeks each month, though some physicians do recommend daily use to avoid withdrawal bleeding.

If you are self-medicating with progesterone cream in an effort to block the cancer-promoting effect of estrogen on the uterus, you need to make sure you are taking enough progesterone for it to be protective. Blood or saliva testing of progesterone levels will help to determine if the level of supplemental progesterone you're using is in the therapeutic range.

The cream is used twice daily in ¼–½ teaspoon amounts, generally upon rising in the morning and before going to bed at night. The cream can be applied to any area of the skin. Many women rub it into their chest, abdomen, arms, or back. If the cream is absorbed rapidly (under two minutes), it means that the body needs a higher dose, and a slightly higher amount may be used.

Note: Some reputed progesterone creams that contain wild yam extract contain only the precursor compound—diosgenin—and little to no progesterone. Also, progesterone delivered as a cream must suspend the hormone in a proper medium or it will not be effective.

A cream containing mineral oil will not allow the progesterone to be absorbed properly. Some products have not stabilized the progesterone and, as a result, the hormone deteriorates over time.

Transdermal Sprays

Transdermal sprays work much like the creams, but without the mess. They are also quickly and efficiently absorbed into the skin with little need for rubbing. The spray also has a unique delivery system which makes it easier to absorb than the cream.

A typical dosage of the spray is 5 to 10 sprays per day, usually upon rising in the morning and before going to bed at night. Like the cream, the spray can be applied to any area of the skin. I find that most women prefer to spray it on their arms, thighs, or abdomen. **I am particularly partial to the ProgestEase brand of progesterone spray.**

Sublingual Drops

Progesterone is available in a vitamin E oil base. This is held under the tongue for at least one minute so that it is absorbed, rather than swallowed. This results in a quick rise in hormone levels, followed by a drop three to four hours later. It is necessary to take the drops three to four times a day to maintain stable blood levels.

Suppositories

Progesterone can also be taken as a rectal or vaginal suppository. Vaginal suppositories allow for excellent local intake of progesterone into the uterus, and may be helpful for pre- or perimenopausal women with heavy and irregular bleeding.

In a study published in 1995 in the *Journal of Assisted Reproduction and Genetics*, 25 women with severe PMS and seventeen reproductive-age females participated in a controlled trial. Treatment consisted of a 200 mg vaginal progesterone suppository, taken twice daily. The researchers observed that the women receiving the progesterone reported significant improvement in mood symptoms and nervousness.

A randomized, double-blind, placebo-controlled study published in *American Journal of Obstetrics and Gynecology* also found that the use of a vaginal progesterone suppository reduced the risk of preterm labor. Researchers gave 142 high-risk pregnant women either 100 mg of progesterone a day (administered by vaginal suppository) or a placebo. All were monitored for uterine contraction once a week for 60 minutes, between weeks 24 and 34 of gestation. They found that those women taking the progesterone had less uterine contractions that those receiving the placebo. They also found that less than 14 percent of the women in the progesterone group delivered early, and less than three percent delivered before 34 weeks, as compared to more than 18 percent of the placebo group delivering before 34 weeks. Researchers concluded that progesterone suppositories reduce the frequency of uterine contractions and the threat of preterm delivery in high-risk women.

THE BONE-A-FIDE BENEFITS OF PROGESTERONE

A number of studies have suggested that natural progesterone may be effective in protecting women from osteoporosis. John R. Lee, M.D., has done much research into the use of progesterone to reverse osteoporosis. The results of one of his studies were published in the *International Clinical Nutrition Review*. Dr. Lee selected 100 Caucasian, postmenopausal women between the ages of 38 and 83. The average age was 65.2 at the beginning of the study. The majority of the women had already experienced some loss of height due to osteoporosis. They were instructed to use conjugated estrogen (0.3 to 0.625 mg per day for three weeks each month) and progesterone (a 3 percent topical cream applied daily to the skin for 12 days each month or during the last two weeks of estrogen use). The women were also given a dietary and exercise program to follow, as well as vitamin and mineral supplements. Alcohol consumption was limited, and no smoking was allowed. The bone health of the women was followed for at least three years.

All the women in the study experienced some degree of progressive increase in bone mineral density, as well as improvement in such clinical symptoms as height stabilization, pain relief, and an increase in physical activity. During the course of the study, there were also no fractures due to osteoporosis. These improvements occurred independent of the women's ages. The women commonly had an increase in the density of vertebral bone of 10 percent in the first six to 12 months of treatment. This increase was purportedly followed by additional yearly increases of 3 to 5 percent. This degree of bone remineralization over a relatively short period of time constitutes an exceptionally good therapeutic response.

* * *

Maintaining adequate progesterone levels benefits your mood, your sleep, and your overall health. By following the program I've outlined here, you can maintain this balance for years to come by simply following the three easy steps I've described:

1. Stimulating progesterone production at the central nervous system level with 5-HTP, vitex, maca, and glandulars.
2. Promoting progesterone production in the ovaries with lutein, beta-carotene, flaxseed, and fish oil.
3. Using biochemically identical natural progesterone.

Next, we will take a look at testosterone deficiency. As a woman, you also make small amounts of male hormones, and like estrogen and progesterone, they play a crucial role in helping you maintain your overall health.

You'll learn why this male hormone plays a key role in female health. Plus, you'll be able to determine if you are in need of a testosterone boost, and how to get that boost with some little-known nutrients.

feminine benefits of testosterone   16

If you are like most women, you probably don't spend much time thinking about your testosterone levels. While testosterone is typically thought of as a "male hormone," it is just as critical to your health as the more feminine hormones estrogen and progesterone. You simply produce testosterone in much smaller amounts.

Like estrogen and progesterone, testosterone is also critical for your reproductive health. It also plays a key role in several other health functions, including heart and bone health, the strength of your tissues, and your mood. Let's take a closer look at this "male" hormone and how it benefits female health.

What is Testosterone?

Testosterone is the predominant male sex hormone, and is responsible for the development of male sexual characteristics. Women make small amounts of testosterone in the ovaries and adrenal glands via the precursor hormone androstenedione.

Similar to the female hormones, testosterone production is also stimulated through the hypothalamus. As I've indicated before, the hypothalamus is the master endocrine gland contained within your brain that regulates your production of all sex hormones. This gland produces a precursor hormone called gonadotropin releasing hormone (GnRH). When it is released, it travels to your anterior pituitary gland, where it stimulates the secretion of the follicle stimulating (FSH) and luteinizing hormones (LH). These hormones then travel to the adrenals and ovaries, where they stimulate the production of testosterone and androstenedione, as well as estrogen and progesterone.

Like estrogen and progesterone, the level of androstenedione varies throughout your menstrual cycle. The level rises at mid-cycle, when androstenedione is secreted from the ovarian follicle (the structure in your ovary containing a female reproductive cell), and during the second half of the menstrual cycle, when it is produced by the corpus luteum (the structure that develops within the ruptured ovarian follicle after ovulation or the release of the egg from the ovary).

Because LH controls the production of the androgens such as androstenedione and testosterone, low levels of LH often correlate to low levels of these androgens. In fact, research has shown that if you can increase your body's production of LH, you can better support your own production of testosterone.

I'll discuss how you can accomplish this in the next chapter. In the meantime, let's discuss how healthy levels of testosterone keep you healthy, active, and vital throughout your life.

Testosterone's Role in Your Body

Testosterone plays an important role in normal female sexual development. The initiation of menstruation and puberty is, in part, triggered by testosterone production. Additionally, testosterone stimulates libido. Levels of the hormone rise and decline during the menstrual cycle to insure that sexual desire increases just before ovulation, when a woman is fertile and chances are greatest for conception.

Testosterone also restores vitality and energy levels, helps reduce depression, balances mood and, in part, engenders attributes such as optimism, assertiveness, and aggressiveness that are usually associated with male behavior. Testosterone also benefits female health by helping to relieve menopausal symptoms such as hot flashes, nervousness, vaginal dryness, and the strength of vaginal tissues. It can also help to prevent osteoporosis.

How Testosterone Deficiency Occurs

You normally produce about 0.3 mg of testosterone per day. Total production is about one-tenth the amount produced by men. Production peaks around age 20, and by the time you reach age 40, it will have declined by about half. Additionally, older women exhibit a circadian variation in their androstenedione (and thus testosterone) levels, with the greatest concentration mid-morning and the least mid- to late-afternoon. This is due to adrenal activity, which affects (in part) testosterone production.

As is the case with all sex hormones, testosterone production from both the adrenal glands and the ovaries also decreases after menopause. Most circulating testosterone is bound to sex hormone–binding globulin (SHBG), with only a small percentage that is biologically active. Because estrogen increases the concentration of SHBG, natural fluctuations in estrogen levels, as well as estrogen replacement therapy, can further diminish available testosterone.

Interestingly, postmenopausal women seem to express the physical signs of their testosterone production more after menopause than before. For example, subtle signs of masculinization many occur after post-menopause, which can be distressing for many women. This can include hair growth on the chin and chest, thinning hair on the scalp, and more sparse pubic hair. The reason for this is that while testosterone production drops after menopause, estrogen levels drop even more drastically. Normally, your high levels of estrogen block this male pattern of hair growth (or loss) from occurring. However, after menopause, this unusual growth (or loss) of hair is stimulated by the action of the male hormones on the follicle.

Symptoms of Testosterone Deficiency

Even the small amount of testosterone that a woman produces can have a significant effect on her performance and influence her quality of life. If levels are below normal, you can experience a wide range of emotional symptoms, including decreased energy, depression, and anxiety. You'll also notice a few physical effects as well, such as loss of libido, osteoporosis, and insomnia.

Menopausal Symptoms

As you pass through menopause, you may experience a variety of symptoms initiated by the drop in hormone production that occurs at this time, including hot flashes, mood swings, and vaginal atrophy. While estrogen replacement therapy is successfully used to treat many of these symptoms, there is also a growing body of clinical and experimental research that indicates that testosterone may also be beneficial in reversing some of these symptoms, especially when combined with estrogen therapy.

Loss of Libido

Testosterone levels in women are associated with sexual drive. As I indicated above, your testosterone levels decline during menopause. About 30 to 50 percent of menopausal women experience a drop in libido soon after ceasing menstruation, because the ovaries stop making testosterone as well as estrogen. For others, the decline may be less rapid.

Many of my patients describe this decrease in desire as "something missing from their relationship with their sexual partner," or that their interest in sex just evaporated after menopause. This speaks to the first of four phases of sexual response—desire. The other three—excitement, orgasm, and resolution—are equally important, and can be equally problematic if testosterone levels are low.

In these cases, many women say that pain during sex due to vaginal dryness and atrophy significantly decreases arousal. This is often due to decreased blood flow to the vaginal tissues, changes in lubrication, and shrinkage of the vagina itself, due to atrophic changes in the tissue. If you experience difficulties with either desire or arousal, orgasm may not readily occur.

Fortunately, supplementing with testosterone can significantly increase all three phases. In fact, I've had a number of women patients who have been placed on testosterone therapy after a hysterectomy or for the treatment of certain gynecologic conditions. Many of these women found that their libido went into a higher gear. These women reported that they thought and fantasized about sex more often and requested more frequent sexual activity with their partner if they were currently in a relationship. In fact, several of my patients even told me that such intense sexual desire was a problem since their partners simply did not have the sexual stamina to keep up with their demands!

Depression and Anxiety

While estrogen therapy is often prescribed in postmenopausal women as a mood elevator, it is not the only hormone to produce this benefit. Low levels of testosterone also impact your emotional well-being.

Studies have shown that testosterone has beneficial effects on emotional well-being, perhaps just as striking as those noted with estrogen replacement therapy. Additionally, testosterone may be even more effective than certain anti-depressants in lifting mood and managing depression in menopausal women.

This can have a life-changing impact. If testosterone is able to elevate mood, you are far more likely to get up in the morning with a seize-the-day attitude and participate fully in and enjoy family, social, and business activities.

Osteoporosis

Scientists are now discovering that testosterone also plays a more important role in female bone health than was previously thought. The use of combined estrogen and testosterone therapy may be more effective at preventing osteoporosis than estrogen therapy alone. While estrogen slows down the rate of bone loss, testosterone helps promote formation of new bone. This can be of great benefit even for women in whom osteoporosis has already begun.

Arthritis

As you age, your testosterone production begins to decline. This can be bad news for your hips, knees, ankles, and wrists, as this hormone has a proven anti-inflammatory effect on the joints. In fact, according to a study from the *Annals of the New York Academy of Sciences*, people with rheumatoid arthritis have significantly decreased levels of testosterone (as well as pregnenolone and DHEA).

Even worse, as you enter mid-life, these declining hormone levels also thin the cartilage, tendons, and ligaments of your joints. As the muscles surrounding the joints try to help out your failing joints, they begin to clench and contract. This can lead to aches, pain, and stiffness throughout your entire body.

As the joints and surrounding muscles work overtime to compensate for this reduction in movement and ease, you begin to experience less flexibility and increased friction. This quickly sets the stage for increased wear and tear on your joints and the onset of arthritis.

Decreased Energy

Several studies have demonstrated that women taking just estrogen replacement have lower levels of energy than those who also use testosterone replacement. Additionally, women who engage in regular exercise have more energy because of it. This results in an increase in oxygen reaching the tissues and a greater production of beta-endorphins (natural mood elevators). Because higher testosterone levels can increase strength, such an increase in physical ability can mean that you find exercise easier to do and are more likely to spend time in energy-generating physical activity.

The Cosmetic Effects of Testosterone Imbalance

In the last two decades, I've had more and more women come to me for advice in treating adult acne. In addition to treatment options, many want to know why this teenage condition is plaguing them in their later years. The answer is simple. It's the same reason you broke out in your teens—hormones and stress.

The cause of acne can be found deep in your hair follicles. Each hair follicle has a sebaceous gland connected to it. This gland secretes sebum, an oil and wax mixture that keeps your skin moist and lubricated. During hormonal changes (such as puberty, menstruation, and perimenopause) and times of stress, you experience an increase in male hormones (androgen). This causes changes in the pH of the skin and overstimulates the sebaceous gland, which responds by secreting excess sebum. This in turn creates the skin lesions we call acne.

Acne can go through three stages. Blackheads are the first stage. They occur when sebum and oil block skin pores. Most of the oil in the pores is white, but the oil that is exposed to the air on the skin surface turns black. As the pore becomes clogged, bacteria multiplies and inflammation sets in, setting up stage two—whiteheads.

With this stage, the oil has no pore opening to the outside and drainage cannot occur. Cysts form underneath the skin and become infected. Your body responds to this by sending white blood cells to fight the infection. The result is a whitehead on the surface of the skin. If the cysts are too deep to be seen through the skin's layers, they can cause the third stage—cystic acne. These cysts are hard and deep and can be extremely painful to the touch.

In order to treat adult acne, I often recommend that women try a variety of approaches: diet, supplements, or topical treatments.

The first thing I recommend is to avoid refined sugar and foods high in sugar. Sugary foods over-stimulate the sebaceous glands and can trigger excess oil production. Refined sugar can also contribute to blood sugar imbalances, which can worsen symptoms of anxiety and stress, both of which can lead to breakouts.

Next, include vitamin A in your diet. It not only helps improve the overall health of your skin, it is especially helpful in suppressing oily skin and acne. In fact, one study found that high doses of vitamin A helped clear up even the most severe cases of acne in 90 percent of people treated with the vitamin. Since too much vitamin A can adversely affect liver function, I recommend that you take its water-soluble precursor—beta-carotene. **Dosages between 15,000 and 25,000 IU daily should provide you with adequate skin protection.**

If you do break out, I suggest treating the blemish with tea tree oil. Its antiseptic properties have been used for centuries to clean and treat wounds. Even the early settlers of Australia and metal workers during the Second World War used this camphorous-smelling essential oil to treat cuts and insect bites. After washing the infected area, place one drop of Australian tea tree oil directly on blemishes. Read the product label carefully to be sure the oil contains 50 to 60 percent terpenes (preferably terpin-4-ol) and no more than 15 percent cineole. You can find tea tree oil in Whole Food Markets and most health food stores. A $5 jar will most likely last longer than your acne!

Finally, I suggest using blue light to treat breakouts. It is well known that sunlight is beneficial in clearing up acne. By isolating only the blue portion of the visible light spectrum and eliminating the potentially more dangerous invisible bands of ultraviolet light, blue light devices help clear up acne without negative side effects, such as sun burns, skin aging, cataracts, or increased risk of skin cancer. (See more in this on page 311.)

I Have Hair Where?

Another common occurrence related to testosterone imbalance, particularly too much, is the growth of facial hair. While changes in hair structure and growth are common during menopause, the unusual growth of darker, coarser hair in areas where hair may never have been before (chin, upper lip, chest, or abdomen) is due to the stimulation of hair follicles by low amounts of androgens. High estrogen levels block the action of these male hormones on hair follicle receptors.

However, after menopause, the effect of these low amounts of androgens is unmasked as your production of estrogen decreases. The development of facial hair occurs when the enzyme 5-alpha reductase (which exists in the facial hair follicles) converts all of this biologically active testosterone to a locally active form called dihydrotestosterone (DHT). DHT directly stimulates the follicle to switch from producing its usual baby-fine peach fuzz hair to the thick, dark facial hair that's associated with postmenopausal facial hirsutism.

Standard Treatment Options

Postmenopausal facial hirsutism is temporary and lasts until your body adjusts to its new hormonal composition—typically three to 10 years. Some women can get by with occasional tweezing during that adjustment period. But others find that they can't tolerate the facial hair, no matter how temporary it is.

Therefore, many women resort to all sorts of bleaches and depilatory creams to lighten or remove facial hair. However, these methods contain harsh chemicals that can irritate delicate facial skin. Another popular hair removal option is waxing, which temporarily (and painfully) removes all facial hair, including peach fuzz. While there's nothing particularly harmful about waxing, a lot of my patients have found that they simply do not like how different their face looks without that baby-fine peach fuzz. Plus, waxing can also be irritating to the skin.

Some women turn to electrolysis and laser treatments, thinking they are permanent solutions—but unfortunately, they are not. Using an electrical charge or a pulsed laser beam, these methods damage—but don't destroy—hair follicles. Electrolysis treats one follicle at a time, which is impractical for women who have a lot of facial hair. Laser treatment zaps a dime-sized area, but the beam targets dark pigment on the hair shaft, so it can't be used on light-colored hair or dark skin. Plus, it's painful and can cause burns and permanent skin discoloration. Not to mention, it typically takes six or more sessions to obtain noticeable results. And according to David Larson, M.D., Professor and Chairman of Plastic and Reconstructive Surgery at the Medical College of Wisconsin, the hair usually grows back in about six months.

There is also a prescription cream available that helps reduce facial hair. It's called Vaniqa® (eflornithine hydrochloride), and it blocks the enzyme ornithine decarboxylase, which is involved in the synthesis of hair. However, the side effects—redness, stinging, burning, acne, or rash—make this option less than desirable.

Saving the Best for Last

While all the treatments I've mentioned so far are viable options, they are not the best options because they can be painful, irritating, and in most cases, temporary solutions. However, the following strategies are free of side effects and address the underlying problem so that the growth of facial hair actually stops.

Because hair grows in cycles, these treatments require about two to three months of use before you see results. In the interim, you can remove the worst of the hair by plucking or sugaring. Like waxing, sugaring removes hair at the root, but it doesn't damage the surrounding skin. And it's painless!

I am particularly fond of the MOOM brand of sugaring. MOOM has only four ingredients: sugar, chamomile, lemon, and tea tree oil. While the sugar works to remove the hair, the tea tree oil acts as a mild anesthetic, and the chamomile and lemon function as natural antiseptics. Plus, MOOM is resin-free, hypoallergenic, lasts up to two months, and costs about $25.00 for a six-ounce jar. For more information on MOOM, call 800-492-9464 or visit *www.imoom.com*.

There are also natural botanicals that, when used topically on the face, are known to inhibit 5-alpha reductase—the enzyme that activates testosterone in facial follicles. These substances have significant efficacy, especially when they're used together.

- **Green tea extract** (epigallocatechin gallate, or EGCG), a phytochemical from the green tea plant, inhibits 5-alpha reductase, and also has been shown to reduce skin inflammation in women suffering from rosacea.

- **NDGA** (nordihyroguaiaretic acid), an extract of chaparral, blocks receptor sites for 5-alpha reductase and also inhibits the skin's pro-inflammatory cascade.

- **Zinc, azelaic acid, and vitamin B$_6$:** Even at low doses, zinc and azelaic acid (from the yeast *Pityrosporum ovale*) are potent 5-alpha reductase inhibitors because they work synergistically. Vitamin B$_6$ enhances their activity and their ability to penetrate the skin. In a French study, when very low doses of these agents were applied together, their combined activity blocked 5-alpha reductase by an amazing 90 percent.

Luckily, I have found a product called "Acne Recover Repair Lotion Pod B" that contains all five of these nutrients. It was developed by Dr. Randall Wilkinson, M.D. If you'd like to order it, call the company at 800-539-5195 so they can adjust the packaging to exclude the rest of their acne treatment system.

TOO MUCH TESTOSTERONE?

Like sunshine, which can burn if you get too much, testosterone must also be used carefully. While too little can cause or exacerbate a whole host of health conditions, excess levels can lead to masculinization, including deepening of the voice, abnormal hair growth, acne, and even hair loss. (See page 184 for treatment solutions.)

The areas that tend to be the most affected by excess hair growth are in those areas that have the greatest concentrations of androgens such as testosterone. These include the chin, upper lip, cheeks, just below the navel, and around the nipple. For similar reasons, women at the opposite end of the spectrum (hair loss) will notice the greatest decrease in hair on the top of their head, at the crown, or at the temples.

If you are exhibiting any of these symptoms, work with your doctor to evaluate your hormones, including your testosterone levels.

Are You Testosterone Deficient?

The following checklist will give you an idea of whether you are experiencing the effects of inadequate testosterone production. If you answer yes to three or more of these questions, you very likely need to increase your testosterone levels.

- ✓ I am over the age of fifty.
- ✓ I experience menopausal symptoms such as hot flashes, mood swings, and vaginal dryness.
- ✓ I lack interest in sex.
- ✓ I have a tendency toward depression.
- ✓ I often feel withdrawn.
- ✓ I have experienced a decline in the frequency of my sexual activity and orgasms.
- ✓ I suffer from persistent fatigue.
- ✓ I have osteoporosis and suffer from frequent bone fractures.
- ✓ I have rheumatoid arthritis.
- ✓ I lack stamina.
- ✓ I have experienced a decline in my level of assertiveness.
- ✓ I typically have little desire to take risks.
- ✓ I have poor muscle tone or weak muscles.

If your responses suggest that your testosterone level is low, you may want to get your hormone levels tested.

Testing for Testosterone Deficiency

Total testosterone production is somewhat difficult to assess, as the amount varies during the day, with higher levels occurring in the morning. Additionally, there are seasonal variations. Furthermore, a normal testosterone reading may mask a testosterone deficiency because the majority of testosterone in the bloodstream is bound to the protein SHBG and the protein carrier albumin.

Only about four percent of testosterone in the bloodstream is free and unbound and available to body tissues, where it can perform its functions. As you age, an increasing amount of testosterone remains bound, so in an older person, a normal reading of circulating testosterone does not necessarily indicate that adequate amounts of testosterone are bioavailable. Routine laboratory testing measures total hormone concentration, so special assays are required to measure the amount of active free testosterone.

When it comes to measuring testosterone, I highly recommend saliva testing, since the testosterone in the saliva is the type that is unbound. Best of all, saliva hormone testing is accessible. Even physicians who still don't routinely order saliva hormone testing will usually write an order when a patient requests it. You can even order a limited saliva hormone test kit on your own directly from a laboratory, without a doctor's order.

Get Tested

If you think saliva hormone testing is right for you, consider consulting your physician. Having your doctor order the test has two advantages: The profile is more extensive, and your insurance may cover the cost. Several laboratories perform the test; in the event your physician does not have a preference, I recommend Genova Diagnostics (formerly Great Smokies Diagnostic Laboratory) at *www.gdx.net* or 800-522-4762, as well as ZRT Laboratory (*www.zrtlab.com* or 866-600-1636). If your doctor doesn't order the test, or you simply want insight to help you develop your own self-care regimen, you can order a test kit from several sources. Aeron Laboratories has a wonderful Life Cycles saliva test kit (*www.aeron.com* or 800-631-7900).

When testing testosterone levels, you'll need to submit 2–5 ml of saliva. Samples remain viable for up to seven days, but must be analyzed within that time. A person submitting a saliva sample must note the time of day it was taken, as hourly levels vary. Also, if you are already using testosterone cream that you apply to the skin, you will likely have a very high reading.

Ranges of Testosterone Levels:

Blood: 20 to 80 ng/dL*
Saliva: 20 to 50 pg/mL**

If your results indicate that you are deficient in testosterone (or if you scored high on the questionnaire), there is a solution. Let's take a look at the many ways you can restore your testosterone levels safely and effectively, and start feeling better than ever!

---

* figures from MedlinePlus (a service of the US National Library of Medicine and the National Institutes of Health)
** figures from womenshealth.com

restoring testosterone 17

Over the years, I've had countless women of all ages come to me seeking ways to increase their sex drive, especially prior to the onset of menopause. Even after the onset, many women have told me that their interest in sex just seemed to "evaporate." As you now know from the preceding chapter, low sex drive—along with low energy and vitality, and even osteoporosis—are linked to a deficiency in testosterone.

In this chapter, I'll share with you my amazing program to help you restore your testosterone levels. We'll discuss how you can restore this critical hormone at the central nervous system level, with the help of some key neurotransmitters, as well as a few little-known herbs. You'll also discover the role your ovaries and adrenals play in testosterone production, and how you can slow the breakdown of testosterone in the liver.

Next, we'll explore the nutrients that serve as hormone mimics that greatly help restore functions such as libido, that testosterone normally supports. These include yang herbs and nutrients that help promote nitric oxide production. Finally, you'll learn how supplemental, natural, biochemically identical testosterone can help to restore low levels of this vital hormone.

Let's get started!

Restore Your Own Hormones

As with all hormones, testosterone production begins in the brain. However, it's not as simple as it may seem. We've been traditionally taught that human beings have one brain that is divided into many different parts. But more and more research is putting the "one brain" idea to the test. In fact, it's starting to be widely accepted that the human skull actually houses not one brain, but three—the reptilian brain, the limbic brain, and the neocortical brain.

The reptilian brain is the oldest part of the brain. It controls basic bodily functions like heart rate, breathing, body temperature, hunger, and fight-or-flight responses. Basic drives and instincts, such as defending territory and keeping safe from harm, are other functions of the reptilian brain. The structures in the brain that perform these functions are the brain stem (which controls breathing, heart rate, and blood pressure) and the cerebellum (which controls movement, balance, and posture).

The limbic, or mammalian, brain developed once mammals started roaming the earth. It includes the hippocampus, which controls memories and learning; the amygdala, which controls memory and emotions; and the hypothalamus, which controls emotions (among many other things). Therefore, the limbic brain allows mammals to learn, retain memories, and show emotions.

The neocortical brain, or neocortex, is the complex maze of grey matter that surrounds the reptilian and limbic brains, and accounts for about 85 percent of brain mass. It is found in the brains of primates and humans, and is responsible for sensory perception, abstract thought, imagination, and consciousness. It also controls language, social interactions, and higher communication.

The Chemistry of the Brain

Like the three parts of the brain, there are also three key types of brain chemicals: neuropeptides, neurohormones, and neurotransmitters.

Neuropeptides are responsible for the cell-to-cell communication system in your body. A peptide is a short chain of amino acids connected together, and a neuropeptide is a peptide found in neural tissue. Neuropeptides are widespread in the central and peripheral nervous systems and different neuropeptides have different excitatory or inhibitory actions.

Neuropeptides control such a diverse array of functions in the body. When they work together properly, the wonderful results in your body include elevated mood and other positive behaviors and emotions, stronger bones, better resistance to disease, glowing skin, and boosted metabolism. Conversely, if your neuropeptides function abnormally, the result can be an increased tendency towards neurological and mental disorders such as Alzheimer's disease, epilepsy, and schizophrenia.

There are several types of neuropeptides. Some of the most common include endorphins and beta-endorphins. Endorphins are opiod peptides, meaning they have morphine-like effects within the body. They produce feelings of well-being and euphoria, and a rush of endorphins can lead to feelings of exhilaration brought on by pain, danger, or stress. Endorphins also may also play a role in memory, sexual activity, and body temperature. Beta-endorphins are another form of opiod peptides, but they are stronger than endorphins. They are composed of 31 amino acids and work in the body by numbing pain, increasing relaxation, and promoting a general feeling of well-being.

While there are many, many hormones and hormonal interactions that occur in the brain and body, the most widely known neurohormone is melatonin. (I discussed melatonin in more detail on page 125.)

Neurotransmitters are naturally occurring chemicals that relay electrical messages between nerve cells throughout your body. While all three types of neurochemicals are important for hormone and overall health, neurotransmitters are particularly important for the production of sex hormones.

In the aggregate, all three types of neurochemicals help to regulate the brain's endocrine glands, specifically the hypothalamus and pituitary gland. Your brain's hypothalamus regulates the production of all sex hormones. Specifically, the hypothalamus produces a precursor hormone called gonadotropin releasing hormone (GnRH). When it is released, it travels to your anterior pituitary gland, where it stimulates the secretion of the follicle stimulating (FSH) and luteinizing hormones (LH). These hormones then travel to your adrenals and ovaries, where they stimulate the production of androgens (male hormones), especially androstenedione and testosterone (as well as estrogen and progesterone).

The neurotransmitters norepinephrine, epinephrine, dopamine, and serotonin regulate the hypothalamus' release of GnRH. Without proper production and balance of these neurotransmitters, you cannot have proper balance of the sex hormones, including testosterone.

This is critical, as the inhibitory neurotransmitters (those in the serotonin pathway) help with insomnia and anxiety. On the reverse side, the excitatory neurotransmitters—namely dopamine, norephinephrine, and epinephrine— have powerful antidepressant effects. They also support arousal, alertness, optimism, zest for life, and sex drive.

The amino acids phenylalanine and tyrosine are precursors for these excitatory neurotransmitters. Phenylalanine is an essential amino acid that must be taken in through the diet, while tyrosine is produced from phenylalanine. Without proper levels of these nutrients, your dopamine, norephinephrine, and epinephrine levels will most likely be decreased. This can lead to low libido, depression, and other conditions also associated with low testosterone levels.

To ensure you have adequate levels of these vital amino acids, I recommend that you take either 500–1,000 mg of tyrosine per day or 500 mg phenylalanine once or twice a day. (Phenylalanine is a precursor of tyrosine.) In addition to taking it in supplement form, you can increase your levels of phenylalanine by consuming soybeans, fish, meat, poultry, almonds, pecans, pumpkin and sesame seeds, lima beans, chickpeas, and lentils.

Be sure to take tyrosine in divided doses, half in the morning and half in the afternoon. Do not take in the evening, as it may interfere with sleep. Also, I generally don't recommend going over 1,000 mg a day of tyrosine. Do not take tyrosine in conjunction with MAO inhibitors, and taper off if you start having headaches. Be sure to take phenylalanine and tyrosine with 25–100 mg of vitamin B_6 and a small amount of protein.

Note: I strongly advise that you undertake a program to restore and properly balance your neurotransmitter levels under the care of a complementary physician, naturopath, or nutritionist. You should also have your neurotransmitter levels tested regularly, as dosage needs vary from woman to woman.

THE TESTOSTERONE-ESTROGEN HYBRID

While this may seem like the title of a bad B-movie, it is actually a pretty accurate description of polycystic ovarian syndrome (PCOS). If you suffer from PCOS, you can attest that it is a very frustrating and difficult condition. On one hand, you suffer with the effects of too much testosterone, including acne and increased growth of hair on the face, abdomen, upper thighs, chest, and back. Plus, you must contend with excess estrogen issues, such as infertility and menstrual irregularities. As if that wasn't bad enough, PCOS is also linked to insulin resistance, which can cause many sufferers to become severely overweight, and puts them at risk for developing diabetes.

Part of the difficulty of working with PCOS is that it has multiple underlying causes, namely a number of different hormonal imbalances. Specifically, the production of the pituitary's luteinizing hormone (LH) is significantly elevated in women with PCOS, while the production of the pituitary's follicle-stimulating hormone (FSH) is normal or slightly diminished. The imbalances in these hormones upset the normal production of estrogen, progesterone, and testosterone by the ovaries and adrenal glands, disrupting the healthy balance between all three of these sex hormones. Moreover, 50 percent of the women with PCOS have elevated levels of prolactin and decreased levels of dopamine.

Fortunately, by following the nutrient and lifestyle recommendations laid out in this book, most women with PCOS can find relief quickly and effectively.

The Mighty Mucuna Bean

Like phenylalanine and tyrosine, the tiny mucuna bean has also been shown to increase your libido and restore your sex drive. This power-packed legume can be traced as far back as Medieval times, and was first described in the English literature in 1804. While every part of the plant is full of medicinal promise, the greatest benefits come from the seeds and root.

The key to mucuna's reputation lies in its rich store of L-dopa, one of the few natural sources of the precursor to dopamine—your brain's neurotransmitter responsible for energy, alertness, and libido.

As I indicated above, dopamine is normally made from the amino acids phenylalanine and tyrosine. Up until age 45, levels of dopamine remain fairly stable in your body. However, after 45, levels decrease by about 13 percent every 10 years.

The aphrodisiac qualities of mucuna have been known for centuries. In fact, it is one of two primary treatments for low libido in India. An animal study from the journal *Fitoterapia* confirmed this benefit. Researchers found that the mucuna bean can produce "striking improvement in normal mating behavior, potency, and libido and substantiates its use as a sexual function improver."

replacement therapy (HRT) and even phytoestrogens, all of which work to mimic your body's hormones, maca helps your body produce its own unique balance of hormones. It does this by encouraging your ovaries and adrenals to produce the hormones you need, in the levels you need them, apparently more toward the progesterone and testosterone side of the equation.

This was shown in a study from the *Journal of Veterinary Medical Science*. Researchers tested the effects of maca on mouse sex hormones. They found that while progesterone and testosterone levels increased significantly in those mice that received the maca, their estradiol levels were not increased. In other words, the maca helped to raise the levels of progesterone and testosterone to offset the blood levels of estradiol.

If you are interesting in trying maca, a traditional dosage is 2–10 grams; however, dosages are unique to each woman, so you will need to determine which dosage works for you. There have been no acute toxic effects of maca, even at very high doses. In fact, many Peruvians eat it every day! I am particularly fond of Whole World Botanicals' Royal Maca (*www.wholeworldbotanicals.com* or 888-757-6026).

Note: If you are naturally sensitive or allergic to herbs, you may want to avoid maca altogether, or at least use it cautiously. In any event, I suggest starting with the low end of the recommended dosage, as *too* much can cause increased hot flashes, breast tenderness, or headache. It is also recommended that you avoid maca if you have a hormone-related cancer (due to lack of formal studies), liver disease, if you are pregnant or nursing, or if you are currently taking conventional HRT.

SPICE UP YOUR SEX LIFE

Researchers have shown that certain scents have particularly strong aphrodisiac-like qualities, especially cinnamon, cloves, ginger, and nutmeg. In addition to using these spices when cooking, place potpourri or essential oils that include these scents in your bedroom, bathroom, or wherever tickles your fancy.

Keep in mind that these herbs support the yang in Chinese medicine. They are heating and drying. Therefore, if you are having hot flashes, vaginal dryness, etc., you should not use these herbs. Conversely, if you are bloated, carry excess weight, and need to "contract," then these spices are just what the doctor ordered.

- **Cinnamon**—When the Crusaders returned to Western Europe from the Far East, they brought a reputed sexual stimulant with them—cinnamon. Today, this spice is one of the most common herbs across the globe.
- **Cloves**—The Persians, Egyptians, Europeans, and Arabians all considered this spicy scent to be an aromatic aphrodisiac. In the Sudan, women concoct a wedding potion that consists of clove mixed with musk, cherry, and sandalwood. They then wear the blend to the party so its aroma will drift in the air as they dance the night away.

continued

- **Ginger**—The ancient Persian physician Avicenna used to mix this fragrant spice with honey as a cure for impotence. Whether its benefits are due to its pungent aroma or its ability to increase circulation, ginger soon grew to be known as the spice of "burning desire." Today, women in Senegal wear ginger in their belts in order to attract men, while female New Guineans can't say no to a man who emits ginger's strong scent.
- **Nutmeg**—While this spice has a strong smell, it is actually a relaxing scent that relieves anxiety and stress, and even reduces blood pressure. The Chinese are particularly fond of nutmeg's aphrodisiac qualities. They have found that it can elicit a feeling of rapture and invigoration. In North America in the 1700's, men and women often added nutmeg to their nightcaps. Maybe our ancestors were onto something!

Great Glandulars

Glandular therapy is also helpful in boosting testosterone levels. The success of glandular therapy lies in their ability to help restore hormone function by supporting the health of your endocrine glands themselves.

Glandulars are often comprised of purified extracts from the secretory endocrine glands of animals. Most commonly, extracts are drawn from the thyroid and adrenal glands, as well as the thymus, pituitary, pancreas, and ovaries. Most extracts come from cows, with the exception of pancreatic glandular preparations usually drawn from sheep.

In the past, experts believed that glandulars could not be effective because the intestinal lining of a healthy person was impenetrable, and that proteins and large peptides could not breach its barrier. However, recent evidence has shown that large macromolecules can and do pass completely intact from the intestinal tract into the bloodstream. In fact, there's further evidence to suggest that your body is able to determine which molecules it needs to absorb whole, and which can be broken down.

Both animal and human studies alike have proven this theory. In some cases, several whole proteins taken orally, including critical enzymes, have been shown to be absorbed intact into the bloodstream. Additionally, many smaller proteins and numerous hormones have also been found to be absorbed intact into the bloodstream, including thyroid, cortisone, and even insulin. In essence, it means that the active properties of the glandulars stay active and intact, and are not destroyed in the digestive process.

There are multi- and single-glandular systems available from companies like Standard Process—a leader in the field. However, they do require a prescription from a health care practitioner. Other good products are also available in health food stores and should be used as part of a nutritional program to support healthy menstruation.

Examples of widely used and accepted glandulars involve the thyroid and the adrenals. Natural thyroid medications such as Armour Thyroid, Naturthyroid, and Bio-Thyroid have been the preference of complementary physicians for decades. Unlike many of the commonly prescribed brands of thyroid therapy that only replace a synthetic form of T4, these natural thyroid replacements contains the whole animal-derived thyroid gland, including T3 *and* T4. This is a significant difference. T3 is more physiologically active than T4, and is critical in regulating normal growth and energy metabolism. Without the use of glandulars, this type of natural thyroid replacement wouldn't be possible. However, the thyroid glandulars sold in the health food stores have the hormone removed and are used to support the function of your own gland.

Adrenal glandular preparations are even more common. With the stress epidemic in this country, the majority of Americans are walking around with depressed adrenal function. This can also manifest as fatigue, susceptibility to infection, allergies, and infection.

Fortunately, whole adrenal extracts have been found to help restore the health and function of comprised adrenal glands. They have also been shown to possess cortisone-like properties that help treat asthma, eczema, rheumatoid arthritis, and even psoriasis.

To help support healthy testosterone levels, I suggest taking a good multi-glandular or single glandular product from a company like Standard Process. These could include glandulars such as hypothalamus, pituitary, ovary, adrenal, and thyroid, depending on the specific needs of each individual woman. I also highly recommend that you consider taking a whole brain glandular, if appropriate. To further support your adrenal function, I recommend taking 1,000–3,000 mg of a mineral-buffered vitamin C each day with a meal, 25–100 mg of a vitamin B complex a day, and an additional 250 mg of B$_5$ (pantothenic acid) twice a day.

Testosterone Production in the Ovaries and Adrenals

In addition to stimulating testosterone production at the central nervous system level, you can also increase this vital hormone in your ovaries and adrenals with the help of certain important nutrients. I've found that DHEA, boron, and ginseng are critical for increasing testosterone production in your endocrine glands.

Multi-Faceted DHEA

DHEA is the precursor hormone to the major sex hormones testosterone and estrogen (but not progesterone). It is produced mainly by the adrenal glands, with smaller amounts also produced by the brain, skin, and ovaries. Once DHEA is produced by the adrenals, it travels through your bloodstream to cells throughout your body, where it's converted into testosterone, and then estrogen (in the form of estrone) in your adrenals and, subsequently, your ovaries and fatty tissues. Therefore, by increasing your DHEA levels, you can increase your body's production of testosterone.

If you choose to use DHEA, start with the lowest possible dosage. It is better absorbed when taken with food and it's best to take it in the morning, because it can have a stimulating effect. Begin with a daily dosage of 5–15 mg in capsule form and monitor the effect. You can increase the dose by 5–10 mg each day, but do not exceed 25 mg daily.

Note: Before taking DHEA, have your hormone levels tested and consult an informed health care professional who can monitor your response to the hormone. Not all women are good candidates for DHEA therapy, as some may experience such side effects as anxiety and nervousness. Additionally, women should have a mammogram and Pap smear test done before beginning DHEA supplementation to avoid the risk of stimulating a preexisting cancer of the reproductive tract, as DHEA will increase the levels of the major sex hormones.

JENNIFER'S STORY

When "Jennifer" came to see me, her most distressing complaint was her lack of libido and difficulty enjoying sex with her husband. She had gone through menopause at age 49, and now, one year later, she complained that her sex drive had not only evaporated, but intercourse was painful because her vaginal tissues would tear a bit during penetration.

Besides a powerful libido-enhancing nutritional program of DHEA, PABA, arginine, and other important nutrients, Jennifer began using bioidentical estrogen and progesterone, as well as testosterone creams to build up her tissues. Within no time, sex became much more pleasurable once again.

Beneficial Boron

While the trace mineral boron is most commonly associated with increasing estrogen levels, it has been found to increase testosterone as well. This may be one reason it is so beneficial in the fight against osteoporosis.

According to a study published in *Nutrition Today*, boron reduced urinary excretion of calcium by 44 percent and significantly reduced excretion of magnesium as well. It also found that it increased levels of both testosterone and beta-estradiol.

To help boost testosterone levels and prevent osteoporosis, I suggest taking 3 mg of boron a day.

Glorious Ginseng

The herb ginseng has an almost legendary reputation for treating nearly every ailment known to man. In the 1950's, scientists began to test these claims and found that when high quantities of standardized extracts were administered, ginseng could be a very beneficial tonic and therapy. As an adaptogen, it has been shown to improve testosterone levels, and help maintain normal biological functions such as stamina and immunity.

The most widely used and studied type of ginseng is panax ginseng, which is either of Chinese, American, or Korean origin. When processed in its mature form, after at least six or eight years of growth, panax ginseng should contain 13 or more hormone-like compounds called ginsenosides. Clinical studies have shown that panax ginseng minimizes the harmful effects of stress on the body, protects against damage caused by radiation, and improves liver function.

Besides these actions, ginseng also has an effect on reproductive function. Traditionally, panax ginseng was taken to enhance virility and fertility. Human studies assessing this function have yielded mixed results, but animal studies, such as one published in the *American Journal of Chinese Medicine*, have demonstrated ginseng's ability to increase sexual and mating activity. Another study from the *Archives of Andrology* found that a five percent preparation of ginseng resulted in a significant increase in blood testosterone levels. Based on its traditional use and these modern studies, ginseng appears to be a suitable treatment to improve sexual function.

If you are interested in trying ginseng, I suggest taking 4–6 grams of a high-quality panax ginseng root per day. Ginseng and extracts of ginseng vary greatly in type and quality. The most valued are wild roots that are old and well formed, which have a high proportion of active substances. The lowest grade comes from the smaller roots of cultivated plants. They may contain various parts of the plant as well as additives. For this reason, **it is important to use a standardized preparation that has guaranteed amounts of certain of the active ingredients.** The dosage is then based on the potency of the ginseng preparation being administered. As with many therapies, it is best to start with a small dosage and increase gradually. One regimen recommends taking ginseng on a repeating schedule, with two to three weeks of ginseng followed by two weeks with no treatment. Women do best on American or Chinese ginseng, as they are better suited for the female body.

Note: Side effects of ginseng include nervousness, hypertension, morning diarrhea, skin problems, insomnia, and euphoria. That's why it's important that you monitor yourself for these symptoms. Additionally, it's best to avoid red Korean ginseng, which is too heating and drying for most menopausal women.

Slow Down the Breakdown

In the same way you want to maintain your levels of circulating estrogen during menopause, you also want to preserve testosterone. One of the best ways to do this is by preventing the breakdown of the hormone in the liver.

The fat-soluble B vitamin PABA (para-aminobenzoic acid) is a critical part of this plan. Studies indicate that PABA helps to safely and effectively slow down the breakdown of sex hormones, including testosterone, in the liver. Research has shown that higher levels of PABA are associated with better mood and outlook, better vaginal lubrication, and improved sex drive—all of which are also indicative of higher testosterone levels. In fact, PABA is the only vitamin that has been shown to increase libido!

To restore libido and help impede the breakdown of testosterone, I recommend taking 400–500 mg of PABA a day.

Support the Effects of Testosterone with Hormone Mimics

In addition to increasing testosterone production and slowing down the breakdown of the hormone, you can also use nutrients that help boost libido and sexual responsiveness. Two highly effective ways to accomplish this is to use yang herbs or certain nutrients that promote the production of nitric oxide.

Key Herbs Support Testosterone

Herbs have long been the province of traditional and folk medicine, but many Western doctors are just now paying attention to their many uses. In recent years, several major universities such as UCLA and Columbia have hosted conferences on how to incorporate both European and Chinese herbs into standard treatment protocols.

In my practice, I've used herbs to help improve a wide variety of hormone-related complaints. When it comes to using herbs to restore libido and sex drive (which are testosterone-supported health benefits), I've found that damiana, *Rhodiola rosea*, Siberian ginseng, and *gingko biloba* are the most effective. These herbs also contain a wide variety of chemicals that help you increase vitality and stamina, generate assertiveness, gain energy, boost libido and sexual responsiveness, ease anxiety, and even generate feelings of optimism.

Dynamic Damiana

Damiana is a yellow, flowering bush indigenous to hot and humid climates such as Central America, Mexico, and the southwestern U.S. It has a long history as an aphrodisiac for women, dating all the way back to the Mayan civilization. Women typically use the leaves to make a libido-lifting elixir to drink before intercourse.

In recent times, damiana has been used to increase sex drive and treat impotence. While no clinical trials have been performed on this herb, animal studies have shown that it does increase sexual desire and frequency of sex. Additionally, most herbalists agree that the alkaloids found in damiana are responsible for this mild, testosterone-like effect on the body.

The recommended dosage is 100–200 mg of damiana per day. To date, there are no known negative interactions or side effects associated with the herb.

Remarkable Rhodiola Rosea

Rhodiola rosea is a popular plant indigenous to Eastern Europe and Asia. The ancient Greeks used the herb medicinally as far back as 100 A.D. Named for the rose-like odor of the rootstock when newly cut, *Rhodiola rosea* has been used for centuries in China to prolong life and enhance wisdom. Siberian healers believe that people who drink *Rhodiola* tea on a regular basis will live to be more than 100 years old. And in the former Soviet Union, *Rhodiola* has been used to diminish fatigue and increase your body's resistance to stress.

Rhodiola works to support testosterone (and other hormone production) by easing stress and fatigue—both killers of healthy hormone production. According to the journal *Phytomedicine*, *Rhodiola* is particularly effective in fighting stress-induced fatigue. In one study, researchers tested 40 male medical students during exam time to determine if the herb positively affected physical fitness, as well as mental well-being and capacity. The students were divided into two groups and given either 50 mg of *Rhodiola rosea* extract or a placebo twice a day for 20 days. Researchers found that those students who took the extract had a significant decrease in mental fatigue and increase of psychomotor function, with a 50 percent improvement in neuromotor function. Plus, scores from exams taken immediately after the study showed that the extract group had an average grade of 3.47, as compared to 3.20 for the placebo group.

To ease fatigue, stress, or anxiety—all of which can play havoc with your testosterone production—and boost your energy and stamina (which testosterone supports), I recommend taking 50–100 mg of *Rhodiola rosea* three times a day, standardized to 3 percent rosavins and 0.8 percent salidrosides. While the herb is generally considered safe, some reports have indicated that it may counteract the effects of antiarrhythmic medications. Therefore, if you are currently taking this type of medication, I suggest you discuss the use of *Rhodiola rosea* with your physician.

Regain Your Sex Drive With Ginkgo

The *Ginkgo biloba* tree originated about 250 million years ago, and a single tree can live as long as 1,000 years. It is often planted in urban settings, lining fashionable streets and decorating parks, as it resists disease, insects, and pollution.

Modern science is finding that this ancient plant has a wide range of benefits, including improving blood flow, preventing the brain from aging, and improving all four stages of sexual response—desire, excitement (lubrication), orgasm, and resolution. It has even been shown to reverse sexual dysfunction in women taking certain antidepressants.

When it comes to helping improve blood flow, there is no debate as to ginkgo's benefits. Three hundred published scientific papers and 40 double-blind studies have proven its efficacy. This is due, in large part, to the rich store of antioxidant bioflavonoids found in ginkgo. This also allows this amazing herb to help improve circulation and fight inflammation in just about every organ system in the body, as well as scavenge free radicals.

As for your brain health, ginkgo increases blood flow and energy production, as well as improves production of neurotransmitters, chemicals that help transmit nerve signals. Plus, ginkgo protects brain and nerve cells from deteriorating by stabilizing cell walls and scavenging free radicals that can destroy delicate cell structures. It also helps maintain the brain's supply of energy in the form of glucose and oxygen. This is beneficial, as it supports healthy neurotransmitter- and brain-based hormone production.

I suggest taking 30 mg of *Ginkgo biloba* extract (standardized to 24 percent flavonoid glycosides and 6 percent terpene lactones) three times a day. Ginkgo is extremely safe and side effects are uncommon.

Promote Nitric Oxide Production

Another way to further support the effects of testosterone in your body and promote healthy sexual functioning is to promote the production of nitric oxide. Nitric oxide is a gaseous molecule produced in the body from the amino acid arginine. As a potent vasodilator, nitric oxide enhances the flow of blood through the arteries and veins to all the tissues and cells of your body. It not only improves the health and functional capability of your heart, but also helps to support the health of your respiratory, neuroendocrine, immune, reproductive, and other systems because of its beneficial effect on circulation.

Impaired circulation due to diminished nitric oxide production can also lead to diminished physical and mental energy and immune-system function, diminished sexual responsiveness, poor or slow recovery from exertion and injury, and impaired wound healing. Furthermore, levels of nitric oxide tend to decrease with age. In fact, high nitric oxide producers typically have healthy skin and hair and well-developed muscles. In contrast, elderly individuals (and even younger individuals with diminished nitric oxide production) often have thinner hair and paler, thinner skin. Nitric oxide is particularly important for healthy sexual function and responsiveness.

In my experience, there are five key nutrients that promote nitric oxide production: arginine, citrulline, ginseng, alpha lipoic acid, and vitamin C.

Amazing Arginine

L-arginine—an amino acid found primarily in protein sources such as red meat, dairy products, eggs, poultry, and fish—is used within your body to produce nitric oxide. As a result, it helps to promote blood flow and vascular relaxation, and works to make tissues firmer and more elastic. In fact, research studies have shown that intravenous administration of arginine can increase nitric oxide production. Additionally, a nutraceutical research and development company has been able to orally administer small amounts of arginine combined with other nutrients, allowing the body to increase its production of nitric oxide.

The L-arginine/nitric oxide pathway has been shown to be responsible for sexual arousal and heart protection. While most of the research surrounding L-arginine and sex drive has been focused on men, there have been a few intriguing studies involving women.

In one randomized, double-blind, placebo-controlled, three-way crossover clinical trial, 23 women with documented Female Sexual Arousal Disorder (FSAD) were given L-arginine (as well as a few other nutrients) for six months. The women were shown a non-sexual movie, as well as a sexual film. The degree of each woman's sexual reaction was documented by changes in vaginal pulse amplitude. The women also filled out a self-report questionnaire. Researchers found that women taking the L-arginine had a significant and rapid increase in vaginal pulse amplitude response after watching the sexually charged film.

In a separate study presented at the Ninth Annual Congress on Women's Health & Gender-Based Medicine, researchers determined that L-arginine increased sexual desire and satisfaction. This double-blind, placebo-controlled study looked at 93 women between the ages of 22 and 73, all of whom reported a lack of sexual desire. Half of the group was given L-arginine daily, while the other half received a placebo. After four weeks, 64 percent of the women taking L-arginine reported improved satisfaction with their sex life, and 64 percent reported greater sexual desire.

I can also speak to the positive effects L-arginine has on sex drive that I've seen in my own practice. In one case, a 38-year old woman began taking this amino acid to help regulate her periods. On a subsequent appointment, she told me that her libido was stronger since she started taking the supplement. Another patient taking L-arginine described an increased intensity during sex, a sensation she attributed to the nutrient.

Not only does it improve the health and functional capability of the heart and boost libido, but arginine also helps to support the health of the respiratory, neuroendocrine, immune, reproductive, and other systems because of its beneficial effect on circulation.

If you would like to try L-arginine, I recommend taking 1,000 mg in capsule form once or twice a day, in combination with 250 mg of B5 and 250 to 350 mg of choline once a day to promote better blood flow to your organs and tissue. L-arginine is readily available in most health food stores.

Note: Women taking lysine for a serious herpes infection should avoid supplemental use of L-arginine, as it may counteract any potential benefits of the lysine. Additionally, women with diabetes may want to check with their physicians before using L-arginine, as it may interfere with insulin and carbohydrate metabolism.

Spectacular Citrulline

Another amino acid—citrulline—also increases nitric oxide production, thus relaxing blood vessels and improving blood flow. Latin for watermelon (from which the nutrient was first discovered), citrulline is needed by your liver to detoxify ammonia.

In fact, citrulline is produced from a combination of ammonia and carbon dioxide. The byproduct (ornithine) is then combined with aspartic acid, and later metabolized into arginine.

Beyond its nitric oxide-producing effects, citrulline also increases energy and boosts your immune system. **To receive all of these benefits, I suggest taking 500–1,000 mg of citrulline a day.**

Other Key Nutrients

While they play a much lesser role, the antioxidants alpha lipoic acid and vitamin C help to fight free radical damage that may occur with increased nitric oxide production.

Alpha lipoic acid (ALA) is a universal antioxidant, working in both water- and fat-soluble parts of your cells. It recycles other antioxidants in your body and scavenges more types of free radicals than any other known antioxidant.

Similarly, vitamin C is an important antioxidant. It not only helps prevent the oxidation of "bad" low-density lipoprotein (LDL) cholesterol and increases "good" high-density lipoprotein (HDL), it also helps maintain vitamin E levels and helps absorb iron. Plus, vitamin C has an antihistamine effect, meaning that it may shorten the length and severity of infections, including colds. Vitamin C is also plays an important role in the production of glutathione, a powerful substance that helps to increase nitric oxide production.

Most importantly, ALA and vitamin C work synergistically to protect you from free radical damage. One study in particular from the *International Journal of Cosmetic Science* looked at the effects ALA and other antioxidants had on women with sun damage. They gave the women either a supplement that contained 5 mg of ALA, 10 mg of vitamin E, 90 mg of vitamin C, and 6 mg of lutein, or a placebo. After two months, the women who took the antioxidant-rich supplement had lower levels of free radicals in their blood, as well as better skin hydration than women who took the placebo.

To receive the full benefits of these outstanding antioxidants, I recommend taking 50–100 mg of ALA and 500–3,000 mg of a mineral-buffered vitamin C per day, in divided doses.

Supplementing With Testosterone

The final step in my program is to supplement your nutrient regimen with natural, biochemically identical testosterone, if needed, for the "heavy lifting" that the use of actual hormone replacement therapy provides. Now that estrogen and progesterone hormone replacement therapy has become more generally accepted, countless numbers of women have also begun to supplement with testosterone. At about age 20, a woman produces peak levels of estrogen, progesterone, and testosterone, but by the time she reaches midlife and passes through menopause, production of these hormones is greatly diminished. To remedy this, estrogen and progesterone are routinely prescribed to restore a woman to youthful hormone status. However, testosterone, which was very much a part of her original hormonal makeup, is much less commonly added into the mix.

Among those women who do decide to take this hormone, the most common reasons are its ability to help prevent vaginal discomfort and soreness while increasing sex drive. In my practice, I've seen testosterone rapidly restore libido (though not for all women), which is an issue for many of my patients, as it affects the pleasurable aspects of intimate relationships. Testosterone is also prescribed for postmenopausal women who are troubled by abnormally low body weight, poor musculature, poor coordination, and osteoporosis.

Physicians who practice conventional medicine prescribe testosterone in the form of capsules. However, there are other forms of testosterone to consider, including testosterone creams and gels.

Synthetic Testosterone

The two forms of synthetic-testosterone administration for women are by capsule and subdermally.

Capsules
The synthetic androgen methyltestosterone has been used clinically for many years. Taken orally as a capsule, the product name is Android®, from ICN Pharmaceuticals. Each capsule contains 10 mg of the hormone. Replacement therapy starts at 10 mg a day and can be gradually increased, with a limit of 50 mg per day.

Testosterone is also marketed combined with estrogen, in a product called Estratest®. The full-strength capsule contains 1.25 mg of esterified estrogen and 2.5 mg of methyltestosterone. There is also a half-strength capsule. Combined estrogen/testosterone therapy is not appropriate for all women. It is probably most useful in women who have undergone surgical removal of their ovaries or whose ovaries have stopped producing even small amounts of testosterone and estrogen soon after menopause. Estratest is recommended for more short-term use, to treat moderate to severe hot flashes associated with menopause. The hormone replacement should be taken for three weeks on and one week off. Medication should be stopped or reduced at three- to six-month intervals.

The drawback of orally administered testosterone is that it is poorly absorbed once in the digestive tract. Another option is subdermal testosterone.

Subdermal Administration
While this delivery method is more common for men, some women have had testosterone pellets implanted beneath the skin. These contain 75 mg of testosterone USP and provide sustained release of the hormone. One pellet can be used for three to six months.

Natural, Bioidentical Testosterone

Natural testosterone is produced by compounding pharmacies, which are able to formulate a wide range of dosages. These can be prepared as a cream or a gel (the two most popular forms), or as sublingual tablets or oral capsules.

Creams
Most women's health-prescription compounding pharmacies suggest using creams containing 0.5 mg/g to 1 mg/g of testosterone. One-quarter teaspoon provides 1 g of cream and 0.5 mg of testosterone. A typical dose is ⅛–¼ teaspoon, used daily in the morning. The cream is applied to various sites, which are rotated, including the inner thigh, the back of the hand, the abdomen, and the arm. An advantage of testosterone cream is that, once absorbed through the skin, it immediately enters the general circulation and travels directly to target cells. Only later does the testosterone pass through the liver, which then begins to metabolize, or break down, the hormone.

Gels
The gel is normally applied to vaginal tissue, from which the testosterone is absorbed into the bloodstream.

Sublingual Tablets

Sublingual tablets are well absorbed. Women usually begin with doses of 2–5 mg, but even a dose of only 0.5 mg may be sufficient. A reduced dose may be appropriate for a woman who is also taking estrogen, because estrogen activates testosterone receptor sites and strengthens its hormonal effect.

Oral Capsules

Capsules can be prepared with no preservatives, which some people prefer. However, capsules do have a disadvantage in that, once absorbed, the testosterone must first pass through the liver before entering the general circulation. Because the liver metabolizes the hormone, a smaller quantity of less active testosterone reaches target cells.

Injections

In a double-blind, placebo-controlled trial of 107 women with active rheumatoid arthritis, weekly supplemental testosterone injections brought significant improvement in comfort and quality of life (November 1996, *Annals of the Rheumatic Diseases*).

The Proof is in the Research

As you can imagine, much research has been done on the use of supplemental testosterone. Unfortunately, for reasons of money and shareholders, most of this research is performed using synthetic versions of the hormone. However, I and other like-minded alternative and complementary medicine physicians believe that biochemically identical testosterone has the same benefits found with the synthetic versions, but is a healthier hormonal option.

One study published in the *American Journal of Obstetrics and Gynecology* found that women who had received a total hysterectomy, including removal of their ovaries, benefited greatly from testosterone supplementation. As the ovaries make one-third of the testosterone in the female body, their removal causes a significant decline in testosterone production. The women were divided into four groups and given combined estrogen and androgen, one or the other of the hormones alone, or a placebo. The treatments were administered for three months, followed by a differing treatment for another three months. There was also a control group of ten women who underwent hysterectomy, but retained their ovaries. The women receiving androgen therapy, alone or with estrogen, and the women with ovarian function intact reported significantly higher ratings of energy and well-being than those women not receiving androgens.

Another study cited in a review article appearing in the *Journal of Clinical Endocrinology and Metabolism* found that testosterone cream or the oral estrogen/testosterone combination therapy can significantly increase sex drive. Women who had had their ovaries surgically removed were injected with testosterone enanthate (a synthetic) and reported an increase in the intensity of sexual arousal, sexual interest, and frequency of sexual fantasies above the effect they experienced taking only estrogen. Similarly, a study from the *Journal of Clinical Endocrinology and Metabolism* cited several controlled studies also documenting an increased intensity of sexual drive, sexual arousal, and frequency of sexual fantasies in women receiving testosterone supplementation.

Additionally, testosterone has a positive effect on a variety of psychological symptoms. In a study from the *American Journal of Obstetrics and Gynecology*, patients completed a daily questionnaire, rating such items as feeling blue and depressed, crying spells, needless worry, and loss of interest in most things. Those women receiving testosterone reported negative feelings significantly less frequently than women not receiving the hormone.

Research from the journal *Menopause* confirms these findings. The study tested the effects of an SSRI (selective serotonin reuptake inhibitor) antidepressant versus a combination of various hormonal therapies. Researchers divided 72 postmenopausal, depressed women into four groups. One group received the antidepressant alone, another received the antidepressant with a synthetic estrogen/progesterone combination, the third took a synthetic testosterone with the antidepressant, and the fourth received a combination of all four drugs. At the end of 24 weeks, only 48 women were still involved in the trial. Of the remaining women, researchers found that they all enjoyed relief from their menopausal symptoms. However, only those women who took the antidepressant with the testosterone reported an improvement in mood.

Testosterone supplementation can also improve your physical health, including menopausal symptoms and osteoporosis. A small study, reported in American Family Physician and presented at the sixth annual meeting of the North American Menopause Society, monitored two groups of women experiencing menopausal symptoms. One group of 12 women were each given 1.25 mg of estrogen daily, while a second group of 13 women were each given the same dosage of estrogen and 2.5 mg of methyltestosterone. While both treatments had a positive effect on vaginal dryness and hot flashes, only the combined therapy helped relieve associated nervousness, irritability, fatigue, and insomnia. Other studies have shown that combined hormone therapy is also more effective in improving sleep quality and energy levels.

In another study from *Obstetrics and Gynecology*, 66 women who had undergone surgical menopause were given estrogen either alone or combined with testosterone. While both treatments prevented loss of bone in the spine and hip, only the combined therapy produced a significant increase in bone mineral density in the spine.

DON'T OVERDO

The downside of supplementing with testosterone is that, when taken in high amounts, masculinization can occur. Your voice may deepen, you may develop more facial hair, and there may be clitoral enlargement. Acne may develop, and existing skin problems can worsen. You may also experience changes in your menstrual cycle, and if you are pregnant and take testosterone, a female fetus can develop male sexual characteristics. However, these effects are not likely to happen when testosterone is administered in the smaller, safer dosages appropriate for women.

There is also a possibility that testosterone may increase your risk of heart disease, and if taken with estrogen, testosterone may neutralize some of the benefits of estrogen therapy. Testosterone lowers "good" HDL cholesterol, a risk factor for cardiac problems. There is some evidence that testosterone given by injection, rather than given orally, is able to maintain more healthful levels of HDL.

It is important for anyone taking testosterone to be monitored closely by a physician so that any adverse effects can be recognized and dealt with promptly.

* * *

Maintaining optimum testosterone levels not only improves your libido and enhances your mood, it also protects your heart and bones. By following the program I've outlined in this chapter, you can maintain proper testosterone balance for years to come.

1. Support testosterone production at the central nervous system level with tyrosine, phenylalanine, macuna, *Tribulus terrestris*, maca, and glandulars.
2. Support testosterone production in the ovaries and adrenals with DHEA, boron, and ginseng.
3. Slow the breakdown of testosterone in the liver with PABA.
4. Use herbs such as *Damiana*, Siberian ginseng, *Rhodiola rosea*, and *Ginkgo biloba* to support the effects of testosterone in your body.
5. Boost nitric oxide production with arginine, citrulline, alpha lipoic acid, and vitamin C.
6. Using biochemically identical natural testosterone.

Next, we take a look at pregnenolone—the "mother" of all your sex hormones. You'll learn why this little-known hormone is making such a splash in the health world. Plus, you'll learn how to increase your production of this vital hormone and support its beneficial effects throughout your entire body.

18 pregnenolone: the mother hormone

It's very possible that you have never heard of the hormone pregnenolone, because it is rarely prescribed, or even discussed, by conventional physicians. However, it is the most important of the five primary sex hormones, as it plays a pivotal role in the production of all the others. As the "mother hormone" or precursor to all the major sex hormones, pregnenolone has a widespread effect throughout your body. However, pregnenolone does far more than simply act as a precursor to the other sex hormones. In animal and human studies, as well as decades of clinical use, pregnenolone has been shown to relieve symptoms of PMS and support hormonal health of women during the menopause transition. It also helps to heal a myriad of hormone-related conditions, like memory loss, rheumatoid arthritis, and other autoimmune diseases that occur much more commonly after menopause. It also increases energy, improves cognitive function, and stabilizes moods. Other studies suggest that pregnenolone may be useful in reducing symptoms due to inflammation (which may explain why it is beneficial for treating rheumatoid arthritis), spinal-cord injuries, and possibly Alzheimer's disease.

Pregnenolone was first synthesized in Germany in 1934, and by the 1940's, researchers had begun to study its many uses, including reducing fatigue, increasing physical and mental endurance, and treating various inflammatory conditions. However, this research came to a halt in the 1950's when synthetic cortisone became the therapy of choice for such diseases as rheumatoid arthritis.

Cortisone relieved symptoms quickly, while pregnenolone sometimes required weeks to produce results. Furthermore, synthetic cortisone could be patented, turning it into a highly lucrative drug, so pharmaceutical companies were far more motivated to develop cortisone as a product, and research on pregnenolone was abandoned. Subsequently, patients on cortisone began to suffer its harmful side effects, including a weakening of the immune system and a deterioration of bone mass leading to osteoporosis. Unfortunately, by the time these side effects were fully known, cortisone was established as a widely accepted treatment, and pregnenolone therapy, although known to be nontoxic, was forgotten.

Thankfully, pregnenolone is again being studied, thanks to the widespread, renewed interest in natural therapies. Researchers are investigating pregnenolone in relation to a wide range of topics, including memory, mood, enzyme activity, joint function, premenstrual syndrome, and the aging process. Given the exciting results of these studies, the potential benefits that pregnenolone can provide in the area of health deserves greater attention.

What is Pregnenolone?

Sex hormones are produced through a series of chemical reactions, beginning with cholesterol. Of the total cholesterol in your body, about 75 percent is produced in your liver. The remaining 25 percent is supplied in the diet by foods such as meat and dairy products. On average, a person's body contains about one-third of a pound of cholesterol (150 g), mostly as a component of cell membranes. There is also about seven grams of cholesterol that circulates in the blood.

Cholesterol is first converted into pregnenolone, a steroid hormone that is the precursor to all the other sex hormones. Because of its precursor role, pregnenolone is considered the mother sex hormone, thus inspiring its name. Pregnenolone is then converted into a variety of other hormones, following two pathways. By one route, pregnenolone leads to DHEA, which is then converted into testosterone and subsequently estrogen. This pathway is operative in women during the first half of the menstrual cycle, when estrogen is the dominant hormone. In the second pathway, pregnenolone is converted into progesterone. The progesterone is then converted into testosterone and, finally, into estrogen. In females, this second pathway predominates during the second half of the menstrual cycle, when progesterone and estrogen are dominant.

Pregnenolone's Role in Your Body

Although much of the body's pregnenolone is converted into other sex hormones, a certain portion of it remains unchanged and can produce a variety of beneficial effects on your health. In fact, a study published in the *Journal of Steroid Biochemistry and Molecular Biology* found that pregnenolone accumulates in the brain, independent of sources in other areas of the body. This may have great significance, given the beneficial effects that pregnenolone seems to have on maintaining physical energy as well as stabilizing mood.

Research studies have also demonstrated that pregnenolone plays a role in increasing physical stamina and productivity when a person is working under stress, as well as enhancing mental acuity, concentration, and memory. Pregnenolone can also increase a person's productivity on the job and improve leisure skills that require spatial thought, such as playing bridge or figuring out how to repair a dining room table. Plus, pregnenolone has been found to stabilize mood, thereby benefiting social relationships.

On the whole, pregnenolone has a whole host of health benefits, both physical and mental. The proper levels of this primary hormone have been found to help treat symptoms of PMS and premenopause, enhance mental clarity and acuity, balance mood, and even help in the treatment of Alzheimer's disease. The hormone is also associated with increased physical vitality and stamina, decreased discomfort from arthritis and other autoimmune diseases, quicker recovery from spinal-cord injuries, and treatment of multiple sclerosis.

How Pregnenolone Deficiency Occurs

A variety of factors can decrease pregnenolone production, as noted in an article published in *Biochemical Pharmacology*. Stress and disease can lower levels of pregnenolone throughout your body and in specific tissues. Pregnenolone production also naturally decreases with age. Blood serum levels of pregnenolone can drop as much as 60 percent between ages 35 and 75. Obviously, as pregnenolone levels diminish, the production of all the other sex hormones arising from pregnenolone also declines.

In order to maintain adequate production of pregnenolone, many systems of the body must function properly. Good digestion is required so that hormone precursors such as amino acids (the smallest units of digested protein), protein fragments, and fat molecules can be absorbed and enter the system. Liver health also is important for pregnenolone production. When liver enzyme systems are impaired and the detoxification function is inadequate, hormone production can be affected. For instance, poor liver function can prevent the conversion of pregnenolone into DHEA. Your cholesterol profile is another factor in pregnenolone production. When the level of HDL ("good" high-density lipoproteins) is low, because it is a carrier molecule for hormones, pregnenolone production can become blocked.

Symptoms of Pregnenolone Deficiency

Because pregnenolone is the "mother hormone," deficiencies can have a wide-reaching effect on your health. If levels are below normal, you can experience PMS symptoms, low energy, unstable mood, and poor memory. You may also notice a worsening of pre-existing physical conditions such as rheumatoid arthritis and possibly even multiple sclerosis.

PMS and Perimenopause

Premenstrual syndrome (PMS) is thought to be a result of hormonal changes. Because pregnenolone is the precursor to all sex hormones, deficiencies in this vital hormone will surely disrupt the production of other key hormones, including estrogen and progesterone, which have been linked to PMS. This can lead to a whole host of PMS-related symptoms, including fluid retention and congestion, irritability, anxiety, and depression.

> ### CONNIE'S STORY
>
> When "Connie" came to see me, she was 46 years old. She had always had severe PMS symptoms, complete with moodiness, headaches, breast tenderness, and menstrual cramps. Although she had always had regular menstrual periods, she was now in the early stages of premenopause and had begun experiencing irregular periods and her premenstrual mood swings had worsened. She was also experiencing joint pain and inflammation, and was told by her doctor that she had early signs of rheumatoid arthritis.
>
> Connie started using pregnenolone, the precursor to progesterone, along with a very strong nutritional program, to help her deal with her PMS and premenopause symptoms. Within a few short weeks, she began to feel significantly better. Over a period of several months, her joints became less sore, her periods were more regular, and she had an even, balanced mood.

Unstable Mood

Because pregnenolone may play an important role in stabilizing mood due to its effect on balancing nervous-system function, deficiencies may lead to mood swings and irritability. Additionally, research studies estimate that about five to 10 percent of the population is affected by feelings of helplessness, low self-esteem, and poor motivation. Such a state of mind can act as an emotional barrier, preventing someone from even thinking about setting goals, let alone trying to reach them. When these feelings are caused by a deficiency of brain steroid hormones, pregnenolone supplementation may potentially help.

Low Energy

Women who have pregnenolone deficiency appear to be at risk for symptoms of low energy and fatigue. This can impair your ability to perform complex tasks and/or operate under stressful conditions.

Poor Memory

Pregnenolone stimulates key receptors in your brain that regulate the function and formation of synapses on certain neurons that affect learning and memory. Therefore, a deficiency in pregnenolone may hinder your ability to maintain mental clarity and memory. Fortunately, several recent studies in the arena of human cognitive research suggest that pregnenolone may enhance memory in humans.

Alzheimer's Disease

A review article on pregnenolone suggested that it may one day be proven useful in the treatment of Alzheimer's disease. This degenerative brain disease is characterized by loss of memory and other cognitive functions. The progression of the disease is believed to involve a low-grade inflammatory process that is self-perpetuating and interferes with the body's ability to repair itself.

Pregnenolone may prove to be an effective anti-inflammatory therapy for the treatment of this disease. As pregnenolone is nontoxic and readily absorbed, it has great potential as a treatment and deserves further investigation in this capacity.

Arthritis and Autoimmune Disease

Women who are deficient in pregnenolone are at higher risk for rheumatoid arthritis, as well as other inflammatory diseases such as systemic lupus erythematosus (an autoimmune condition), ankylosing spondylitis (a chronic inflammatory disease of the joints in the spine that causes back stiffening and pain), scleroderma (a rigidity and hardening of the skin and even fibrosis of internal organs), and psoriasis. While much more research needs to be done in this area, pregnenolone may eventually prove to be an exciting new and effective therapy for these disabling chronic conditions.

Multiple Sclerosis

Multiple sclerosis is a disease of the central nervous system involving progressive destruction of the myelin sheath surrounding the nerves. This disease commonly affects young and middle-aged adults, causing symptoms such as weakness, loss of coordination, unsteady gait, and visual deterioration. Researchers have found that both pregnenolone and progesterone play a role in the healing of damaged nerves.

Spinal Cord Injuries

Pregnenolone is useful in reducing the inflammation that occurs at the time of accident in spinal-cord injuries. The inflammation that occurs as a result of these injuries can cause tissue damage and may even lead to permanent functional impairment and paralysis. By reducing inflammation, pregnenolone speeds recovery and helps prevent further health problems. Because so many factors are involved in recovery from a spinal-cord injury, any single therapy is usually not effective in reversing this process.

Are You Pregnenolone Deficient?

The following checklist will give you an idea of whether you are experiencing the effects of low pregnenolone. If you answer yes to four or more of these questions, you very likely need to increase your pregnenolone levels.

- ✓ I have a history of PMS.
- ✓ I am in perimenopause.
- ✓ I am in menopause.
- ✓ My sleep quality is poor; I tend to wake up intermittently during the night.
- ✓ I have a negative state of mind.
- ✓ I have unstable moods, am irritable, and/or tend to be depressed.
- ✓ I am unable to work efficiently and effectively under stress.
- ✓ I have low energy and lack stamina.
- ✓ I have a poor memory.
- ✓ I have poor verbal recall.
- ✓ I'm at risk for Alzheimer's disease.
- ✓ I have a history of autoimmune disease, including rheumatoid arthritis, systemic lupus erythematosus, ankylosing spondylitis, scleroderma, and/or psoriasis.
- ✓ I have a history of multiple sclerosis.
- ✓ I have a history of spinal cord injury.

If your responses suggest that your pregnenolone level is low, then your next step is to get your hormone levels tested.

Testing for Pregnenolone Deficiency

Pregnenolone levels are assayed by measuring the amount of pregnenolone sulfate in the blood. Pregnenolone sulfate is a more water-soluble than pregnenolone itself and is therefore more easily transported through the circulatory system. In adult men, blood levels of pregnenolone sulfate are about 10 mcg per 100 ml. Average daily production of pregnenolone is about 14 mg a day, a relatively small amount (30,000 mg equals about one ounce). However, these amounts may vary significantly among individuals.

Levels of pregnenolone can be measured in the blood and the saliva. Tests can be ordered to assess the quantity present of pregnenolone, pregnenolone-sulfate, and 17-hydroxy-pregnenolone. The latter is the intermediary hormone in the conversion of pregnenolone to DHEA. Health care practitioners who place patients on pregnenolone therapy recommend especially close monitoring of levels, since taking this hormone as a supplement is somewhat new.

Experts caution on the usefulness of such tests. There is not a lot of information on what consists of a normal reading in different age groups. It is also not known how accurately blood levels represent tissue levels of the hormone. Various tissues may also make use of pregnenolone in different ways, so that a blood reading would tell little about its eventual activity level.

Ranges of Pregnenolone Levels:

Taking these questions into consideration, the following ranges for blood levels of pregnenolone are currently used by several labs:

Pregnenolone production in adult women: 10 to 230 ng/dl
Pregnenolone production in postmenopausal women: 5 to 100 ng/dl

If your results indicate that you are deficient in pregnenolone (or if you scored high on the questionnaire), help is just a few pages away. Let's take a look at the many ways you can restore your pregnenolone levels quickly and effectively, while helping to ultimately improve the production of *all* your sex hormones.

restoring
pregnenolone

19

Low levels of the mother hormone can throw all of your sex hormones out of balance. In this chapter, I'll share with you my program to help you restore and maintain proper pregnenolone levels. We'll discuss how you can restore this critical hormone at the central nervous system level, with the help of some key neurotransmitters and glandulars, as well as a few little-known herbs.

You'll also discover the how vital vitamins and nutrients can help to keep your pregnenolone levels in the healthy range by optimizing adrenal and ovarian function. Finally, you'll learn how supplemental, natural, biochemically identical pregnenolone can help to restore low levels of this vital hormone.

Let's get started!

Boost Adrenal and Ovary Function

Pregnenolone itself is made primarily in the adrenal glands, but it is also produced in the cells of the liver, skin, ovaries, and brain. It is manufactured in the mitochondria, the energy-producing factories of the cells. In the mitochondria, nutrients from our diet are converted into usable energy, and cholesterol is also converted into pregnenolone. The pituitary gland regulates the amount of pregnenolone produced.

For this reason, you need to keep your adrenals and ovaries operating at peak performance to ensure that you have proper pregnenolone health and balance. You can do this at the central nervous system level, as well as the adrenal and ovarian level.

Support Production from the Central Nervous System

As I've indicated in earlier chapters, all sex hormone production begins in the brain, and pregnenolone is no exception. While women are surprised to learn that you can increase progesterone production through the brain or central nervous system, the truth is that all hormone production begins in the brain.

We've been traditionally taught that human beings have one brain that is divided into many different parts. But more and more research is putting the "one brain" idea to the test. In fact, it's starting to be widely accepted that the human skull actually houses not one brain, but three—the reptilian brain, the limbic brain, and the neocortical brain.

The reptilian brain is the oldest part of the brain. It controls basic bodily functions like heart rate, breathing, body temperature, hunger, and fight-or-flight responses. Basic drives and instincts, such as defending territory and keeping safe from harm, are other functions of the reptilian brain. The structures in the brain that perform these functions are the brain stem (which controls breathing, heart rate, and blood pressure) and the cerebellum (which controls movement, balance, and posture).

The limbic, or mammalian, brain developed once mammals started roaming the earth. It includes the hippocampus, which controls memories and learning; the amygdala, which controls memory and emotions; and the hypothalamus, which controls emotions (among many other things). Therefore, the limbic brain allows mammals to learn, retain memories, and show emotions.

The neocortical brain, or neocortex, is the complex maze of grey matter that surrounds the reptilian and limbic brains, and accounts for about 85 percent of brain mass. It is found in the brains of primates and humans, and is responsible for sensory perception, abstract thought, imagination, and consciousness. It also controls language, social interactions, and higher communication.

The Chemistry of the Brain

Like the three parts of the brain, there are also three key types of brain chemicals: neuropeptides, neurohormones, and neurotransmitters.

Neuropeptides are responsible for the cell-to-cell communication system in your body. A peptide is a short chain of amino acids connected together, and a neuropeptide is a peptide found in neural tissue. Neuropeptides are widespread in the central and peripheral nervous systems and different neuropeptides have different excitatory or inhibitory actions.

Neuropeptides control such a diverse array of functions in the body. When they work together properly, the wonderful results in your body include elevated mood and other positive behaviors and emotions, stronger bones, better resistance to disease, glowing skin, and boosted metabolism. Conversely, if your neuropeptides function abnormally, the result can be an increased tendency towards neurological and mental disorders such as Alzheimer's disease, epilepsy, and schizophrenia.

There are several types of neuropeptides. Some of the most common include endorphins and beta-endorphins. Endorphins are opiod peptides, meaning they have morphine-like effects within the body. They produce feelings of well-being and euphoria, and a rush of endorphins can lead to feelings of exhilaration brought on by pain, danger, or stress. Endorphins also may also play a role in memory, sexual activity, and body temperature. Beta-endorphins are another form of opiod peptides, but they are stronger than endorphins. They are composed of 31 amino acids and work in the body by numbing pain, increasing relaxation, and promoting a general feeling of well-being.

While there are many, many hormones and hormonal interactions that occur in the brain and body, the most widely known neurohormone is melatonin. (I discussed melatonin in more detail on page 125.)

Neurotransmitters are naturally occurring chemicals that relay electrical messages between nerve cells throughout your body. While all three types of neurochemicals are important for hormone and overall health, neurotransmitters are particularly important for the production of sex hormones.

In the aggregate, all three types of neurochemicals help to regulate the brain's endocrine glands, specifically the hypothalamus and pituitary gland. The hypothalamus is the master endocrine gland contained within your brain that regulates your production of sex hormones. This gland produces a precursor hormone called gonadotropin releasing hormone (GnRH).

The neurotransmitters norepinephrine, epinephrine, dopamine, and serotonin regulate the hypothalamus' release of GnRH. Without proper production and balance of these neurotransmitters, you cannot have proper production and even balance of the sex hormones. Neurotransmitters also support the production of hormones by the pituitary gland. These processes are supported by precursor amino acids such as tyrosine, phenylalanine, and 5-HTP. Neurotransmitters themselves are produced by the conversion of these amino acids. This occurs in the presence of essential vitamins and minerals such as vitamin C, vitamin B_6, and magnesium.

To understand this more fully, let's take a more detailed look at neurotransmitters in action.

The Key to Unlocking Hormone Production

There are two crucial neurotransmitter pathways that help to support your overall health and well-being. The first leads to the production of inhibitory neurotransmitters like serotonin and GABA. The second leads to the production of excitatory neurotransmitters such as dopamine, norepinephrine, and epinephrine, as well as glutamate.

Generally speaking, the inhibitory neurotransmitters quiet down the processes of your body, while the excitatory neurotransmitters speed them up. Thus, the brain chemicals produced through these two pathways oppose and complement one another. Within your brain, serotonin often inhibits the firing of neurons, which dampens many of your behaviors. In fact, serotonin acts as a kind of chemical restraint system.

Of all your body's chemicals, serotonin has one of the most widespread effects on the brain and physiology. It plays a key role in regulating temperature, blood pressure, blood clotting, immunity, pain, digestion, sleep, and biorhythms. Along with another inhibitory neurotransmitter—GABA (gamma-aminobutyric acid)—serotonin also produces a relaxing effect on your mood. Taurine, a type of amino acid, is often used in a similar fashion as these two neurotransmitters due to its therapeutic, inhibitory effects in your body.

Dopamine, norepinephrine, and epinephrine make up the excitatory neurotransmitter pathway. Glutamate is another important excitatory neurotransmitter, though it is not part of the pathway. Unlike serotonin, which has a relaxing effect on your energy and behavior, excitatory neurotransmitters energize and elevate your mood. In addition to their powerful anti-depressant effects, they support alertness, optimism, motivation, zest for life, and sex drive. Plus, the excitatory neurotransmitters are particularly important for the production of progesterone.

In order to ensure that you have adequate neurotransmitter levels for healthy hormone production, you need to supplement with key amino acids, vitamins, and minerals. All neurotransmitters are produced from amino acids found in the protein that you eat. The essential amino acid tryptophan is initially converted into an intermediary substance called 5-hydroxytryptophan (5-HTP), which is then converted into serotonin.

While tryptophan is available as a supplement and is abundant in turkey, pumpkin seeds, and almonds, I've found that 5-HTP is a more effective and reliable option for boosting your neurotransmitter production. Numerous double-blind studies have shown that 5-HTP is as effective as many of the more common antidepressant drugs and is associated with fewer and much milder side effects. In addition to increasing serotonin levels, 5-HTP triggers an increase in endorphins and other neurotransmitters that are often low in cases of depression.

The excitatory neurotransmitters are derived from tyrosine, an amino acid produced from phenylalanine, another amino acid. A variety of vitamins and minerals, such as vitamin C, vitamin B_6, and magnesium, act as co-factors and are necessary for the conversion of these amino acids into neurotransmitters.

To maintain proper serotonin levels, it is helpful to take 50–100 mg of 5-HTP once or twice a day, with one of the dosages taken at bedtime. Be sure to start at 50 mg and increase as necessary. If needed during the day, use carefully, as too much serotonin can interfere with your ability to drive or concentrate.

To maintain optimum dopamine levels, take 500–1,000 mg of tyrosine per day. Be sure to take in divided doses, half in the morning and half in the afternoon. Do not take in the evening, as it may interfere with sleep.

As I recommend with all nutritional supplements, you should start at the lower to more moderate dosage, such as 500 mg a day of tyrosine and 50 mg a day of 5-HTP. Stay on this dosage for two weeks. If you don't notice a reduction in your symptoms, gradually increase the dosage by 500 mg for tyrosine and 50 mg for 5-HTP every two weeks until you have either noticed a reduction in your symptoms or have reached the maximum dosages. I generally don't recommend going over 1,000 mg a day of tyrosine, although you may find that you need as much as 100–200 mg of 5-HTP once or even several times a day.

Additionally, be sure to use a high potency multivitamin/mineral nutritional supplement so that you are taking in all of the co-factors needed to produce neurotransmitters. These include vitamin C, vitamin B_6, folic acid, niacin, magnesium, and copper.

Note: I strongly advise that you undertake a program to restore and properly balance your neurotransmitter levels under the care of a complementary physician, naturopath, or nutritionist. You should also have your neurotransmitter levels tested regularly, as dosage needs for the amino acids I've described often vary from woman to woman (see below).

TEST YOUR NEUROTRANSMITTER LEVELS

State-of-the-art neurotransmitter testing is currently available and can accurately pinpoint your exact levels of these essential brain chemicals. NeuroScience, Inc., (888-342-7272 or *www.neurorelief.com*) is a leader in the development of neurotransmitter testing. They have developed sensitive testing for these neurochemicals that can be done through your urine. The test is simple to do, non-invasive, and can be done in the privacy of your own home. In addition to NeuroScience, there are many other similar laboratories that offer neurotransmitter testing.

I would strongly recommend that you consider such testing if you suspect that you suffer from a moderate to severe neurotransmitter deficiency. Your health care provider will need to order these tests for you.

Support Production in the Ovaries and Adrenals

While hormone production begins in your brain, the actual production of pregnenolone takes place primarily in your adrenals and ovaries, making it critical that you keep these glands functioning at their optimal level. To do this, I highly recommend using the following key nutrients: glandulars, beta-carotene, vitamin C, vitamin B_5, zinc, and magnesium.

Transforming Glandulars

Glandular therapy involves the use of purified extracts from the secretory endocrine glands of animals. Most commonly, extracts are drawn from the thyroid and adrenal glands, as well as the thymus, pituitary, pancreas, and ovaries.

In the past, most experts believed that glandulars could not be effective because the intestinal lining of a healthy person was impenetrable, and that proteins and large peptides could not breach its barrier. However, recent evidence has shown that large macromolecules can and do pass completely intact from the intestinal tract into the bloodstream. In fact, there's further evidence to suggest that your body is able to determine which molecules it needs to absorb whole, and which can be broken down.

Both animal and human studies alike have proven this theory. In some cases, several whole proteins taken orally, including critical enzymes, have been shown to be absorbed intact into the bloodstream. Additionally, many smaller proteins and numerous hormones have also been found to be absorbed intact into the bloodstream, including thyroid, cortisone, and even insulin.

In essence, it means that the active properties of the glandulars stay active and intact, and are not destroyed in the digestive process. This is key to the success of glandular therapy, and explains why they clearly help to restore hormone function by supporting the health of your endocrine glands themselves.

There are multi- and single-glandular systems available from companies like Standard Process—a leader in the field. However, they do require a prescription from a health care practitioner. Other good products are also available in health food stores and should be used as part of a nutritional program to support healthy menstruation.

One of the most widely used and accepted glandulars is for your adrenal glands. Whole adrenal glandular preparations are not only beneficial in treating stress and fatigue, they have been shown to possess cortisone-like properties that help treat asthma, eczema, rheumatoid arthritis, and even psoriasis. They have also been found to help restore the health and function of comprised adrenal glands. In one research study, eight women suffering from morning sickness (nausea and vomiting) who took oral adrenal cortex extract found relief within four days. A similar study gave both injected and oral adrenal cortex extract to 202 women also suffering from morning sickness. More than 85 percent of the women completely overcame their nausea and vomiting or showed significant improvement.

Another study looked at the use of adrenal glandulars to treat patients with chronic fatigue and immune dysfunction syndrome (CFIDS), as well as fibromyalgia. Researchers found that 5–13 mg of an adrenal glandular preparation significantly reduced pain and discomfort. Moreover, after six to 18 months, many of the patients were able to reduce and eventually discontinue treatment, while still enjoying relief.

Clearly, glandulars work. **To help support healthy pregnenolone levels, I suggest taking a good multi-glandular or single glandular product from a company like Standard Process. These could include glandulars such as adrenal, ovary, hypothalamus, and pituitary, depending on your specific needs. To boost pregnenolone production even further than the endocrine glands of the brain, you may also want to focus on adrenal and ovarian support specifically. I also highly recommend that you consider taking a whole brain glandular, if appropriate.**

Boost Hormone Production With Key Nutrients

In addition to powerful glandulars, there are several vital nutrients that are critical to the health of your adrenal glands and ovaries. By supporting the function of your adrenals and ovaries, these important nutrients ensure the proper production and balance of adrenal and ovarian hormones, including pregnenolone.

Beta-carotene is the plant-based, water-soluble precursor to vitamin A. It is very abundant in the adrenal glands and is important for the healthy functioning of the ovaries. It is particularly plentiful in the corpus luteum of the ovary. After ovulation, the follicle that contained the egg that was expelled from the ovary during ovulation is then converted into a new structure called the corpus luteum. The purpose of the corpus luteum is to switch from the estrogen production, which predominates during the first half of the menstrual cycle (days 1 to 14) to the production of progesterone and estrogen during the second half of your cycle (days 15 to 28). This is called the luteinizing process. Some research studies even suggest that a proper balance between carotene and the retinal form of vitamin A is necessary for proper luteal function.

To ensure that you have adequate amounts of vitamin A (as beta-carotene) in your system, I suggest taking 25,000–50,000 IU of beta-carotene a day. You can also eat foods rich in beta-carotene, such as spinach, squash, carrots, cantaloupe, pumpkin, and sweet potatoes.

Vitamin C is very well known for its cold- and flu-fighting properties, but most people don't realize that it is an integral part of the structure and function of the adrenal glands. Your adrenals have the highest concentration of vitamin C in your entire body. These glands use the vitamin to synthesize a variety of hormones and neurotransmitters, namely norepinephrine, epinephrine, and serotonin.

Furthermore, the adrenals use vitamin C to produce cortisol, which is released in times of stress. In fact, studies have shown that when you are under extreme stress, your vitamin C stores a rapidly depleted. This means that your entire body suffers from vitamin C deficiency due to acute stress, with your adrenal glands taking the biggest hit.

To be sure your adrenal glands have adequate amounts of vitamin C, take 1,000–3,000 mg of a mineral-buffered vitamin C each day, in divided doses. Also increase your consumption of vitamin C-rich foods, including citrus fruits, strawberries, peaches, broccoli, tomatoes, and spinach.

B vitamins, especially B_5 (pantothenic acid), play a crucial role in adrenal function. They are critical for stress management, neurotransmitter synthesis, and hormone regulation. In particular, B_5 is the primary nourishing nutrient of your adrenal glands. It is necessary to stimulate the adrenal glands to begin hormone production. B_5 is also needed to produce glucocorticoids, including cortisol. Not surprisingly, the symptoms of vitamin B_5 deficiency—fatigue, headaches, sleep issues—mimic those of adrenal exhaustion.

For proper adrenal function, be sure to take 50–100 mg of a vitamin B-complex a day, with an additional 250–500 mg of B$_5$ daily. You can also increase your intake of foods high in B vitamins, including liver, wheat germ, whole grains, legumes, egg yolks, salmon, royal jelly, sweet potatoes, and brewer's yeast.

Zinc not only supports healthy adrenal function, but it helps to manufacture testosterone and progesterone by promoting proper pregnenolone production. This essential trace mineral also helps in a variety of enzymatic functions, aids in vitamin A metabolism, and keeps your immune system strong.

To ensure that your adrenal glands have adequate amounts of zinc, I suggest taking 10–25 mg of zinc a day. You can also eat foods rich in zinc, such as oysters, pumpkin seeds, and eggs.

Magnesium is one of the basic building blocks needed by your adrenals to produce hormones. Adequate amounts of this vital mineral are also necessary to keep your adrenals balanced and functioning properly. Research has shown that low levels of magnesium can often indicate an overly stressed adrenal system. In fact, depressed and suicidal people have been found to be magnesium deficient.

You can maintain healthy adrenal function with 600–1,000 mg of magnesium a day, as well as eating foods like meat, nuts, whole grains, and dairy, all of which are high in magnesium.

Maintain Adrenal Health With Amazing Herbs

Like key vitamins and minerals, adaptogenic herbs also support the adrenals, ovaries, and other endocrine glands, thereby preventing the long-term adrenal burnout and exhaustion that occurs with chronic stress. (An adaptogen is a substance that is innocuous, is able to increase resistance to a wide range of adverse physical, chemical, and biochemical factors, and promotes a normalization between extremes.) These herbs also contain a wide variety of chemicals that help the body recover more quickly from hard physical labor, athletic exertion, and even convalescence from surgery.

Rhodiola rosea was used medicinally by the ancient Greeks as far back as 100 A.D. Named for the rose-like odor of the rootstock when newly cut, Siberian healers believe that people who drink *Rhodiola* tea on a regular basis will have the potential to live to be more than 100 years old. And in the former Soviet Union, *Rhodiola* has been used to diminish fatigue and increase your body's resistance to stress.

Rhodiola works to support all hormone production by easing stress and fatigue—both killers of adrenal function and, therefore, healthy sex hormone production, including pregnenolone. According to the journal *Phytomedicine*, *Rhodiola* is particularly effective in fighting stress-induced fatigue. In one study, researchers tested 40 male medical students during exam time to determine if the herb positively affected physical fitness, as well as mental well-being and capacity. The students were divided into two groups and given either 50 mg of *Rhodiola rosea* extract or placebo twice a day for 20 days. Researchers found that those students who took the extract had a significant decrease in mental fatigue and improved psychomotor function, with a 50 percent improvement in neuromotor function. Plus, scores from exams taken immediately after the study showed that the extract group had an average grade of 3.47, as compared to 3.20 for the placebo group.

To ease fatigue, stress, or anxiety—all of which can play havoc with your pregnenolone production—I recommend taking 50–100 mg of *Rhodiola rosea* three times a day, standardized to 3 percent rosavins and 0.8 percent salidrosides. While the herb is generally considered safe, some reports have indicated that it may counteract the effects of antiarrhythmic medications. Therefore, if you are currently taking this type of medication, I suggest you discuss the use of *Rhodiola rosea* with your physician.

Panax ginseng has been used in Chinese herbal medicine for more than 4,000 years. While the wild form is now rare, panax ginseng widely cultivated.

Ginseng has a balancing, tonic effect on the systems and organs of the body involved in the stress response. It contains at least 13 different saponins, a class of chemicals found in many plants, especially legumes, which take their name from their ability to form a soaplike froth when shaken with water. These compounds (triterpene glycosides) are the most pharmaceutically active constituents of ginseng. Saponins benefit hormone production, as well as cardiovascular function, immunity, and the central nervous system.

During times of stress, the saponins in the ginseng act on the hypothalamus and pituitary glands, increasing the release of adrenocorticotrophin, or ACTH (a hormone produced by the pituitary that promotes the manufacture and secretion of adrenal hormones). As a result, ginseng increases the release of adrenal cortisone and other adrenal hormones, and prevents their depletion from stress. Other substances associated with the pituitary are also released, such as endorphins. Ginseng is used to prevent adrenal atrophy, which can be a side effect of cortisone drug treatment. Ginseng's ability to support the health and function of the adrenal glands during times of stress, as well as the improved hormone health that occurs with the use of ginseng, clearly supports the production of DHEA itself by the adrenal glands.

In a double-blind study published in *Drugs Under Experimental and Clinical Research*, two groups of volunteers suffering from fatigue due to physical or mental stress were given nutritional supplementation over a 12-week period. One hundred sixty-three volunteers were given a multivitamin and multimineral complex, and 338 volunteers received the same product, plus a standardized Chinese ginseng extract. Once a month, the volunteers were asked to fill out a questionnaire during a scheduled visit with a physician. This questionnaire contained 11 questions that asked them to describe their current level of perceived physical energy, stamina, sense of well-being, libido, and quality of sleep.

While both groups experienced similar improvement in their quality of life by the second visit, the group using the ginseng extract almost doubled their improvement, based on their questionnaire responses, by the third and fourth visits. Thus, ginseng, when added to a multivitamin and multimineral complex, appears to improve many parameters of well-being in individuals experiencing significant physical and emotional stress.

There is also evidence that ACTH (the hormone that stimulates the adrenal cortex) and adrenal hormones, which ginseng stimulates, are known to bind to brain tissue, increasing mental activity during stress.

For maximum benefit, take a high-quality preparation, an extract of the main root of a plant that is six to eight years old, standardized for ginsenoside content and ratio. Companies manufacturing ginseng products may mention the age of the plants used in their products as a testimony to their products' quality. **Take a 100 mg capsule twice a day. If this is too stimulating, especially before bedtime, take the second dose mid-afternoon, or take only the morning dose.**

Siberian ginseng (*Eleutherococcus senticosus*) belongs to the same family as panax ginseng, but the exact composition differs considerably. The most pharmacologically active constituents in Siberian ginseng are eleutherosides, some of which are similar in structure to the saponins contained in Asian ginseng. Siberian ginseng has been used in Asia for nearly 2,000 years to combat fatigue and increase endurance. The medicinal properties of this plant have been studied in Russia, with a number of clinical and experimental studies demonstrating that eleutherosides are adaptogenic, increasing resistance to stress and fatigue.

According to a review of clinical trials of more than 2,100 healthy human subjects, ranging in age from 19 to 72, published in *Economic Medicinal Plant Research*, Siberian ginseng reduces activation of the adrenal cortex in response to stress, an action useful in the alarm stage of the fight-or-flight response. It also helps lower blood pressure. In this same study, data indicated that the eleutherosides increased the subjects' ability to withstand adverse physical conditions including heat, noise, motion, an increase in workload, and exercise. There was also improved quality of work under stressful work conditions and improved athletic performance.

Herbalists have also long prescribed Siberian ginseng for chronic-fatigue syndrome. One way in which ginseng may be effective in this capacity is through its ability to facilitate the conversion of fat into energy, in both intense and moderate physical activity, sparing carbohydrates, and postponing the point at which a person may "hit the wall." This occurs when stored glucose is depleted and can no longer serve as a source of energy.

Siberian ginseng is also used to treat a variety of psychological disturbances, including insomnia, hypochondriasis, and various neuroses. The reason Siberian ginseng is effective may be its ability to balance stress hormones from the adrenals and neurotransmitters such as epinephrine, serotonin, and dopamine, all of which support healthy hormone production by the adrenal glands and ovaries, including pregnenolone.

Though Siberian ginseng has virtually no toxicity, individuals with fever, hypertonic crisis, or myocardial infarction are advised not to use it. **A standard dosage of the fluid extract (33 percent ethanol) ranges from 3–5 ml, three times a day, for periods of up to 60 consecutive days. An equivalent dosage of dry powdered extract (containing at least one percent eleutheroside F) is 100–200 mg three times a day. Take in multiple-dose regimens with two to three weeks between courses.**

TAKE CARE WHEN CHOOSING GINSING

I have had a number of patients over the years who have bought inexpensive ginseng, either as a root or in capsule form, expecting miraculous results, given ginseng's venerable reputation. Unfortunately, these cheaper grades of ginseng rarely, if ever, deliver the punch that individuals expect—that is, the chemical equivalent of an auxiliary set of adrenal glands, testicles, or ovaries.

However, I have seen some remarkable results with high-grade ginseng purchased from reputable Chinese pharmacists that sell top-of-the-line herbs or American companies selling herbs of equivalent quality. Given that the potency of the therapeutic chemicals takes many years to develop within the ginseng root, it is no surprise that with ginseng, you get what you pay for. If you have a serious interest in using ginseng for its adaptogenic properties, I strongly suggest that you search out the reputable dealers.

The Benefits of Bioidentical Pregnenolone

As described in the preceding chapter, pregnenolone is the precursor hormone from which all other sex hormones are made. In the last few years, this powerful compound has become available over the counter and is sold in pharmacies and natural-food stores. It can also be ordered by a physician from a compounding pharmacy.

Pregnenolone is often made from either soy or the Mexican wild yam, both of which belong to the *Dioscorea* species. (The Mexican wild yam is not related to the yams and sweet potatoes found in the supermarket, and eating these does not increase hormone levels.)

The active steroid compound used in manufacture is diosgenin, which has a chemical structure closely related to the structure of the hormones in our own body. To make pregnenolone, diosgenin must be converted in a laboratory. For this reason, when purchasing pregnenolone, it is important to note if the container specifically states that the product contains pregnenolone, rather than just an unprocessed extract of wild yam.

Many people take pregnenolone rather than DHEA, which is also a powerful precursor hormone, because a much lower dose of pregnenolone can enhance the central-nervous-system function. Other advantages of pregnenolone are that it has more potent anti-inflammatory effects and is less likely than DHEA to cause side effects such as skin problems and facial hair.

Prove It to Me

In today's busy work environment, many women are experiencing a great deal of stress around the need to not only maintain a high level of energy, but also their productivity to do the very best they can with their assigned tasks. This, on top of all the other demands that women face in terms of caring for their homes and families, means that the ability to be energetic and revitalized is crucial. Research done many years ago suggests that pregnenolone can be a real help to the hundreds of thousands of women who are exceedingly busy and perhaps overwhelmed. Let's spend some time reviewing these amazing studies.

Researchers conducted several experiments using pregnenolone in the 1940's, as reported in an article in *Aviation Medicine*. In one experiment, 14 volunteers were trained to operate a machine designed to simulate airplane flight. The goal of the exercise was to operate the equipment properly in order to avoid obstacles and prevent crashes. Of the volunteers, seven were pilots, while the others had no flying experience. These volunteers were tested for their flying ability many times over several weeks. Before each test, a volunteer was either given a 50 mg capsule of pregnenolone or left untreated. The results of this test showed that pregnenolone improved performance for all the volunteers. The pilots participating in the experiment also reported that their actual flying on the job improved and that they felt less tired when taking the hormone.

In another experiment reported in the same article, the researchers measured levels of a stress hormone (17-ketosteroid) in the urine of pilots. The amount of 17-ketosteroid normally increased in direct relation to the number of flights completed by the pilots. However, pilots taking pregnenolone had only half the increase in stress hormone excretion as compared with pilots not receiving pregnenolone. Based on these results, the researchers suggested that pregnenolone can help sustain competent performance over a period of time, which could benefit anyone who must work long hours and perform tasks that require coordinated mental and physical activity.

The same research team conducted three other experiments, cited in a review article in *Biochemical Pharmacology*, in which they gave pregnenolone to three groups of skilled workers: leather cutters, lathe operators, and optical workers. The benefits of pregnenolone were assessed by monitoring units of work produced, wastage of material, and number of flaws in the finished product. They found that when workers received a fixed wage and the work was unhurried and stress-free, pregnenolone had no effect on productivity. But when workers were paid by the piece and worked under pressure, pregnenolone was associated with an increased output above their usual levels. Given the amount of stress in the contemporary workplace, having a sufficient amount of pregnenolone appears to be essential for peak performance. Of particular interest in this study is that some of the volunteers taking pregnenolone also reported a sense of well-being and felt better able to cope with the requirements of their jobs.

Most people work under constant stress, doing high-precision work. Think of technicians producing computer chips under sterile conditions or surgeons performing microscopic laser surgery. The requirements and complexity of modern economic life are extraordinarily stringent. Food and nutritional products must be processed and delivered free of disease-causing microorganisms, products must arrive at retailers at almost the same time the sale is made, and airplanes must operate perfectly. All of this economic complexity requires precision and great concentration. The stresses are found throughout the economy, from automobile and computer manufacturing and repair to people performing stressful mental jobs such as physicians, accountants, and book editors. Many professions require after-hours reading just to keep up with new developments in the field. Given these stresses and the fact that the population is aging, it is exciting to know that pregnenolone can support productivity and decrease stress, especially after midlife, when your body's natural production begins to decline.

Treat Insomnia

Not only does the job stress take its toll on productivity, but many women are engaged in work that causes them to be sleep deprived. Research studies have shown that sleep deprivation can lower productivity through the interruption of normal biological cycles. Pregnenolone also offers promise in this area.

In a study published in *Brain Research*, 12 healthy male volunteers (aged 20 to 30) who were given pregnenolone experienced improved sleep quality and were also somewhat less likely to wake intermittently during the sleep period. These results are particularly impressive since the effects seen in this study were achieved using a dosage of only 1 mg of pregnenolone, given orally before sleep.

Another study found that when participants were given 1 mg of pregnenolone, they had an increase in stage IV delta sleep. With just five stages of sleep (one being the shallowest and five being REM or dream-state sleep), the fact that pregnenolone induced such deep sleep is great news for women suffering from insomnia.

Improve Memory

We all want to keep our cognitive function and memory working well into old age. Fortunately, some very exciting research has been done on pregnenolone's benefits in the area of cognitive function. Researchers designed an animal study, published in *Proceedings of the National Academy of Sciences, USA*, that assessed the effectiveness of pregnenolone in improving the memory of mice trained to avoid electric shock as they proceeded through a maze. Some of the mice were then given individual dosages of various steroid hormones, including pregnenolone, pregnenolone sulfate, DHEA, and testosterone. One week later, the mice were again placed in the maze to test if they remembered the correct way out. While all the hormones improved memory to some extent, pregnenolone and pregnenolone sulfate had the most potent effect.

This same team of researchers conducted another experiment, also published in *Proceedings of the National Academy of Sciences, USA*, that demonstrated that even remarkably small dosages of pregnenolone can improve memory. In this study, mice were given dosages containing fewer than 150 molecules of pregnenolone sulfate, and again memory processes improved. The investigators injected pregnenolone into various regions of the brain, with the amygdala (a portion of the brain believed to play an important role in arousal and alertness) proving the most sensitive. These researchers concluded that the effectiveness of pregnenolone treatment in improving memory, when given after learning trials, may indicate that the hormone has an effect on memory storage and retrieval processes.

In the arena of human cognitive research, several recent studies suggest that pregnenolone may also enhance memory in humans. Rahmawhati Sih, a specialist in geriatrics and an associate professor of medicine at Loyola University Medical School in Chicago, conducted several trials to explore this possibility. In the study, 13 healthy older adults—five men and eight women over the age of 65—were given pregnenolone in randomly assigned quantities. Dosages were 10 mg, 50 mg, 200 mg, and 500 mg. Every 14 days, the volunteers received a single dose and were asked to complete a variety of memory tests. The results of this study were promising, with memory improving somewhat as the dosage increased.

In a second trial, the volunteers were again given a range of dosages between 10 and 500 mg and asked to complete a second set of memory tests. In general, the men showed more improvement in visual/spatial tasks, while the women showed improvement in verbal recall. Dr. Sih hypothesized that the difference in these results reflects the different metabolic pathways pregnenolone follows in men and women. In males, pregnenolone metabolizes to testosterone, which is associated with visual/spatial memory, whereas in women, pregnenolone metabolizes to estrogen, which is associated with verbal recall.

Additionally, several animal studies have conclusively shown that pregnenolone (as well as DHEA) significantly improved both short- and long-term memory performances in rats. While more study is needed, these trials suggest that for older persons with diminished pregnenolone production, supplementation may prove an effective memory enhancer.

Balance Mood

A deficiency in pregnenolone has also been linked to unstable moods in patients with emotional (affective) illness. In a study published in *Biological Psychiatry*, researchers analyzed the pregnenolone present in the cerebrospinal fluid (CSF) of 27 mood-disordered patients and 10 healthy volunteers as a way of measuring levels of pregnenolone. Pregnenolone normally circulates throughout the brain and spinal column and is seen as an indicator of changes in brain chemistry. The investigators found that those patients with affective illness had lower levels of pregnenolone in the CSF compared to the healthy volunteers. Levels were especially low among those patients who were depressed on the day the CSF was drawn.

Similarly, a study reported in the journal *Molecular Pharmacology* discusses the role pregnenolone plays in regulating the delicate balance between excitation and inhibition in the central nervous system. As discussed in earlier chapters, there needs to be a balance between the excitatory neurotransmitters (which increase nerve activity), and the inhibitory neurotransmitters (which decrease nerve activity). This is not only necessary for female hormone health and balance, but also for balanced mood and energy. This becomes more and more difficult for women to achieve as they reach their 40's and beyond.

A person in the excitatory state will experience a heightened mood and feel energized. In contrast, in the inhibitory state, an individual will feel relaxed and calm. For normal human functioning, it is important that a balance exists between these two nervous states to avoid the extremes of anxiety and depression. And pregnenolone may play an important role in maintaining that balance.

Ease Health Conditions

On the more "physical" front, early research studies suggest that pregnenolone may be effective in treating patients in the early stages of rheumatoid arthritis, lessening symptoms associated with inflammation. In fact, pregnenolone was first studied in the 1940's as a way to treat various inflammatory conditions, including rheumatoid arthritis. While the treatment soon gave way to synthetic cortisones, it is clear that pregnenolone plays a major role in protecting the joints.

When your body has adequate amounts of the hormone, inflammation is kept at bay. However, if your body is deficient in pregnenolone, inflammation and its nasty sidekicks, including rheumatoid arthritis, show up. To this point, a study from the *Annals of the New York Academy of Sciences* found that people with rheumatoid arthritis have significantly depleted levels of pregnenolone (as well as DHEA-S and testosterone). Therefore, researchers have concluded that supplemental pregnenolone can help ease rheumatoid arthritis symptoms.

Several studies have tested this theory. One in particular followed the results of pregnenolone treatment of 11 patients with rheumatoid arthritis. Of these men and women, ranging in age from 34 to 65, six experienced moderate to marked improvement, and some of the others showed slight improvement. Furthermore, between the third and seventh day of therapy, patients noted a sense of well-being and improved appetite. And between the fourth and eighth days, patients reported a noticeable reduction in joint pain. This improvement allowed greater joint mobility and reduced muscular atrophy. In some of the patients, there was also less swelling in the joints.

Another study had similar results. Researchers gave 21 patients an injection of pregnenolone (100 mg) every day for five to 30 days, followed by 100 mg one to three times a week. They found that eight of the patients had significant improvement, four had moderate improvement, and four enjoyed a slight improvement. Only five of the participants reported no benefit from the treatment.

Additional research has indicated that combining pregnenolone with other therapeutic agents may lead to treatments for multiple sclerosis (MS), as well as improved recovery from spinal cord injuries. A study published in *Science* found that when progesterone and pregnenolone were administered, myelin sheath development around the nerves progressed normally. This is key for MS, as destruction of the myelin sheath is a hallmark of the disease. However, much more research on the use of pregnenolone as a treatment for multiple sclerosis remains to be done.

An animal study published in the *Proceedings of the National Academy of Sciences, USA*, looked at pregnenolone's role in treating spinal cord injuries. In this study, investigators combined several treatments including pregnenolone; dehydroepiandrosterone (DHEA); indomethacin (IM), an anti-inflammatory compound; and bacterial lipopolysaccharide (LPS), a substance that stimulates cytokine secretion (cytokines are intercellular messengers that regulate many cell functions, especially those related to immunologic and inflammatory responses). This combination of therapies was given to animals that had undergone injury. Within 21 days after the injury, 11 of 16 animals were able to stand and walk. Of all the therapies administered, the combination of IM, LPS, and pregnenolone produced notably significant improvements. This treatment was far more effective than any of the treatments given independently or in any combination of two.

Supplementing With Pregnenolone

Pregnenolone is available as an oral pill or capsule, in a micronized form, as a sublingual tablet, as an ointment or cream, and in a liposome-based oral spray. The degree to which pregnenolone is absorbed and the amount that eventually enters the general circulation depends on which route of delivery is used.

Pregnenolone in capsule form, taken orally, first travels to the liver, which metabolizes it into other hormones. As a result, the amount of pregnenolone in circulation will be less than what was consumed. In contrast, micronized pregnenolone—in the form of tiny particles, taken as a capsule—is absorbed from the intestines directly into the lymphatic system, with most of it initially bypassing the liver. Another way to bypass the liver is by taking a sublingual tablet, which is absorbed through the tissue under the tongue. There is a spray, a chewing gum, and a liquid—all of which can deliver pregnenolone through the mouth—as well as a topical cream.

In retail stores, pregnenolone is available in capsule form in various dosages, including 10, 15, 25, 30, and 50 mg. It can also be found in combination with DHEA, vitamin C, vitamin E, and herbs such as ginkgo biloba. Compounding pharmacies working with physicians can prepare pregnenolone in doses from 2 to 100 mg. These pharmacies offer pregnenolone as a pill, a sublingual tablet, a cream, and a micronized capsule. Different delivery systems produce markedly different rates of assimilation and absorption. Be careful not to overdose if you switch from one method to another. Also, most dosages you will read about are based on pregnenolone in capsule form. Use the information below as a guideline for using a different delivery system. This information was supplied by VitalSource Nutrition.

Capsules

The assimilation and absorption rate is between 30 and 50 percent, because the pregnenolone is first processed through the liver before going into the bloodstream. Higher absorption rates may be attained by opening a capsule and releasing the contents under the tongue; hold this for a minute or two before swallowing.

Liquid Sublinguals

Assimilation and absorption rates run as high as 90 to 95 percent. This is because these are held under the tongue and the absorption is directly into the bloodstream, avoiding the liver. Sublinguals usually provide 5 mg of pregnenolone per drop, while liposome sprays usually contain 7.5 mg per spray.

Creams

The assimilation and absorption rate is between 50 and 85 percent. Absorption is also directly into the bloodstream, again avoiding the liver. The absorption rate depends on the quality of the cream, what carriers are present, where on the body the cream is applied (areas where skin is thinner or areas of fatty tissue), the cleanliness of the skin, and the humidity.

When pregnenolone is used for hormone replacement therapy, the dosage depends largely on age. In general, any regimen of pregnenolone supplementation should begin at the lower end of the dosage range. The range of dosages for women in their 40's is 5–10 mg, taken in the morning. For postmenopausal women, dosages range from 10–15 mg, taken in the morning, before or with breakfast. Women over 65 may need from 10–20 mg daily, taken in the morning. Do not take it in the evening, as it can increase your level of alertness and interfere with sleep.

If you are also taking progesterone as part of your hormone replacement program, the dosage may need to be reduced, as pregnenolone is converted into progesterone, adding to the overall supply of the body.

When pregnenolone is used to treat chronic health problems such as rheumatoid arthritis, effective dosages used in studies range from 100–200 mg. However, a dosage this high should be taken only under the supervision of a physician.

Side Effects

While animal and human studies have shown that pregnenolone is non-toxic, this powerful hormone should be used carefully, preferably under the supervision of a health care professional. There has been no formal assessment of its safety when used for years, and research on its side effects is only in the early stages. For instance, it is not known with certainty whether it is safe to allow pregnenolone to enter the general circulation without first passing through the liver, where it can be partially broken down.

If you are taking more pregnenolone than your system can handle, side effects such as irritability, anxiety, and anger may be experienced. Although there are no studies available, physicians who prescribe hormones suggest that pregnenolone and DHEA be taken in the morning as the body appears to have its highest concentrations of these hormones at that time. If, however, pregnenolone is taken later in the day, it can cause overactivity and heightened alertness in sensitive individuals and may prevent them from falling asleep.

If you are taking any prescription or over-the-counter drugs, you should check with your physician for any possible negative interactions or dosage changes.

A Caution on Taking Pregnenolone

Individuals under 40, who normally produce sufficient levels of sex hormones, should not take pregnenolone. It is also not recommended during pregnancy, for people with cardiac problems, or for those who are taking multiple medications. Also, if you are using conventional HRT, you must consult with your prescribing physician before supplementing with pregnenolone, as it may affect the HRT dosages. Pregnenolone is a powerful hormone and should be treated as such.

* * *

Maintaining optimum pregnenolone levels not only improves the production and balance of all your sex hormones, but also improves your mental, emotional, and physical health. By following the program I've outlined in this chapter, you can maintain proper overall hormone balance for years to come.

1. Maintain pregnenolone production at the central nervous system level with 5-HTP and tyrosine, as well as other supportive nutrients.

2. Support pregnenolone production in the adrenals and ovaries with glandulars, beta-carotene, vitamin C, vitamin B$_5$, zinc, and magnesium.
3. Support adrenal health with herbs such as *Rhodiola rosea*, Panax ginseng, and Siberian ginseng.
4. Use biochemically identical natural pregnenolone.

Next, we take a look at DHEA—the key to testosterone and estrogen production. This hormone is gaining more and more popularity among alternative health care practitioners as its benefits for easing menopausal symptoms and boosting heart and bone health become increasingly apparent. You'll not only learn how to increase your own production of this critical hormone, but also how you can support its valuable effects throughout your entire body.

20

the unsung benefits of dhea

I first became aware of DHEA as a medical student more than 30 years ago while reading textbooks on reproductive medicine. However, it was barely mentioned, since no one seemed to know what it actually did. DHEA was always described as a hormone produced abundantly by the adrenal glands, the production of which appeared to diminish significantly with age.

During my early years in the medical field, I thought it odd that the body would produce so much of a hormone that seemed to have no purpose. As subsequent research studies on DHEA began to receive attention, both in the medical literature and in the popular press, it became apparent that this hormone actually has great importance in maintaining many aspects of health. In fact, it is also a very important marker of aging. Research studies suggest that it is a veritable "fountain of youth" when DHEA levels are balanced and healthy in the body.

What is DHEA?

DHEA is the abbreviation for a long and complicated-sounding hormone—dehydroepiandrosterone. DHEA is very important to your health, since it is one of the primary steroid sex hormones from which your body produces testosterone and estrogen. Until about 10 years ago, scientists thought that DHEA had little use beyond its role as a precursor for other hormones. Only recently have studies begun to reveal its many physiological activities that benefit both performance and health. Ninety percent of DHEA is produced by the adrenal glands, while some is also made in the ovaries, brain, and skin tissue.

Adrenal hormones such as DHEA are primarily produced from a substance called acetyl coenzyme A (acetyl CoA), as well as cholesterol. Acetyl CoA is a chemical produced in the liver, made from fatty acids and amino acids. It provides an important source of energy for the body as well as being a building block from which hormones are made. Cholesterol is a waxy, white, fatty material, widely distributed in all body cells. The cholesterol in the body is supplied by animal foods in the diet, such as eggs and organ meats. Your liver also produces a certain amount of cholesterol.

Once DHEA is produced by the adrenals, it travels through the bloodstream to cells throughout the body. Within the glands and sex organs, it is converted to testosterone and estrogen in both men and women. However, the conversion is predominantly to testosterone in males and to estrogen in females. Some DHEA is also converted in the liver to a sulfur compound when a molecule of sulfate (sulfur plus oxygen) is added to it. This new substance is referred to as DHEA-S. It is thought that DHEA is predominantly produced in the morning. This form of the hormone is rapidly excreted through the kidneys. In contrast, DHEA-S is eliminated slowly, so levels remain more constant in the body. Because of the two different rates of excretion, of the total amount of this hormone in the blood, about 90 percent is DHEA-S.

As discussed in the previous chapters, pregnenolone is converted to many other hormones via two pathways; the first stage in one of these pathways is the creation of DHEA. Curiously, not all animals make DHEA in significant amounts. It is produced in abundance by just the primates, including humans, monkeys, apes, and gorillas.

DHEA's Role in Your Body

DHEA works at many levels in your body, supporting physical as well as mental and emotional functions. It has been shown to lessen the symptoms of menopause; increase stamina, improve mood, mental outlook, and your ability to handle stress; reduce body fat; and treat diabetes. It also enhances mental clarity and acuity, promotes confidence and assertiveness, and may even improve libido!

Plus, DHEA may help to decrease your risk of heart disease and cancer; promote healthy bones; strengthen your immune system; ease autoimmune diseases such as rheumatoid arthritis, systemic lupus erythematosus, and ulcerative colitis; and treat conditions as varied as multiple sclerosis, asthma, and burns. This quite a long and positive list of benefits that this awesome hormone provides!

How DHEA Deficiency Occurs

Of all the steroid hormones in your body, DHEA is the most prevalent and circulates in the bloodstream in the highest concentrations. Women produce about 1–2 mg of DHEA-S per day. This production declines with age. A fetus has relatively high amounts of DHEA, which functions to ease the birth process. However, by the time an infant is six months old, DHEA production all but ceases, and only revives at age six to eight in preparation for puberty. Peak DHEA production is between the ages of 25 and 30; after this, production declines by as much as 10 percent per year. A person may feel the effects of this by their mid-40's. At age 80, you make only about 15 percent of what you produced in your 20's.

A study appearing in the *Annals of the New York Academy of Sciences* documents this. Sixty-four volunteers, between the ages of 20 and 40, had four times the levels of DHEA-S as 138 volunteers over age 85. Patients with major diseases such as atherosclerosis, cancer, and Alzheimer's also have significant deficiencies.

As explained in the chapters on pregnenolone, when various functions such as digestion and detoxification by the liver are impaired, or if you have elevated levels of HDL cholesterol, this can have an impact on the production of precursor hormones such as DHEA.

The physical and psychological well-being enjoyed in youth may well depend in part on having sufficient levels of DHEA. For many years, little attention was given to the effect of DHEA on humans, especially in terms of aging and the decline of performance functions. Most of the research on DHEA had been done on rodents and focused on disease. Then a study by Morales et al. investigating the effects of DHEA in older individuals was published in the *Journal of Clinical Endocrinology and Metabolism*. Volunteers in the study described a list of benefits that made DHEA seem like a fountain of youth. They reported increased energy, improved mood, better sleep quality, and a greater ability to remain calm and handle stress.

Poor lifestyle habits—especially excess stress and a lack of exercise—can also affect DHEA levels. In addition to producing DHEA, your adrenal glands manufacture other hormones, including cortisol. Cortisol is released during times of extreme stress, be it physical, emotional, or mental. When you produce too much cortisol and not enough DHEA, you can throw your adrenal glands out of balance, and eventually strain them to the point of exhaustion. Because DHEA levels are already naturally decreasing as you get older, this imbalance can aggravate both perimenopausal and menopausal symptoms.

Additionally, too little exercise may be linked to decreased DHEA levels. Fortunately, a study from *Age and Ageing* found that regular, moderate aerobic exercise such as walking, swimming, or biking increased DHEA production in older people. This is another one of the many health benefits that regular exercise provides for women (and men) of all ages. For more detailed information on the important aspects of all forms of exercise on hormonal health, read Section Five of this book.

Symptoms of DHEA Deficiency

A wealth of research on DHEA has begun to accumulate, particularly during the past few decades. These studies have examined many of the different physiological effects that DHEA produces within the body. Let's take a look at some of the more common ones.

Menopausal Symptoms

As estrogen production declines in menopause, many women experience a variety of symptoms due to this deficiency. Supplementing with DHEA can help remedy these complaints.

Once it is absorbed, DHEA is converted to estrone, a form of estrogen, so DHEA supplementation can become a natural form of estrogen therapy for many women. Women in menopause may experience a thinning of the vaginal tissue and a decline in vaginal secretions. At this time in life, a woman's skin becomes drier. DHEA has been found to revive vaginal tissues; it also activates oil glands in the skin, restoring a youthful texture to the hands and face.

Stress and Anxiety

The natural stress-reducing aspect of DHEA is another one of its amazing benefits. Animal studies suggest that DHEA may have a modulating effect on stress hormones, thereby lessening the impact of stress on the body. The stress response involves an increase in the production of stress hormones, or corticosteroids. DHEA can lessen the strength of this stress response so that corticosteroid levels do not increase as dramatically.

Depression

Many individuals and studies report that DHEA has the ability to enhance psychological well-being, a state of mind in which all seems right with the world. Having a sense of well-being predisposes a person to having an optimistic approach to life and encourages visionary thinking. Because DHEA fosters this general state of mind, having higher levels of DHEA may allow an individual to live a fuller, more positive, and enjoyable life.

Insomnia

DHEA plays a role in reducing fatigue by improving the quality of sleep. Women with insufficient levels of DHEA often miss out on this crucial benefit. They can experience either difficulty falling asleep or staying asleep. Fortunately, supplementing with DHEA has been shown to be effective in treating insomnia.

Loss of Libido

Not only does DHEA help maintain physical energy and muscle mass through its conversion to testosterone, it also affects behavioral traits linked to male hormone production, such as assertiveness and the maintenance of libido. Specifically, I have found DHEA to be useful not only for men with loss of libido but also for women. This is definitely a benefit of DHEA that has been reported by many patients using this hormone.

"Laura," a 51-year-old office manager, consulted me for treatment of her perimenopausal symptoms. As her periods began to be lighter and more irregular, she also found that her sex drive began to diminish. She had a high-stress diet. She drank too much red wine and ate too much white-flour pasta with butter and cream sauces. She definitely needed to start eating a healthier diet, to which she reluctantly agreed. She also started a nutritional supplement program that included DHEA.

After a few weeks on this program, her interest in sex returned, and she became a more enthusiastic participant in sexual activity with her husband.

Poor Memory and Mental Fog

Having a good memory is one of the most fundamental skills required in all areas of life. And there is both anecdotal and scientific evidence that DHEA enhances memory. DHEA improves the brain's ability to process and store information.

The mechanism by which DHEA may benefit memory is not known. However, DHEA has been added to tissue cultures of brain cells from mice, which has stimulated the growth of certain structures that allow communication between nerves. Older mice injected with DHEA completed a memory test as easily as younger mice and retained this information at a second testing.

People taking DHEA find that it aids two specific types of memory: (1) incidental memory (the ability to recall details of recent events), and (2) semantic memory (the ability to retrieve more general types of stored data). These two types of memory tend to decline with age and are the first aspects of memory to deteriorate in patients with Alzheimer's disease. Various studies have been conducted to determine whether DHEA may be useful in treating Alzheimer's. Current research is focusing on the most effective dosages and on whether DHEA is best used in the early stages of the disease.

Osteoporosis

Osteoporosis and osteopenia are so prevalent in women today, it is critical to find and use safe, natural therapies that can help to support bone mass. Unfortunately, thinning bones are another common occurrence associated with menopause and low levels of estrogen, as well as progesterone and testosterone. Animal studies have found that DHEA increases bone mineral density. And human studies are also showing that DHEA can increase bone mineral density at various bone sites. This is very important news for women, given the significant problems and side effects of both conventional hormone replacement therapy and drugs used to treat osteoporosis and osteopenia.

Cardiovascular Disease

Heart disease is currently the leading cause of death among Americans. In younger women, coronary-heart disease (CHD) is rare, but by the time a woman reaches age 65, her probability of having the disease is equal to that of a man.

Healthy levels of DHEA appear to be protective. The majority of research studies on this topic support the conclusion that maintaining healthy levels of DHEA can help prevent heart disease. Conversely, depressed levels of DHEA can be a risk factor for heart disease.

Many theories of how DHEA protects against heart disease are now being investigated. Both laboratory and human studies have indicated that DHEA helps prevent blood clots that can block an artery and trigger a heart attack or stroke. DHEA is known to reduce plaque on the walls of arteries, which can also limit blood flow. It has also been observed that women taking DHEA experience a decline in cholesterol levels. DHEA may produce this effect by facilitating the breakdown of cholesterol in the liver.

In a healthy person, DHEA is able to counteract these risk factors for heart disease. But various conditions, such as stress, can lower DHEA levels and increase the probability of cardiac problems. High levels of the hormone insulin, which manages the metabolism and storage of sugars and starches, can also reduce DHEA levels. To maintain cardiovascular health, there needs to be a balance between these two powerful hormones.

Excess Weight

As people age, their weight can slowly increase to a condition of obesity. As the excess pounds and fat accumulate, self-esteem can plummet, and health problems such as heart disease and diabetes are more likely to occur. It appears that levels of DHEA influence the changes in weight and body composition that occur over time.

Some researchers suggest that DHEA may decrease body fat by blocking the synthesis of fatty acids, which eventually become body fat. Others have noted that DHEA can act as an appetite suppressant and dampen the desire for fatty foods. As the DHEA story unfolds, dieters may someday find that DHEA can help them toward the goal of having a fitter, healthier, slimmer body.

Diabetes

Every woman should be aware of the increasing incidence of diabetes in the Western world. Once this disease has been diagnosed, it often has very dramatic effects that can negatively affect your health, quality of life, and even your longevity. Prevention and effective treatments, including DHEA, are key to fending off diabetes and keeping your blood sugar levels low.

Blood sugar (glucose) is a source of energy used by your cells throughout the body. Normally, the pancreas produces a sufficient amount of insulin, the hormone that manages levels of glucose in the blood and enables the storage of glucose in the cells. The balance between insulin activity and cell uptake determines blood sugar levels. As a person ages, the cells become less responsive to insulin and do not store glucose as readily, a condition called insulin resistance.

However, studies have shown that DHEA causes tissues to be more insulin sensitive. In this way, DHEA may one day become a useful treatment for diabetes (a disease characterized by high levels of insulin and glucose circulating in the blood, coupled with insulin resistance of the cells).

Weakened Immune Function

A compromised immune system often leads to prolonged colds and infection, stress and strain in the body, and impaired hormonal function. By working at the cellular level, DHEA can positively impact immune function. In the immune system, the fighter T cells identify and disarm invading substances that find their way into the body. One type of T cell is the suppressor cell, which detects foreign substances versus those that are a natural part of body tissues. With age, suppressor cells perform these functions less efficiently. DHEA may help prevent this decline and even reverse it.

Another component of the immune system is cytokines. These are hormone-like substances produced by immune cells that determine how your cells respond. Cytokines can either trigger a reaction or inhibit one, and either promote or limit growth. They are the communication system between immune-system cells. With age, however, they begin to send the wrong messages. It appears that DHEA may restore their proper function.

DHEA also suppresses the stress response, which can weaken the immune system and cause a person to be vulnerable to disease. Low levels of stress hormones are associated with higher levels of DHEA.

DHEA strengthens immune-system function, which can ward off a cold and help prevent diseases that can be life-threatening. A variety of laboratory studies, both animal and human, give evidence of DHEA's role in immunity.

Health care practitioners working with DHEA find that patients with adequate levels tend not to have colds or the flu. But there is also indication that DHEA may be a potent tool for combating diseases directly involved with the immune system itself. These include autoimmune diseases such as rheumatoid arthritis, systemic lupus erythematosus, multiple sclerosis, and ulcerative colitis. There is also evidence that DHEA can be of benefit in the treatment of AIDS (which is caused by human immunodeficiency virus).

Cancer

DHEA may have potent anti-cancer benefits. Various laboratory and animal studies suggest that DHEA protects against a wide range of carcinogens and may inhibit the growth of tumors. Whether the initiating carcinogenic substance is cigarette smoke, heavy metals such as lead and cadmium, or radiation, DHEA may be able to block its activation. One theory is that DHEA blocks an enzyme required for certain cancer-promoting chemical reactions to occur. DHEA may also prevent the formation of free radicals, which are unstable atoms that easily bond to other atoms. Free radicals can damage cells and cause them to mutate, resulting in cancerous growth. Additionally, older women with breast cancer have been shown to be deficient in DHEA.

Asthma

The use of DHEA for treating asthma is now being explored. Studies have found that persons with asthma have lower levels of DHEA. Various medications are used to treat the tightening and spasming of the lung tubes (bronchi). It has been noted that when a medication such as prednisone (a potent anti-inflammatory agent) is given to asthma patients, DHEA-S levels rise.

Poor Muscle Strength

DHEA helps increase physical strength by increasing stamina and muscle power, as it is directly converted within the body into testosterone in men, and first testosterone then estrogen in women. Testosterone is the hormone that directly influences muscle mass and strength. The more testosterone a woman has, the more likely she is to be well muscled.

Are You DHEA Deficient?

DHEA is produced in abundance by your body during youth, but its production slows markedly with time. To begin to determine whether your body's supply of this hormone has lessened enough to affect your ability to perform at your best and maintain optimal health, see the following checklist. If you answer yes to four or more of these questions, you very likely need to increase your DHEA levels.

- ✓ I am over the age of 50.
- ✓ I experience symptoms of menopause such as hot flashes.
- ✓ I have low libido.
- ✓ I suffer from insomnia.
- ✓ I am unable to handle stress.
- ✓ I am easily upset.
- ✓ I have a negative outlook on life.
- ✓ I am often unable to recall details of recent events.
- ✓ I have a history of osteoporosis or osteopenia (low bone mass).
- ✓ I have a history of cardiovascular disease.
- ✓ I have significant excess body fat.
- ✓ I am at risk for diabetes.
- ✓ I have a history of autoimmune disease, including rheumatoid arthritis, lupus, multiple sclerosis, ulcerative colitis, and/or AIDS.
- ✓ I have a weak immune system and am prone to colds and flu.
- ✓ I am at high risk for cancer, especially bladder cancer.
- ✓ I suffer from asthma.
- ✓ I lack muscle mass and strength.
- ✓ I tend to tire easily; my level of stamina is low.

If your responses suggest that your DHEA level is low, then your next step is to get your hormone levels tested.

Testing for DHEA Deficiency

The DHEA in the blood is a combination of DHEA sulfate (DHEA-S) and unbound, or free, DHEA. It is generally thought that unbound DHEA is most active and that DHEA-S is not fully metabolically active. Therefore, it is important that any lab assessment distinguish between the two. When a physician is assessing a patient's DHEA levels in relation to specific illnesses, this differentiation takes on special meaning. For instance, research has shown that DHEA levels, but not levels of DHEA-S, can be predictive of the progression of HIV to AIDS.

Levels of DHEA are routinely assessed using a blood test, but salivary testing is also thought to be accurate. DHEA can also be assessed using a 24-hour urine test. If you are taking DHEA supplementation, you need to have initial levels tested and then be tested again every few months, to keep the amount in the upper normal range typical of a young person.

Ranges of DHEA Levels:

As supplementing with DHEA is a relatively new practice, it is a particularly good idea to have levels monitored regularly. However, some physicians believe that this is unnecessary when the dosages used are low. A cautious approach is also advised to monitor metabolites of DHEA such as androsterone and etiocholanolone, as well as hormone metabolites such as testosterone. This can be done using a 24-hour urine test. Some practitioners also think it is important to monitor DHEA levels if an individual has a significant illness, and that at age 40, all people should obtain a baseline reading.

Range of DHEA blood levels in adult men:	180 to 250 ng/dl
Range of DHEA blood levels in adult women:	130 to 980 ng/dl
Ranges of DHEA-S blood levels in adult women:	
Aged 31–50:	2 to 379 µg/dl
Postmenopausal:	30 to 260 µg/dl
Range of DHEA salivary levels in women:	40 to 140 pg/ml

If your results indicate that you are deficient in DHEA (or if you scored high on the questionnaire), then the next chapter is a must-read. You'll discover how you can restore your DHEA levels quickly and effectively.

21 restoring dhea

Like pregnenolone, inadequate levels of DHEA can cause an imbalance in your other sex hormones, namely estrogen and testosterone. In this chapter, I'll share with you my program to help you restore and maintain proper DHEA levels. We'll discuss how you can restore this critical hormone at the central nervous system level with the help of some key neurotransmitters and glandulars, as well as a few little-known herbs.

And since the vast majority of DHEA is produced in your adrenals (with small amounts in your ovaries), you'll also learn about key vitamins and nutrients that help to keep your DHEA levels in the healthy range by optimizing adrenal and ovarian function. Finally, you'll learn how supplemental, natural, biochemically identical DHEA can help to replenish low levels of this vital hormone.

Let's get started!

Boost Your Adrenal Function

Because so much of DHEA's production takes place in the adrenals, with a bit also made in the ovaries, it is critical that you keep these glands operating at peak performance. The best way to accomplish this is to use specific nutrients that support functioning at the central nervous system level, as well as the ovarian and adrenal level.

Support Production from the Central Nervous System

As with all the sex hormones, production begins in your brain. We've been traditionally taught that human beings have one brain that is divided into many different parts. But more and more research is putting the "one brain" idea to the test. In fact, it's starting to be widely accepted that the human skull actually houses not one brain, but three—the reptilian brain, the limbic brain, and the neocortical brain.

The reptilian brain is the oldest part of the brain. It controls basic bodily functions like heart rate, breathing, body temperature, hunger, and fight-or-flight responses. Basic drives and instincts, such as defending territory and keeping safe from harm, are other functions of the reptilian brain. The structures in the brain that perform these functions are the brain stem (which controls breathing, heart rate, and blood pressure) and the cerebellum (which controls movement, balance, and posture).

The limbic, or mammalian, brain developed once mammals started roaming the earth. It includes the hippocampus, which controls memories and learning; the amygdala, which controls memory and emotions; and the hypothalamus, which controls emotions (among many other things). Therefore, the limbic brain allows mammals to learn, retain memories, and show emotions.

The neocortical brain, or neocortex, is the complex maze of grey matter that surrounds the reptilian and limbic brains, and accounts for about 85 percent of brain mass. It is found in the brains of primates and humans, and is responsible for sensory perception, abstract thought, imagination, and consciousness. It also controls language, social interactions, and higher communication.

The Chemistry of the Brain

Like the three parts of the brain, there are also three key types of brain chemicals: neuropeptides, neurohormones, and neurotransmitters.

Neuropeptides are responsible for the cell-to-cell communication system in your body. A peptide is a short chain of amino acids connected together, and a neuropeptide is a peptide found in neural tissue. Neuropeptides are widespread in the central and peripheral nervous systems and different neuropeptides have different excitatory or inhibitory actions.

Neuropeptides control such a diverse array of functions in the body. When they work together properly, the wonderful results in your body include elevated mood and other positive behaviors and emotions, stronger bones, better resistance to disease, glowing skin, and boosted metabolism. Conversely, if your neuropeptides function abnormally, the result can be an increased tendency towards neurological and mental disorders such as Alzheimer's disease, epilepsy, and schizophrenia.

There are several types of neuropeptides. Some of the most common include endorphins and beta-endorphins. Endorphins are opiod peptides, meaning they have morphine-like effects within the body. They produce feelings of well-being and euphoria, and a rush of endorphins can lead to feelings of exhilaration brought on by pain, danger, or stress. Endorphins also may also play a role in memory, sexual activity, and body temperature. Beta-endorphins are another form of opiod peptides, but they are stronger than endorphins. They are composed of 31 amino acids and work in the body by numbing pain, increasing relaxation, and promoting a general feeling of well-being.

While there are many, many hormones and hormonal interactions that occur in the brain and body, the most widely known neurohormone is melatonin.

Neurotransmitters are naturally occurring chemicals that relay electrical messages between nerve cells throughout your body. While all three types of neurochemicals are important for hormone and overall health, neurotransmitters are particularly important for the production of sex hormones.

In the aggregate, all three types of neurochemicals help to regulate the brain's endocrine glands, specifically the hypothalamus and pituitary gland. The hypothalamus is the master endocrine gland contained within your brain that regulates your production of sex hormones. This gland produces a precursor hormone called gonadotropin releasing hormone (GnRH).

The neurotransmitters norepinephrine, epinephrine, dopamine, and serotonin regulate the hypothalamus' release of GnRH. Without proper production and balance of these neurotransmitters, you cannot have proper production and balance of the sex hormones either. And to ensure that neurotransmitter production is being properly supported, and that the neurotransmitters themselves are supporting the production of hormones by the pituitary glands, you need adequate amounts of precursor amino acids such as tyrosine, phenylalanine, and 5-HTP.

All neurotransmitters fall into one of two pathways that help to support your overall health and well-being. The first leads to the production of the inhibitory neurotransmitter serotonin, while the second leads to the production of the excitatory neurotransmitters dopamine, norepinephrine, and epinephrine.

Generally speaking, the inhibitory neurotransmitters quiet down the processes of your body, while the excitatory neurotransmitters speed them up. Thus, the brain chemicals produced through these two pathways oppose and complement one another. Within your brain, serotonin often inhibits the firing of neurons, which dampens many of your behaviors. In fact, serotonin acts as a kind of chemical restraint system.

Of all your body's chemicals, serotonin has one of the most widespread effects on the brain and physiology. It plays a key role in regulating temperature, blood pressure, blood clotting, immunity, pain, digestion, sleep, and biorhythms. Along with another inhibitory neurotransmitter—GABA (gamma-aminobutyric acid)—serotonin also produces a relaxing effect on your mood. Taurine, a type of amino acid, is often used in a similar fashion as these two neurotransmitters because it also has therapeutic, inhibitory effects on your body.

Dopamine, norepinephrine, and epinephrine make up the excitatory neurotransmitter pathway. Glutamate is another important excitatory neurotransmitter, though it is not part of this pathway. Unlike serotonin, which has a relaxing effect on your energy and behavior, excitatory neurotransmitters energize and elevate your mood. In addition to their powerful anti-depressant effects, they support alertness, optimism, motivation, zest for life, and sex drive.

In order to ensure that you have adequate neurotransmitter levels for healthy hormone production, you need to supplement with key amino acids, vitamins, and minerals. All neurotransmitters are produced from amino acids found in the protein that you eat. The essential amino acid tryptophan is initially converted into an intermediary substance called 5-hydroxytryptophan (5-HTP), which is then converted into serotonin.

While tryptophan is available as a supplement and is abundant in turkey, pumpkin seeds, and almonds, I've found that 5-HTP is a more effective and reliable option for boosting your neurotransmitter production. Numerous double-blind studies have shown that 5-HTP is as effective as many of the more common antidepressant drugs and is associated with fewer and much milder side effects. In addition to increasing serotonin levels, 5-HTP triggers an increase in endorphins and other neurotransmitters that are often low in cases of depression.

The excitatory neurotransmitters are derived from tyrosine, an amino acid produced from the essential amino acid phenylalanine. A variety of vitamins and minerals, such as vitamin C, vitamin B_6, and magnesium, act as co-factors and are necessary for the conversion of these amino acids into neurotransmitters.

To maintain proper serotonin levels, it is helpful to take 50–100 mg of 5-HTP once or twice a day, with one of the dosage taken at bedtime. Be sure to start at 50 mg and increase as necessary. If needed during the day, use carefully, as too much serotonin can interfere with your ability to drive or concentrate.

To maintain optimum dopamine levels, take 500–1,000 mg of tyrosine per day. Be sure to take in divided doses, half in the morning and half in the afternoon. Do not take in the evening, as it may interfere with sleep.

As I recommend with all nutritional supplements, you should start at the lower to more moderate dosage, such as 500 mg a day of tyrosine and 50 mg a day of 5-HTP. Stay on this dosage for two weeks. If you don't notice a reduction in your symptoms, gradually increase the dosage by 500 mg for tyrosine and 50 mg for 5-HTP every two weeks until you have either noticed a reduction in your symptoms or have reached the maximum dosages. I generally don't recommend going over 1,000 mg a day of tyrosine, although you may find that you need as much as 100–200 mg of 5-HTP once or even several times a day.

Additionally, be sure to use a high potency multivitamin/mineral nutritional supplement so that you are taking in all of the co-factors needed to produce neurotransmitters. These include vitamin C, vitamin B_6, folic acid, niacin, magnesium, and copper.

Note: I strongly advise that you undertake a program to restore and properly balance your neurotransmitter levels under the care of a complementary physician, naturopath, or nutritionist. You should also have your neurotransmitter levels tested regularly, as dosage needs for the amino acids I've described often vary from woman to woman (see next page).

Support Production in the Ovaries and Adrenals

You now know that hormone stimulation begins in your brain via the neurotransmitters and your brain's endocrine glands. However, the actual production of DHEA takes place primarily in your adrenal glands and ovaries. For this reason, it is crucial that you keep these glands healthy so they can function at peak performance. To do this, you need to make sure you have adequate amounts of the following nutrients: glandulars, beta-carotene, vitamin C, vitamin B$_5$, zinc, and magnesium.

Glorious Glandulars

Many women have had great success with the use of glandular therapy. Glandulars are purified extracts from the secretory endocrine glands of animals, usually the thyroid and adrenal glands, as well as the thymus, pituitary, pancreas, and ovaries.

In the past, most experts believed that glandulars could not be effective because the intestinal lining of a healthy person was impenetrable, and that proteins and large peptides could not breach its barrier. However, recent evidence has shown that large macromolecules can and do pass completely intact from the intestinal tract into the bloodstream. In fact, there's further evidence to suggest that your body is able to determine which molecules it needs to absorb whole, and which can be broken down.

Both animal and human studies alike have proven this theory. In some cases, several whole proteins taken orally, including critical enzymes, have been shown to be absorbed intact into the bloodstream. Additionally, many smaller proteins and numerous hormones have also been found to be absorbed intact into the bloodstream, including thyroid, cortisone, and even insulin.

In essence, it means that the active properties of the glandulars stay active and intact, and are not destroyed in the digestive process. This is key to the success of glandular therapy, and explains why they clearly help to restore hormone function by supporting the health of your endocrine glands themselves.

There are multi- and single-glandular systems available from companies like Standard Process—a leader in the field. However, they do require a prescription from a health care practitioner. Other good products are also available in health food stores and should be used as part of a nutritional program to support healthy menstruation.

One of the most widely used and accepted glandulars is for your adrenal glands. Whole adrenal glandular preparations are not only beneficial in treating stress and fatigue, they have been shown to possess cortisone-like properties that help treat asthma, eczema, rheumatoid arthritis, and even psoriasis. They have also been found to help restore the health and function of comprised adrenal glands. In one research study, eight women suffering from morning sickness (nausea and vomiting) who took oral adrenal cortex extract found relief within four days. A similar study gave both injected and oral adrenal cortex extract to 202 women also suffering from morning sickness. More than 85 percent of the women completely overcame their nausea and vomiting or showed significant improvement.

Another study looked at the use of adrenal glandulars to treat patients with chronic fatigue and immune dysfunction syndrome (CFIDS), as well as fibromyalgia. Researchers found that 5–13 mg of an adrenal glandular preparation significantly reduced pain and discomfort. Moreover, after six to 18 months, many of the patients were able to reduce and eventually discontinue treatment, while still enjoying relief.

Clearly, glandulars work. **To help support healthy DHEA levels, I suggest taking a good multi-glandular or single glandular product from a company like Standard Process. These could include glandulars such as adrenal, ovary, hypothalamus, and pituitary, depending on your specific needs. For an extra boost, you may also want to focus on adrenal and ovarian support specifically. I also highly recommend that you consider taking a whole brain glandular, if appropriate.**

Nutritional Support for Hormone Production

In addition to glorious glandulars, there are several key nutrients that are critical to the health of your adrenal glands. By supporting the function of your adrenals, these important nutrients ensure the proper production and balance of adrenal hormones, especially DHEA.

Beta-carotene is the plant-based, water-soluble precursor to vitamin A. It is very abundant in the adrenal glands and ovaries, and is essential for their healthy functioning. Beta-carotene is particularly plentiful in the corpus luteum of the ovary. After ovulation, the follicle that contained the egg that was expelled from the ovary during ovulation is then converted into a new structure called the corpus luteum. The purpose of the corpus luteum is to switch from the estrogen production, which predominates during the first half of the menstrual cycle (days one to 14) to the production of progesterone and estrogen during the second half of your cycle (days 15 to 28). This is called the luteinizing process. Some research even suggests that a proper balance between carotene and the retinal form of vitamin A is necessary for proper luteal function.

To ensure that you have adequate amounts of vitamin A (as beta-carotene) in your system, I suggest taking 25,000–50,000 IU of beta-carotene a day. You can also eat foods rich in beta-carotene, such as spinach, squash, carrots, cantaloupe, pumpkin, and sweet potatoes.

Vitamin C is very well known for its cold- and flu-fighting properties, but most people don't realize that it is an integral part of the structure and function of the adrenal glands. Your adrenals have the highest concentration of vitamin C in your entire body. These glands use the vitamin to synthesize a variety of hormones and neurotransmitter, namely norepinephrine, epinephrine, and serotonin.

Furthermore, the adrenals use vitamin C to produce cortisol, which is released in times of stress. In fact, studies have shown that when you are under extreme stress, your vitamin C stores a rapidly depleted. This means that your entire body suffers from vitamin C deficiency due to acute stress, with your adrenal glands taking the biggest hit.

To be sure your adrenal glands have adequate amounts of vitamin C, take 1,000–3,000 mg of a mineral-buffered vitamin C each day, in divided doses. Also increase your consumption of vitamin C-rich foods, including citrus fruits, strawberries, peaches, broccoli, tomatoes, and spinach.

B vitamins, especially B_5 (pantothenic acid), play a crucial role in adrenal function. They are critical for stress management, neurotransmitter synthesis, and hormone regulation. In particular, B_5 is the primary nourishing nutrient of your adrenal glands. It is necessary to stimulate the adrenal glands to begin hormone production. B_5 is also needed to produce glucocorticoids, including cortisol. Not surprisingly, the symptoms of vitamin B_5 deficiency—fatigue, headaches, sleep issues—mimic those of adrenal exhaustion.

For proper adrenal function, be sure to take 50–100 mg of a vitamin B-complex a day, with an additional 250–500 mg of B_5 once or twice a day. You can also increase your intake of foods high in B vitamins, including liver, wheat germ, whole grains, legumes, egg yolks, salmon, royal jelly, sweet potatoes, and brewer's yeast.

Zinc not only supports healthy adrenal function, but it helps to manufacture testosterone and progesterone by promoting proper pregnenolone production. This essential trace mineral also helps in a variety of enzymatic functions, aids in vitamin A metabolism, and keeps your immune system strong.

To ensure that your adrenal glands have adequate amounts of zinc, I suggest taking 10–25 mg of zinc a day. You can also eat foods rich in zinc, such as oysters, pumpkin seeds, and eggs.

Magnesium is one of the basic building blocks needed by your adrenals to produce hormones. Adequate amounts of this vital mineral are also necessary to keep your adrenals balanced and functioning properly. Research has shown that low levels of magnesium can often indicate an overly stressed adrenal system. In fact, depressed and suicidal people have been found to be magnesium deficient.

You can maintain healthy adrenal function with 600–1,000 mg of magnesium a day, as well as eating foods like meat, nuts, whole grains, and dairy, all of which are high in magnesium.

Nutrients to Lower Cortisol and Boost Adrenals

In addition to sex hormones such as DHEA, your adrenal glands also produce the stress hormone cortisol. When you are under extreme, chronic stress, your body pours out continual amounts of cortisol. Over time, this excess cortisol can lead to fatigue, weight gain, insomnia, low immune function, and even premature aging. In contrast, low levels of cortisol can indicate that your adrenal glands have become exhausted and are not functioning properly.

Fortunately, DHEA balances the effects of cortisol. In this way, DHEA helps you better deal with all forms of stress, be it physical, mental, or emotional. To this end, many herbs have been shown to improve DHEA levels by helping to lower cortisol and boost adrenal function. I have used these herbs—namely *Rhodiola rosea*, panax ginseng, Siberian ginseng, and licorice root—as well as the vitamin PABA in my practice for many years, and many of my patients have found them to be effective remedies.

Rhodiola rosea has been used medicinally for nearly 2,000 years. The ancient Greeks revered this rose-like rootstock, as did Siberian healers, who believed that people who drank Rhodiola tea on a regular basis would live to be more than 100 years old.

Rhodiola works to support all hormone production by easing stress and fatigue—both killers of adrenal function and, therefore, healthy sex hormone production, including DHEA. According to the journal *Phytomedicine*, *Rhodiola* is particularly effective in fighting stress-induced fatigue. In one study, researchers tested 40 male medical students during exam time to determine if the herb positively affected physical fitness, as well as mental well-being and capacity. The students were divided into two groups and given either 50 mg of *Rhodiola rosea* extract or placebo twice a day for 20 days. Researchers found that those students who took the extract had a significant decrease in mental fatigue and improved psychomotor function, with a 50 percent improvement in neuromotor function. Plus, scores from exams taken immediately after the study showed that the extract group had an average grade of 3.47, as compared to 3.20 for the placebo group.

To ease fatigue, stress, or anxiety—all of which can play havoc with your DHEA production—I recommend taking 50–100 mg of *Rhodiola rosea* three times a day, standardized to 3 percent rosavins and 0.8 percent salidrosides. While the herb is generally considered safe, some reports have indicated that it may counteract the effects of antiarrhythmic medications. Therefore, if you are currently taking this type of medication, I suggest you discuss the use of *Rhodiola rosea* with your physician.

Panax ginseng is an ivy-like ground cover originating in the wild, damp woodlands of northern China and Korea. Its use in Chinese herbal medicine dates back more than 4,000 years. In colonial North America, ginseng was a major export product. The wild form is now rare, but panax ginseng is a widely cultivated plant.

Ginseng has a legendary status among herbs. While extravagant claims have been made about its many uses, scientific research has yielded inconsistent results in verifying its therapeutic properties. However, enough good research does exist to demonstrate ginseng's activity, especially when high-quality extracts, standardized for active components, are used.

Ginseng has a balancing, tonic effect on the systems and organs of the body involved in the stress response. It contains at least 13 different saponins, a class of chemicals found in many plants, especially legumes, which take their name from their ability to form a soaplike froth when shaken with water. These compounds (triterpene glycosides) are the most pharmaceutically active constituents of ginseng. Saponins benefit hormone production, as well as cardiovascular function, immunity, and the central nervous system.

During times of stress, the saponins in the ginseng act on the hypothalamus and pituitary glands, increasing the release of adrenocorticotrophin, or ACTH (a hormone produced by the pituitary that promotes the manufacture and secretion of adrenal hormones). As a result, ginseng increases the release of adrenal cortisone and other adrenal hormones, and prevents their depletion from stress. Other substances associated with the pituitary are also released, such as endorphins. Ginseng is used to prevent adrenal atrophy, which can be a side effect of cortisone drug treatment. Ginseng's ability to support the health and function of the adrenal glands during times of stress, as well as the improved hormone health that occurs with the use of ginseng, clearly supports the production of DHEA itself by the adrenal glands.

In a double-blind study published in *Drugs Under Experimental and Clinical Research*, two groups of volunteers suffering from fatigue due to physical or mental stress were given nutritional supplementation over a 12-week period. One hundred sixty-three volunteers were given a multivitamin And multimineral complex, and 338 volunteers received the same product, plus a standardized Chinese ginseng extract. Once a month, the volunteers were asked to fill out a questionnaire during a scheduled visit with a physician. This questionnaire contained eleven questions that asked them to describe their current level of perceived physical energy, stamina, sense of well-being, libido, and quality of sleep.

While both groups experienced similar improvement in their quality of life by the second visit, the group using the ginseng extract almost doubled their improvement, based on their questionnaire responses, by the third and fourth visits. Thus, ginseng, when added to a multivitamin and multimineral complex, appears to improve many parameters of well-being in individuals experiencing significant physical and emotional stress.

There is also evidence that ACTH (the hormone that stimulates the adrenal cortex) and adrenal hormones, which ginseng stimulates, are known to bind to brain tissue, increasing mental activity during stress.

For maximum benefit, take a high-quality preparation, an extract of the main root of a plant that is six to eight years old, standardized for ginsenoside content and ratio. Companies manufacturing ginseng products may mention the age of the plants used in their products as a testimony to their products' quality. **Take a 100 mg capsule twice a day. If this is too stimulating, especially before bedtime, take the second dose mid-afternoon, or take only the morning dose.**

Siberian ginseng (Eleutherococcus senticosus) has been used in Asia for nearly 2,000 years to combat fatigue and increase endurance. The medicinal properties of this plant have been studied in Russia, with a number of clinical and experimental studies demonstrating that eleutherosides are adaptogenic, increasing resistance to stress and fatigue.

According to a review of clinical trials of more than 2,100 healthy human subjects, ranging in age from 19 to 72, published in *Economic Medicinal Plant Research*, Siberian ginseng reduces activation of the adrenal cortex in response to stress, an action useful in the alarm stage of the fight-or-flight response. It also helps lower blood pressure. In this same study, data indicated that the eleutherosides increased the subjects' ability to withstand adverse physical conditions including heat, noise, motion, an increase in workload, and exercise. There was also improved quality of work under stressful work conditions and improved athletic performance.

Herbalists have also long prescribed Siberian ginseng for chronic-fatigue syndrome. One way in which ginseng may be effective in this capacity is through its ability to facilitate the conversion of fat into energy, in both intense and moderate physical activity, sparing carbohydrates, and postponing the point at which a person may "hit the wall." This occurs when stored glucose is depleted and can no longer serve as a source of energy.

Siberian ginseng is also used to treat a variety of psychological disturbances, including insomnia, hypochondriasis, and various neuroses. The reason this type of ginseng is effective may be its ability to balance stress hormones and neurotransmitters such as epinephrine, serotonin, and dopamine, all of which supports healthy hormone production, including DHEA.

Though Siberian ginseng has virtually no toxicity, individuals with fever, hypertonic crisis, or myocardial infarction are advised not to use it. **A standard dosage of the fluid extract (33 percent ethanol) ranges from 3–5 ml, three times a day, for periods of up to 60 consecutive days. An equivalent dosage of dry powdered extract (containing at least one percent eleutheroside F) is 100–200 mg three times a day. Take in multiple-dose regimens with two to three weeks between courses.**

Licorice root has been enjoyed over the centuries as a candy, but it is also an herb with medicinal properties, featured in the great recorded herbals for 4,000 years. Respected by the ancient Egyptians, licorice was among the treasured items archaeologists discovered (in great quantities) when they opened King Tut's tomb. Sometime around the year 1600, John Josselyn of Boston listed licorice as one of the "precious herbs" brought from England to colonial America.

Licorice is used to treat respiratory conditions, urinary and kidney problems, fatty liver, hepatitis, the inflammation of arthritis, and ulcers. The herb also exhibits hormone-like activity. Licorice root increases the half-life of cortisol (the adrenal stress hormone), inhibiting the breakdown of adrenal hormones by the liver. As a result, licorice is useful in reversing low cortisol conditions, and in helping the adrenal glands rest and restore their function.

A standard dosage is 1 to 2 g of powdered root or 450–600 mg in capsule form three times a day with meals. Licorice has activity similar to aldosterone, the adrenal hormone responsible for regulating water and electrolytes within the body. As a result, taking large doses of licorice (10 to 14 g of the crude herb) can lead to high blood pressure, water retention, and sodium and potassium imbalances. Licorice should not be taken by children under age two. Caution should be used with older children, pregnant and nursing women, and people over 65. Start with low dosages and increase the strength only if necessary.

PABA (para-aminobenzoic acid), a fat-soluble B vitamin, has been shown to safely and effectively slow down the breakdown of sex hormones, including DHEA, in the liver. Plus, PABA has been shown to increase libido!

Research has also shown that higher levels of PABA are associated with better mood and outlook, better vaginal lubrication, and improved sex drive—all of which are also indicative of higher testosterone levels. And since testosterone is made from DHEA, it stands to reason that PABA may slow the breakdown of both testosterone and DHEA.

To help impede the breakdown of DHEA, I recommend taking 400–500 mg of PABA a day.

Beneficial Bioidentical DHEA

Until 1996, DHEA was regulated by the FDA and required a doctor's prescription. Now DHEA can be purchased in health food stores, most drugstores, and by mail order. While DHEA has gained great popularity as its availability has increased, it continues to be considered an alternative therapy.

The majority of DHEA is produced in laboratories from diosgenin. Research on DHEA is far behind that of other sex hormones such as estrogen and testosterone. However, the studies that have been performed show great promise.

Balance Mood

So many of my patients have complained that mood imbalances often disrupt their quality of life, as well as their ability to function effectively. The research suggests that DHEA can be of real benefit for stabilizing mood and mood-related issues in women, especially those in perimenopause and menopause (younger women still produce adequate amounts of DHEA).

According to one study, 13 men and 17 women, ages 40 to 70, were given 50 mg of DHEA nightly for three months. At the end of the period, 67 percent of the men and 82 percent of the women reported an increase in perceived physical well-being. A similar study from the *Lancet* found that 70 percent of those participants who took 50 mg of DHEA a day enjoyed improved feelings of overall well-being.

DHEA also helps alleviate depression. A study appearing in *Biological Psychiatry* observed the effects of DHEA on six older patients. The dosage was 30–60 mg a day of oral DHEA, given for four weeks. Ratings for depression significantly declined, but when treatment stopped, measurements of mood returned to pretreatment levels.

This finding was supported by a similar study published in the *Journal of Clinical Epidemiology*. In this study volunteers, aged 70–79, were assembled into three groups representing various levels of functioning. There were 1,192 persons in the highest-functioning group, 80 in the medium-functioning group, and 82 in the low-functioning group. Values of DHEA-S increased with functional levels, from a value of 48 in the low group to 69 in the top group. Persons in the highest-functioning group felt more effective, had a greater sense of mastery, and were more satisfied with life. Furthermore, these individuals also engaged in more productive activities, exercised more, and engaged more frequently in volunteer activities.

Improve Memory and Brain Health

DHEA has also been shown to improve memory. In a study published in *Biological Psychiatry*, six middle-aged and elderly volunteers were given 30–90 mg a day of oral DHEA so that the hormone was restored to youthful levels. The researchers noted a significant improvement in memory performance.

Similarly, a double-blind study published in *Psychopharmacology* found that 150 mg of DHEA taken twice daily lead to significant improvement in mood and memory on objective mental tests. Brain imaging in the study also suggested that DHEA influenced neurons in the portion of the brain involved in memory processing.

Yet another study, this time published in *Endocrinology*, demonstrated that DHEA not only protects neurons in the brain, but actually stimulates healing after a vascular brain injury such as stroke—by literally rescuing neurons that would have otherwise perished.

Treat Insomnia

A study published in the *American Journal of Physiology* demonstrated that a single 500 mg oral dose of DHEA significantly increased rapid eye movement (REM) sleep in 10 healthy young men. This phase of sleep, when most dreaming occurs, is essential for a person to feel rested. While this is an enormous dose of DHEA, much greater than that normally used in clinical practice, the finding in this study may have important implications in the field of sleep physiology. Obviously, much more research needs to be done in this area. However, DHEA is converted into estrogen in women, which is linked to sleep quality. Therefore, healthy DHEA levels are important for healthy sleep for this reason, as well as its own possible, independent benefits.

Reduce Stress and Lower Cortisol

Research has also shown that stress can lower levels of DHEA. This has been shown in several studies. In one notable study, appearing in the *European Journal of Endocrinology*, a group of 18 Norwegian cadets were given a five-day military training course. They participated in continuous heavy physical activities and had almost no food or sleep. DHEA-S blood levels were measured for 10 of the cadets at the start of the test and at completion. During the five days, the normal hourly changes in DHEA output were diminished, and while DHEA levels did increase with continued stress, once the training was over, DHEA-S levels remained low during the recovery period.

According to another study, appearing in *Experimental and Clinical Endocrinology*, DHEA levels in patients undergoing thyroid surgery continued to decline during the two days following the operation. This decline in DHEA levels can lead to a situation in which stress hormones dominate. Older persons are more likely to experience this oversensitivity to stress hormones, as they are in a period of their lives where DHEA levels naturally decline.

In a study appearing in the *Journal of Clinical Endocrinology and Metabolism*, researchers measured DHEA and cortisol levels in 62 volunteers, aged three to 85, and found that the ratio of cortisol to DHEA in the brain increased with age. High levels of cortisol are known to cause brain damage in animals. This imbalance of cortisol to DHEA may permit normal levels of cortisol to become toxic.

Improve Bone Health

There is much research surrounding the effectiveness of DHEA on bone health. One such study from the Journal of *Clinical Endocrinology and Metabolism* found that DHEA supplementation improved bone density. Researchers gave 70 women and 70 men aged 60 to 88 years old either 50 mg of DHEA or a placebo every day for one year. They found that those participants taking DHEA had significantly greater bone mineral density in their hips, thigh bone (femoral shaft), and top of thigh bone (trochanter). The women taking DHEA also enjoyed greater bone density in their lower back (lumbar spine).

A controversial study from the *New England Journal of Medicine* had similar results. Researchers evaluated the effect of DHEA supplementation on elderly women and men. They found that of the eight bone sites they tested (mostly spine, hip, thigh, and wrist), DHEA significantly increased bone mineral density at the wrist in women and the femoral neck (where the hip connects to the thigh) in men. There was also an increase in three other sites in those people taking DHEA. Of the three remaining bone sites tested, two others also showed a slight increase in bone mineral density in those participants taking DHEA. In other words, DHEA supplementation significantly improved bone health in two bone sites, was helpful in five others, and was of no benefit in just one site tested. Clearly, the use of DHEA can help to improve bone mineral density.

Prevent Heart Disease

There is a plethora of research on the benefits of DHEA to help prevent heart disease. A study reported in the *New England Journal of Medicine* studied 242 men, aged 50–79. Increases of DHEA-S levels by 100 µg per deciliter of blood were associated with a 48 percent reduction in death from cardiovascular disease. While another study contradicted this result, there is still considerable evidence that having higher levels of DHEA protects against heart disease, especially in men.

Conversely, depressed levels of DHEA can be a risk factor for heart disease. An article appearing in the *Journal of Internal Medicine* referred to a study conducted in Poland in which women with coronary heart disease had significantly lower levels of DHEA-S than women with no heart disease. In another study, published in *Circulation*, DHEA-S blood levels were measured in 49 men who had survived premature heart attacks and compared with an equal number of men who had not suffered heart attacks. DHEA-S levels were significantly depressed in the cardiac patients.

Other studies indicate that DHEA helps keep your blood clot-free. In an animal study published in the *Journal of Clinical Investigation*, rabbits with severe atherosclerosis were treated with DHEA, and plaque size was reduced by almost 50 percent. It has also been observed that women taking DHEA experience a decline in cholesterol levels. DHEA may produce this effect by facilitating the breakdown of cholesterol in the liver.

Balance Thyroid Levels

According to a study from *Clinical Chemistry*, DHEA levels may affect the levels of thyroid hormone in your body. Researchers found that 24 patients with hypothyroidism (low thyroid function) also had significantly lower levels of DHEA than those found in the healthy participants. Similarly, 22 participants with hyperthyroidism (high thyroid function) also had significantly elevated levels of DHEA as compared to the healthy patients. Thus, maintaining healthy, balanced DHEA levels appears to be helpful in supporting healthy thyroid function.

Lose Weight and Fend Off Diabetes

During the early stages of diabetes, insulin levels rise and DHEA activity is blocked. This was observed in a study published in the *FASEB Journal*. The researchers observed that insulin lowers blood concentrations of DHEA and DHEA-S by decreasing production of these hormones and by increasing their breakdown and excretion. They suggested that the well-known association between high levels of insulin in the blood (hyperinsulemia) and heart disease may be through insulin's effect on DHEA. Gaining a great deal of weight, as well as normal aging, is also associated with increased insulin levels. In this way, both obesity and aging can also lower DHEA.

There is even evidence that DHEA may promote weight loss. In one such study, published in the *International Journal of Obesity*, 19 dogs were given increasing doses of DHEA daily. Over the six months of the study, 68 percent of these animals lost an average of three percent of their total body weight each month, without any reduction in food intake. This suggests that DHEA may affect metabolism, the process by which food is turned into energy, causing more calories to be used.

Similarly, a study published in the *Journal of Clinical Endocrinology and Metabolism* monitored 10 men for body fat. The men, in their early 20's and matched for weight, were divided into two groups. One group was treated with DHEA, a 400 mg dosage four times a day for 28 days, and the other group was left untreated. The men reported no changes in their regular activities or diet. At the end of the treatment period, it was found that among the five men receiving DHEA, their average percentage of body fat dropped 31 percent. However, there was no drop in weight, suggesting that while there was a decline in fat, muscle mass increased. No change in these measurements occurred in the untreated men.

Boost Immunity

A variety of laboratory studies, both animal and human, give evidence of DHEA's role in immunity. One such study, appearing in the *Journal of Steroid Biochemistry and Molecular Biology*, analyzed the amount of DHEA by-products present in various tissues in mice. The results suggested that in tissues involved in the immune response, locally produced DHEA metabolites, or breakdown products, may participate in the regulation of the immune response.

Another study published in the *Journal of Infectious Diseases* measured levels of DHEA in 41 men who were asymptomatic HIV-1-seropositive who subsequently progressed to AIDS. They also monitored DHEA in 41 similar men who did not develop AIDS, and in an equal number of men who were HIV-1-seronegative. The researchers found that among the men who developed AIDS, DHEA levels were lower five months before progressing to AIDS than in the other two groups.

Prevent Cancer

Low levels of DHEA have even been linked to cancer prevention. A retrospective study published in *Cancer Research* compared 35 individuals who developed bladder cancer with 69 others who remained cancer-free. The cancer patients had significantly lower levels of DHEA and DHEA-S. Another study, of 37 male lung cancer patients at the Gujarat Cancer and Research Institute, in Ahmedabad, India, found that these patients also had lower levels of DHEA-S, as compared with the control group; the research was published in *Neoplasma*.

Studies have also shown that women with breast cancer have low DHEA levels. While researchers are still trying to determine if this is a cause or effect situation, many believe that DHEA's antioxidant benefits may play a role in cancer prevention.

Animal studies indicate that DHEA has been helpful in the healing of burns. Giving DHEA to burn patients may be useful in stopping the progressive destruction of tissue that can occur when blood is unable to reach the damaged area.

Using DHEA

Various preparations of DHEA are on the market, as well as yam extracts, which are sometimes purported to be a substitute for DHEA. It is important to understand the differences between these products. The conversion of the extract to DHEA can be achieved only in the laboratory, not in the human body. Therefore, natural yam extract, while it does have some of its own health benefits, does not increase blood levels of DHEA. This was confirmed in a study published in *Life Science*. Seven men and women, aged 65 to 82, were given yam extract for three weeks with no change in their DHEA level. In contrast, when the same group received 85 mg of DHEA a day, their blood levels of DHEA doubled.

Different delivery systems produce markedly different rates of assimilation and absorption of DHEA. Be careful not to overdose if you switch from one method to another. Also, most dosages you will read about are based on DHEA in capsule form. Use the information below as a guideline for using a different delivery system. This information was supplied by VitalSource Nutrition.

Capsules

The assimilation and absorption rate is between 30 and 50 percent, because the DHEA is first processed through the liver before going into the bloodstream. Higher absorption rates may be attained by opening a capsule and pouring the contents under the tongue; hold this for a minute or two before swallowing it.

Liquid sublinguals

Assimilation and absorption rates run as high as 90–95 percent. This is because these are held under the tongue and the absorption is directly into the bloodstream, bypassing the liver. Sublinguals usually provide 5 mg of DHEA per drop, while liposome sprays usually contain 7.5 mg per spray.

Note: In this method of delivery, the hormone bypasses the liver, and a significant amount of DHEA is able to enter the general circulation. Be sure to adjust your dose for the different absorption rate that sublinguals have from capsules.

Creams

The assimilation and absorption rate is between 50 and 85 percent. Absorption is also directly into the bloodstream, again avoiding the liver. The absorption rate depends on the quality of the cream, what carriers are present, where on the body the cream is applied (areas where skin is thinner or areas of fatty tissue), the cleanliness of the skin, and the humidity.

Supplementing With DHEA

DHEA is most often taken in the form of capsules, which come in 5 mg, 10 mg, 25 mg, and 50 mg dosages. Once absorbed, the DHEA travels to the liver, where much of it is converted into androgens and estrogen. Because of this, not all the DHEA ingested enters the general circulation. Micronized DHEA (the hormone broken into tiny particles) is more efficiently absorbed by the body because the small size of the particles allows them to enter first the lymphatic system and then the general circulation, initially bypassing the liver. Since DHEA is a fat-soluble hormone, it is better absorbed when taken with food. DHEA taken orally is quickly absorbed, and blood levels rise within one hour.

However, much still needs to be learned about optimal dosage, timing, and how the hormone is best administered. There is a question of whether it is appropriate to raise DHEA to youthful levels or simply to a level that is adequate, given a person's age. Clinical trials are under way; in the meantime, clinicians who regularly prescribe DHEA generally agree on a certain range of starting dosages and recommend a gradual increase if needed.

In my experience, I've found that DHEA supplementation may be most beneficial for women after menopause. Beginning dosages should range from 5–15 mg a day, then be increased by 5–10 mg a day, as needed. DHEA dosages in women should not exceed 25 mg per day.

Conversely, there is no reason for women who have not reached menopause or peri-menopause to consider taking DHEA replacement therapy. Women with normal menstrual cycles have no need for supplementing with DHEA since their bodies are making sufficient amounts of this hormone. Occasionally, I have younger female patients who do so, and I strongly advise against it.

Some physicians recommend taking DHEA in the morning to reflect the body's own production of the hormone by the adrenal glands. Taken later in the day, DHEA can have a stimulating effect and sometimes causes insomnia; however, for a person suffering from a condition such as chronic-fatigue syndrome, this energizing effect could be of benefit.

Note: Women should have a mammogram and Pap smear test done before beginning DHEA supplementation to avoid the risk of stimulating a preexisting cancer of the reproductive tract, since DHEA will increase the levels of the major sex hormones.

If you elect to use DHEA without a physician's guidance, buy the lowest-dose products available in your health food store or pharmacy, begin to use it cautiously, and do not go above 25 mg on your own. Let your physician recommend dosages at higher levels, and be sure to carefully monitor the effects on your body.

A CAUTION ON TAKING DHEA

Before starting DHEA supplementation, it is imperative to measure the amount of DHEA in the blood, and during the course of treatment, DHEA levels should continue to be monitored as regularly as every month. In fact, we strongly recommend that any individual considering taking DHEA consult an informed health care professional before starting a regimen. Taking more than 50 mg of DHEA definitely requires supervision.

Side Effects

DHEA is generally considered safe when taken in recommended dosages of 25 mg or less. While some sensitive people may experience side effects with dosages as low as 5 mg, side effects usually occur only when DHEA is taken in much higher amounts. Anyone taking over 50 mg a day of DHEA should be under a physician's supervision. Elevated doses of DHEA can actually prevent the adrenal glands from making the quantity of DHEA they normally produce.

As DHEA is a precursor hormone, which side effects occur in women depends on whether DHEA is being converted to male or female sex hormones. This varies from woman to woman depending on her genetic predisposition. Side effects of DHEA supplementation can include emotional symptoms such as irritability and depression, or physical ones like headaches, menstrual irregularity, and fatigue. DHEA may also have a slight masculinizing effect, especially in older women, who may develop mild acne and, even more rarely, facial hair.

There may also be long-term side effects from using high doses of DHEA. If a person has a family history of certain cancers that are hormone dependent, such as prostate cancer in men and cancers of the ovary, uterus, and breast in women, DHEA supplementation may increase the risk of developing these types of cancer. DHEA may also affect reproduction; therefore, taking the hormone is not recommended for women who are pregnant or breast-feeding.

Physicians who prescribe hormones suggest that DHEA be taken in the morning, as the body appears to have its highest concentrations at that time. If you are taking any prescription or over-the-counter drugs, you should check with your physician for any possible negative interactions or dosage changes.

Recent reports indicate that some individuals who have taken dosages of between 25 and 50 mg for only three to four weeks have experienced irregularities in heart rhythm. This information reinforces the advice that, if you are self-medicating, you should start at very low doses and only attempt higher doses under the supervision of a medical doctor who specializes in hormone therapy.

* * *

By keeping your DHEA levels balanced, you not only improve the production of other important sex hormones, but you improve your overall health and well-being. By simply following the program I've outlined for you in this chapter, you can maintain proper DHEA production for years to come.

1. Maintain healthy DHEA production at the central nervous system level with 5-HTP, tyrosine, and other supportive nutrients.
2. Support DHEA production in the adrenals and ovaries with glandulars, beta-carotene, vitamin C, vitamin B₅, zinc, and magnesium.
3. Support adrenal health with herbs such as *Rhodiola rosea*, panax ginseng, Siberian ginseng, licorice root, and PABA.
4. Use biochemically identical natural DHEA.

Section Three: Summary

For the past 12 chapters, we've explored the causes and treatments of hormone imbalances, especially hormone deficiency, for the five sex hormones (estrogen, progesterone, testosterone, pregnenolone, and DHEA).

We've also discussed the myriad of ways you can restore you own unique brand of hormones with a variety of neurotransmitters, glandulars, herbs, and key vitamins and minerals—all of which work to create healthy hormone levels and function. You've also learned how biochemically identical hormones can give you that extra "oompf" you may need to get back on track.

In Section Four of *Hormone Revolution*, we'll take a look at how energy and frequency medicine can stimulate hormone production. Specifically, we'll explore the benefits of acupuncture and acupressure, color and light therapy, biofeedback, vibrational healing, and other exciting, cutting-edge treatments.

energy medicine for **healthy** hormones

The first section of Hormone Revolution focused on hormones themselves—how they are produced in your body, how they affect your body, and how they deliver their message. We've also discussed the different phases of a woman's life, including the normal menstrual cycle, making the menopause transition (premenopause and perimenopause), and menopause itself.

Next, we looked at the dangers of conventional hormone replacement therapy, and touched on the safe, natural, effective options that you have. Then we examined each one of the major sex hormones in detail, showing how you can restore and balance your own natural hormones with the use of glandulars, neurotransmitters, herbs, vitamins, minerals, and other key nutrients.

While you are likely familiar with the benefits of nutritional therapies and bioidentical hormones, you may not be aware of the incredible benefits that energy medicine has to offer for restoring hormonal health and helping to bring hormones back into balance. I became interested in energy medicine and started to work with and do research on many different types of energy therapies more than 30 years ago. I think that energy medicine therapies are incredibly powerful and offer tremendous benefit for rejuvenating and balancing your entire body, including hormones.

continued

In this section, we'll look at how you can stimulate healthy hormone production with the use of energy medicine. You'll learn how acupuncture, acupressure, color and light therapy, frequency medicine, and other types of energy therapies all work to bring your hormones back into balance. Whether you suffer from estrogen dominance (too yin, too much growth, fluid retention, etc.) or you are an estrogen deficient-fast processor (too yin deficient, too yang, too dry, too thin, too contracted), you can use a variety of energetic techniques to bring you back to balance in the middle range, where hormonal health and well-being exist.

understanding
acupuncture 22

Many of my patients who wanted to combine Eastern and Western healing theories have benefited greatly from this approach. I have utilized many nutritional therapies, sometimes including Chinese herbal products and formulas, as well as Western-based ones, to help bring my patients back into hormonal balance. Some of my patients have also benefited from acupuncture and acupressure. Not only do these treatments help to reduce menopause-related symptoms, PMS, menstrual cramps, and other female hormonal issues without causing any of the negative side effects associated with conventional HRT, but they can be used in conjunction with any other treatments a woman may also be utilizing.

The ancient Chinese art of acupuncture originated over 5,000 years ago. Its tremendous therapeutic benefits have been proven over thousands of years. More recently, many scientific research studies have validated the effectiveness of this treatment for more than a hundred conditions ranging from hormonal imbalances and menopause-related problems such as insomnia, depression, and anxiety to hair loss, food cravings, and even easing the side effects of cancer-related chemotherapy.

The traditional Chinese medicine model maintains that everything in your body is governed by two equally important, but opposing, principles—yin and yang. Yin is associated with the feminine. It regulates the fluids, blood, and tissues of your body, as well as its structural components, such as flesh, tendons, and bones. It is also is associated with coolness, moisture, quiet, calm, and receptivity. Conversely, yang is associated with masculinity. It regulates your body's energy, and is associated with heat, dryness, and assertiveness.

Balance between yin and yang is essential if you are to achieve and maintain optimal health and well-being. In young, healthy women, the balance between these two polar opposites is maintained almost effortlessly, because these women are usually energetically healthy. Because they have such great reserves of yin and yang during youth, they can maintain a state of being either very yin or very yang in response to the stresses and demands of their lives for several years. For example, they can engage in intense, yang-like activities, such as studying hard, working overtime, or long, strenuous periods of exercise, without depleting their yin. However, too many long hours and over-doing it will begin to accumulate and eventually manifest symptomatically.

As you begin to reach the menopause transition and menopause itself, it becomes increasingly difficult to maintain an optimal yin-yang balance. During this time, it is common to lose this balance and go to either end of the spectrum. You may experience yin deficiency and adequate yang or abundant yin with very little yang.

Many women with yin deficiency will begin to experience symptoms as estrogen levels (a yin-like element) begin to decline. As a result, their body starts to feel much more yang. This can show up as hot flashes, night sweats, vaginal and tissue dryness, insomnia, mood swings, and tighter, tenser muscles, as well as thinning of skin, hair, bones, and connective tissue, resulting in painful and achy joints. In fact, women who are extremely yin deficient may find that even the slightest energy imbalances can result in an increased risk of disease and illness.

In contrast, women with abundant yin reserves who start to have a deficiency of yang properties will start to retain fluid and gain weight more readily. While they have a more peaceful and calm temperament, they may lack libido, vitality, joie de vivre, and even mental acuity. This yin/yang duality is similar to what I discussed in Chapter 13 in relationship to how brain and chemical imbalances that occur after menopause can manifest as two distinct body types. In Western medicine, we describe this difference with a chemical and physiological model, while in traditional Chinese medicine, it is described in terms of an energetic imbalance.

Estrogen is such a powerful substance that I have come to think of it as practically synonymous with yin, energetically speaking. Women who are estrogen dominant during the premenopause also face a difficult challenge, as they are combating symptoms of estrogen excess, which can escalate out-of-control as the condition becomes more and more extreme. Fortunately, acupuncture—and its sister healing technique, acupressure—can help to restore the yin-yang balance.

THE POWER OF TOUCH

Acupressure is closely related to acupuncture. Both are used to restore the proper flow of chi. Unlike acupuncture, which requires needles and can only be done by a trained practitioner, acupressure uses the application of gentle finger pressure to specific points on the skin. And you can do it yourself!

The Rivers of Life

Acupuncture is based on the belief that your health is predicated by a balance of chi—or life energy—flowing throughout your body. Both yin and yang energy (or chi) circulate through your body along 12 major pathways called meridians. The meridians move energy through the body like invisible rivers, flowing deep into the interior of the body through organ systems and skin surfaces. When the energy flow stops or is blocked, the corresponding internal organ system manifests symptoms of disease.

The major meridians are the kidney, bladder, heart, small intestine, large intestine, spleen/pancreas, stomach, lung, liver, gall bladder, pericardium (blood vessels), and triple warmer (san jiao). Of these, the kidney, spleen/pancreas, and liver meridians are key for women in any phase of the hormonal cycle, be it menstruation or menopause.

In traditional Chinese medicine, the kidneys are seen as the foundation of the strength and energy of the body. The reserve energy of the body is also contained within the kidneys. As such, the kidneys regulate the sexual organs (ovaries) and their reproductive function. Healthy menstruation, healthy reproduction, and an easy menopause are all dependent on healthy kidney function. The other source of female hormones—the adrenal glands—are also part of the kidney function.

Given their preeminent role as the root source of your body's energy, the kidneys are the foundation of all yin and yang qualities. Similarly to what I described earlier in this chapter, when kidney yin is sufficient, it has a heat-reducing, calming, cooling, moisturizing, and tissue-building effect on your body. When kidney yin is deficient, the tissues of the body are overheated, drier, and more congested. This leads to hot flashes, night sweats, insomnia, and vaginal dryness. The emotions of a menopausal woman suffering from kidney yin deficiency tend toward nervousness, anxiety, irritation, and fear.

When kidney yang is deficient, menopausal women suffer from low libido, urinary incontinence, loss of mental acuity, low back pain, and pale complexion. This indicates that the warming and energizing yang function of the kidneys is out of balance.

The spleen/pancreas meridian supplies the kidney yang by supporting healthy digestion and absorption of nutrients. If your digestive function is weak, you are more likely to lack in kidney yang. You are also likely to have low willpower and be indecisive. If you are still in your active, reproductive years, you may experience menstrual problems, including irregular and heavy periods, due to weak spleen/pancreas energy.

Liver meridian imbalances can also contribute to menstrual, pre- and perimenopausal, and menopausal symptoms. An overheated, congested, or inflamed liver, overtaxed by an unhealthy diet, alcohol, drugs, or toxins, can put additional stress on the kidneys. The kidneys must produce extra yin fluids to act as a coolant or decongestant to the liver. Over time, this drains your body's yin, depleting your kidney's supply of reserve energy. This, in turn, greatly aggravates menopausal symptoms.

Along all the meridians, there are places where the energy surfaces on the skin. These are called acupuncture points. Stimulating these points on the surface of the skin with a fine needle (acupuncture), laser colored light device, electroacupuncture, or by hand pressure (acupressure) can correct the meridian flow and bring your chi back into balance.

Overwhelming Medical Support

Other than supplementation, acupuncture is the most widely studied alternative medicine treatment. When it comes to stimulating healthy hormone production, restoring proper yin-yang balance with acupuncture or acupressure is a critical complement to any supplementation program. It has been found to help a whole host of illnesses and health conditions, ranging from hot flashes and menstrual cramps to bone health and mood disorders.

Let's take a look at the research that exists specifically for treatment from estrogen dominance- and estrogen deficiency-related conditions.

Acupuncture for Estrogen Dominance

Acupuncture and acupressure have been shown to be highly effective treatment modalities for women suffering from estrogen-dominance related issues. These therapies are particularly effective for treating PMS symptoms such as sore and painful breasts, nausea, headaches, menstrual cramps, and anxiety. Acupuncture has also been found to be highly successful in helping women with hormone-related fertility issues to conceive.

According to a study from the *Archives of Gynecology and Obstetrics*, acupuncture was effective in significantly reducing a wide variety of PMS symptoms, including anxiety, insomnia, nausea, gastrointestinal complaints, and premenstrual headaches. In fact, nearly 79 percent of the women receiving acupuncture enjoyed relief, as compared to less than six percent in the control group.

A study from the *Journal of Advanced Nursing* found that acupressure was also helpful in alleviating PMS symptoms, namely menstrual cramps and anxiety. Researchers divided 69 girls into two groups. The first group received 20 minutes of acupressure on a spot three finger-widths above the ankle bone on the inside of the leg. The second group was given 20 minutes of bed rest. For the next four to six week, the participants were asked to either perform the acupressure on themselves or to rest, depending on which group they were in. At the end of the study period, 87 percent of the participants found the acupressure helpful in reducing pain associated with PMS.

A similar study from the *Journal of Traditional Chinese Medicine* also found that acupressure was highly effective for reducing pain associated with menstrual cramps. Researchers divided 216 teenage girls aged 14 to 18 years into three groups. One group received acupressure, the other received ibuprofen, and the third received "false" acupressure. Both the acupressure group and the ibuprofen group enjoyed a 72 percent reduction in menstrual pain, as compared to the "false" group, who saw a 58 percent decrease in pain.

Finally, acupuncture is widely accepted for its ability to support fertility treatments. One such study published in *Fertility and Sterility* found that of the 80 patients undergoing in-vitro fertilization (IVF) who also received acupuncture for six weeks, 42 percent became pregnant, as compared to just 26 percent of those women who did not receive acupuncture.

Acupuncture for Estrogen Deficiency/Yin Deficiency

There is a plethora of research studies on the use of acupuncture/acupressure to treat a myriad of menopause-related conditions, especially hot flashes and insomnia.

In one study from China, 300 women aged 41 to 60 were treated for hot flashes and other menopause-related symptoms. After three 20-minute acupuncture sessions, 51 percent of the women were "cured," 28 percent had "marked improvement," 18 percent were "improved," and just 3 percent of the women felt the treatment was "ineffective."

Another study from Sweden found that the frequency of hot flashes decreased by 50 percent in 24 women who had been treated with electrostimulated or needle-insertion acupuncture. After three months, the women treated with electrostimulation still enjoyed a reduction in their hot flashes, while those treated with needles had a slight rebound in their symptoms. Similarly, a pilot study conducted at the University Hospital of Geneva in Switzerland reported that acupuncture treatments that had been given to 11 women for relief from menopausal symptoms lasted up to three months.

A growing body of clinical evidence also shows that acupressure is effective in treating insomnia and sleep-related issues. A study published in *Neurophysiologie Clinique* reported that stimulus of a specific acupressure point on the wrist resulted in decreased wakefulness and increased total sleep time. A similar study published in the *Journal of Chinese Medicine* reported that 13 night-crying infants all ceased night crying after only three treatment sessions.

Ease Effects of Chemotherapy

Acupuncture, particularly electroacupuncture, has been shown to help prevent and treat nausea and vomiting associated with chemotherapy. According to a study from the *Journal of Alternative and Complementary Medicine*, 27 cancer patients who experienced severe and refractory nausea and vomiting from chemotherapy were given electroacupuncture at their next chemotherapy treatment. More than 96 percent of the patients had significantly less nausea and vomiting, and more than a third of the patients (37 percent) reported no vomiting at all.

Performing Acupressure for Healthy Hormones

All of the exercises in this chapter can be done with acupuncture or electroacupuncture (both of which require a trained professional), laser colored light therapy, even LED colored light therapy as described in Chapter 25, or acupressure (which can be done on a self-help basis).

If you decide to try acupressure at home, be sure you are relaxed and in a warm, quiet room. Your hands should be clean and warm and your body should be comfortable.

When you locate the correct point you are treating, press the point firmly with the tips of both your index and middle fingers. Hold the point for one to three minutes. If you feel any resistance or tension in the area, increase the pressure slightly. If your hands start to tense up or become tired, reduce the pressure a little bit. Also be sure to breathe deeply during your treatment to relax your mind and allow the meridian flow to rebalance itself.

Finally, acupressure should be performed bilaterally. This means if you treat a point on your right side first, you should also treat the same point on your left side. Also, be sure to perform each step in the exercises sequentially.

Acupressure for Estrogen Dominance

To bring your chi back into balance, you must first determine if you are estrogen dominant or estrogen deficient-slow processor and need to restore yang; if you are postmenopausal with plenty of yin reserve, but are deficient in yang qualities such as libido and "get up and go;" or if you are an estrogen deficient-fast processor and need to restore yin (see chapters 11 and 13).

If you are estrogen dominant or an estrogen deficient-slow processor, you can use acupuncture/acupressure to treat a wide variety of ailments, including menstrual cramps, heavy menstrual bleeding, breast disease, and bloating.

Relieve PMS Symptoms

The following exercises help to relieve painful menstrual cramps, irregular menstruation, and heavy menstrual bleeding, as well as bloating and lower back pain. Stimulating this point also helps with the pelvic and abdominal discomfort associated with fibroids and endometriosis.

- Place two fingers from your left hand in the middle of your crease of your left groin, where you bend your leg. Hold for one to three minutes. Switch sides and repeat.
- Lie down on your back. Put your left hand on top of your right hand and place them under your sacrum (the middle of your lower back, at the base of your spine, just above your tail bone). Hold for one to three minutes.
- With your index and middle fingers of your right hand, measure two finger-widths below your belly button. Press on this point for one to three minutes.
- With your index and middle fingers of your right hand, measure four finger-widths below your belly button. Press on this point for one to three minutes.

- Lie down on your back. Measure two finger-widths to the left of your sacrum. Hold for one to three minutes, then repeat in the same location to the right of your sacrum.
- With your right hand, locate the point in the upper arch of your left foot, in your instep, about a thumb-width below the ball of your foot beneath your big toe. Hold for one to three minutes. Repeat on the right foot.

Relieve Heavy Menstrual Bleeding

These exercises balance the spleen meridian, which affects blood formation and menstrual irregularities. They are particularly useful in controlling heavy menstrual bleeding, as well as fluid retention and menstrual cramps.

- Sit upright in a chair or on the floor with your back against the wall. With your right hand, press the inside of your left shin, about four finger-widths above the ankle. Hold for one to three minutes.
- Sit upright in a chair or on the floor with your back against the wall. Hold your big toe on your left foot with your right hand. Press over the nail, on both the front and back of the toe, and hold for one to three minutes.

Ease Depression and Anxiety

These exercises help to reduce PMS-related stress and anxiety, alleviate tension, calm your mind, and ease depression.

- Locate the points one finger-width below and one finger-width to both the right and left of the base of your skull (you should feel a muscle on these points). Hold the points simultaneously for one to three minutes.
- With the index and middle fingers of your right hand, press the point directly between your eyebrows, where the bridge of your nose meets your forehead. Hold for one to three minutes.
- Press the fingers of your right hand on the point three finger-widths above the bottom of your breastbone, in the center of your breastbone, directly over your heart. Hold for one to three minutes.
- Locate the points on the back of your neck, in the hollows about a finger-width to the right and left of the base of your skull. Hold these points simultaneously for one to three minutes.
- Locate the point four finger-widths below your left kneecap, about one finger-width to the outside of your shin. (The point is on the underside of the curve of the bone just below the knee.) Hold for one to three minutes.

Relieve Bloating and Fluid Retention

The following exercises help to relieve bloating and fluid retention, and helps minimize weight gain.

- Sit with your back against a wall and your legs straight out in front of you.
- Place your left hand on your crease of your left groin, where you bend your leg. Place your right hand on your left leg, about two to three inches above the knee. Hold for one to three minutes.
- With your left hand still pressing on the crease of the left groin, place your right hand just below the inside of your left knee. The point is on the underside of the curve of the bone just below the knee. Hold for one to three minutes.

Support Breast Health

Use this exercise to support healthy breasts by stimulating the pituitary gland.

- Sit upright in a chair or on the floor with your back against the wall. With your right hand, press the spot directly between your eyebrows, where the bottom of your forehead meets the top of your nose. Hold for one to three minutes.

Acupressure for Estrogen Deficiency

If you are an estrogen deficient-fast processor, you'll want to use acupuncture and/or acupressure to restore a healthier yin balance.

Reduce Hot Flashes

These exercises help to relieve a wide variety of menopause symptoms, including hot flashes, menopause-related fatigue, and emotional tension.

- Locate the points on the back of your neck, in the hollows about a finger-width to the right and left of the base of your skull. Hold these points simultaneously for one to three minutes.
- With the thumb and index finger of your right hand, press the point located in the webbing between the base of your thumb and pointer finger of your left hand, directly above the muscle. Hold for one to three minutes, then switch hands.
- With the index and middle fingers of your right hand, press the point directly between your eyebrows, where the bridge of your nose meets your forehead. With the index and middle fingers of your left hand, press the point at the top of your head. (There should be a slight indentation.) Hold for one to three minutes.

- Press the fingers of your right hand on the point three finger-widths above the bottom of your breastbone, in the center of your breastbone, directly over your heart. Hold for one to three minutes.

BETTY'S STORY

When "Betty" came to see me, she was in her late 50's. She had been struggling with menopause-related symptoms for nearly three years, and every attempt at therapy had ended in frustration. Her doctor had put her on two different types of conventional hormone replacement therapy (HRT)—Premarin (an estrogen combination) and Provera (a progestin). However, both gave her very unpleasant side effects.

She eventually quit taking conventional HRT altogether and started using black cohosh and vitamin E. While these natural remedies didn't cause any of the negative side effects she had experienced with HRT, they weren't very effective in relieving her symptoms.

I quickly realized she was taking the wrong dosages. I got her on the proper doses, then suggested she add acupuncture or acupressure to her regimen.

Betty gave acupressure a try, and on a follow-up visit, I was delighted to find that she was doing well with her new program. Not only were her menopause symptoms greatly reduced, but she also found the treatments to be calming and relaxing as well as useful in relieving her symptoms.

Treat Insomnia

If you suffer from menopause-related insomnia, these exercises will be a welcome blessing.

- With your left hand, place your index and middle fingers on the middle of the inner side of your right forearm, two and one-half finger widths from your wrist. Hold for one to three minutes.
- With your left hand, place your index and middle fingers on the inside of your right wrist crease, in line with your little finger. Hold for one to three minutes.
- With your left hand, place your index and middle fingers on the inside of your right ankle, in the indentation directly below the anklebone. Hold for one to three minutes, then repeat on the other side.
- With your right hand, place your index and middle fingers on the outside of your right ankle, in the indentation directly below the anklebone. Hold for one to three minutes, then repeat on the other side.

Note: To ensure these points receive slight pressure throughout the night, you can tape a dry bean, such as a kidney bean, to the point you want to stimulate.

Improve Mental Concentration

Stimulating the following point will help to improve memory and mental clarity.

- With the index and middle fingers of your right hand, press the point at the top of your head. (There should be a slight indentation.) Hold for one to three minutes.

Ease Depression and Anxiety

These exercises help to reduce stress and anxiety, alleviate tension, calm your mind, and ease depression.

- Locate the points one finger-width below and one finger-width to both the right and left of the base of your skull (you should feel a muscle on these points). Hold the points simultaneously for one to three minutes.
- With the index and index fingers of your right hand, press the point directly between your eyebrows, where the bridge of your nose meets your forehead. Hold for one to three minutes.
- Press the fingers of your right hand on the point three finger-widths above the bottom of your breastbone, in the center of your breastbone, directly over your heart. Hold for one to three minutes.
- Locate the points on the back of your neck, in the hollows about a finger-width to the right and left of the base of your skull. Hold these points simultaneously for one to three minutes.
- Locate the point four finger-widths below your left kneecap, about one finger-width to the outside of your shin. (The point is on the underside of the curve of the bone just below the knee.) Hold for one to three minutes.

Relieve Vaginal Dryness

Stimulating the following points will help to relieve symptoms of vaginal dryness and insufficient lubrication.

- Sit on the floor with your knees bent, or sit upright in a straight-backed chair. With your right hand, hold the point at the base of the ball on your right foot, between the two pads of your foot. Hold for one to three minutes.
- With your left hand, locate the point halfway between the inside of your right ankle and your Achilles tendon (at the back of your ankle). Hold for one to three minutes.

Boost Libido

This powerful energy point not only restores sex drive, but also improves energy and endurance.

- Sit on the floor with your knees bent, or sit upright in a straight-backed chair. With your right hand, hold the point four finger-widths below your kneecap, toward the outside of the shinbone.
- Gently apply pressure on this point with the index and middle fingers of your left hand.
- Hold for one to three minutes.

Reduce the Appearance of Wrinkles

These simple exercises can reduce wrinkles and restore your skin's natural luster and glow.

- With your index and middle fingers, press the point at the bottom of your cheekbone, directly below your pupil. Hold for one to three minutes.
- With your index and middle fingers, press the indentation found directly below your ear lobe, just behind your jawbone. Hold for one to three minutes.
- With your index and middle fingers, press the point just below the base of your skull, a finger-width away from the spine. Hold for one to three minutes.

Calm Chemotherapy Side Effects

To help prevent and treat nausea and vomiting associated with chemotherapy, press the point about two inches above your wrist crease on the inside of your forearm, and hold for one to three minutes. You can also use this point to relax stomach muscles and nerves and ease seasickness.

Exceptional Healers

In every field of medicine, and of life, there are a few people that stand out above the rest. In the area of Chinese Medicine, two individuals exemplify the best in class—Dr. Zhi Gang Sha and Master Chunyi Lin.

Dr. Zhi Gang Sha

Dr. Sha is a doctor of traditional Chinese medicine in Canada and China. He also holds an MD in China, where he attended Xi'an Jiaotong University. He also holds a master's degree in Hospital Administration from the University of the Philippines. He is the founder of the Institute for Soul Mind Body Medicine, the International Institute of Zhi Neng Medicine, and the Sha Research Foundation.

I first heard about Dr. Sha when my friend "Marie" told me about her brother "Ralph" and his experience with Dr. Sha. Ralph has had a number of very serious health issues. Besides being a diabetic, he also had heart disease, which resulted in the need for bypass surgery. Plus, Ralph had also been diagnosed with liver cancer, as well as cirrhosis of the liver. He was on the list for a liver transplant, though his doctors considered him to be a "hopeless situation."

Ralph began to work with Dr. Sha's healing program, and within a month, he started to feel better. He continued the work, and Ralph has basically transformed his liver back into a healthy liver, with his cancer going into remission. His blood work is healthy and perfect. Even his doctor has said that if he didn't know Ralph was "dying," he'd think he was very healthy, which I found amusing, since his liver is actually in such good shape.

This experience piqued my interest in Dr. Sha. I bought his books and began doing his exercises and chants. I also learned as much as I could about his unique and incredibly effective form of acupuncture.

Dr. Sha's technique involves quickly inserting and removing the needle on only 12 critical acupuncture points. Because of the success he has had with this technique, Dr. Sha was invited by the World Health Organization's International Acupuncture Training Center in Beijing to teach acupuncture and qigong (a blend of exercise and meditation) to visiting foreign physicians.

Currently, Dr. Sha's main focus and mission in life is to help you transform your health by healing your mind, body, and soul. He believes that you can achieve more than just mind over matter—you can learn to live your life through soul over matter. He shows you how you can reach this ideal by teaching three key empowering messages: (1) you have the ability to heal yourself and others; (2) you can use the wisdom of your soul to transform your life and enlighten others; and (3) by providing unconditional, universal service to yourself and others, you become a universal servant.

You can learn more about Dr. Sha and his highly effective approach to soul-based healing and health by visiting his Web site at *www.drsha.com*. While on his Web site, be sure to register for his free weekly Remote Healing teleconferences and free morning calls. I also highly recommend that you pick up one or all of his books, including *Power Healing* and *Soul Mind Body Medicine*.

ARTEMAS' STORY

Artemas met Dr. Sha two to three years after a major head injury. While Artemas was shopping, she was accidentally struck in the head by the top half of a large, wooden Dutch door. The blow was so severe she not only sustained a minor concussion, but the impact sent intense shock waves from her head, down her spine, and into her back, moving five disks out of place and breaking her lower back, just above her tailbone. Within one to two months, she also sustained a stroke due to the accident.

continued on next page

At this time, Artemas couldn't remember small details, such as the names of her children. She could not complete sentences, do simple math, or handle certain noises, like the ringing of a phone. She had severe headaches and excruciating pain all along her back.

When she met Dr. Sha a couple of years later, he performed nothing short of a miracle. He gave her a blessing to open the blood vessels in her brain, suggested select herbs for her to take, and did a deep manipulation behind her right knee to reduce the pain in her back. While the manipulation was quite painful while it was happening, she immediately felt relief in her back. Within a week of the blessing, the swelling in her head decreased and the sharp pain lessened greatly.

Thanks to ongoing treatments, Artemas now enjoys 90 percent fewer headaches and minimal brain swelling. She has energy to burn, enhanced endurance, improved sleep quality, and a great mood. As an alternative healer and soul communicator, Artemas can now help others more effectively and on a deeper level—including her own mother, who is in her early 90's.

Artemas' mother Helen also experienced Dr. Sha's amazing healing abilities. She was driving herself and her husband home from dinner late one night when they struck a car that had stopped in the middle of the road. Helen sustained a myriad of injuries, including a clot in the main artery to her lungs. Artemas asked Dr. Sha to send a blessing to her mother. He sent a Divine order to clear the clot, and on her mother's next x-ray, the clot was gone.

Recently, Helen also suffered from liver failure after a botched attempt to remove all of her teeth due to a gum infection and a loose tooth. Not only did the dentist fail to give Helen an antibiotic prior to the procedure, but he also fitted her with false teeth that fit over the gaping wounds in her mouth. After the trauma of the situation, coupled with free-floating infection and strong antibiotics and pain killers, the shock to her system sent Helen into liver failure.

Once again, Artemas asked Dr. Sha to send her mother a blessing to either heal quickly or pass peacefully. He sent the blessing to heal her liver, and by the next day, Helen's liver enzymes had improved by 33 percent. Today, her enzymes are nearly 100 percent normal.

Artemas is profoundly grateful to Dr. Sha. Not only did he save her mother's life, but she is certain that his blessings helped her avoid future strokes. She knows that her life has been greatly, miraculously enhanced, allowing Artemas to be in service of others.

Master Chunyi Lin

Qigong master Chunyi Lin, author of *Born a Healer*, is internationally recognized as an important qigong master and innovator—a true miracle worker. He has developed an amazing practice called Spring Forest Qigong, which has benefited the health of thousands and thousands of people all over the world.

In case you aren't familiar with qigong (pronounced chee-GONG), it is an ancient Chinese practice that is both an exercise program and an energy therapy. It combines gentle movements, meditation, breathing, and chanting—all with the purpose of freeing the flow of chi that circulates throughout your body.

And the results are nothing short of astounding. Thousands of people practicing qigong have seen relief from a myriad of physical and psychological disorders, including hormone imbalance, fibrocystic breast disease, migraines, heart disease, osteoporosis, diabetes, anxiety, stress, depression, weight gain, emotional eating, and even cancer. There is no doubt in my mind that qigong should be part of everyone's daily routine, like taking a shower or eating breakfast.

In fact, the medical benefits of qigong have been researched extensively. For example, in one study, 56 patients with Parkinson's disease were divided into two groups. The first group received standard treatment, and the other group received the same treatment, plus qigong exercise lessons. Tests compared motor and non-motor functioning at the start of the study, at three months, at six months, and then a year afterward. The patients who practiced qigong showed significant improvement over those who did not perform the exercises.

In other studies, researchers have discovered that just one hour of qigong training immediately lowered cortisol levels (indicating a more effective stress response), increased intracellular signaling, increased concentrations of growth hormone, and increased oxygen production by neutrophils (a type of white blood cell released in response to stress or pathogens).

In addition, a two-month study conducted at the Adler School of Professional Psychology in Chicago found that of 39 patients who used Master Lin's Spring Forest Qigong, all showed improvement, and those with the most serious levels of depression showed significant improvement.

The research and clinical data are so overwhelming that even the conventional doctors at the Mayo Clinic have become believers, and are working with Chunyi to learn qigong. As you can imagine, I believe that's one of the greatest testaments to this extremely powerful form of healing!

You can learn more about Chunyi Lin and Spring Forest Qigong or would like to purchase his Spring Forest tapes or a copy of his book *Born a Healer*, log on to *www.springforestqigong.com* or call 866-292-1861.

My "Heal the World" Exercise

In traditional Chinese medicine (TCM), the organs of your body are made up of five elements: wood, fire, earth, metal, and water. Each of the major organs is linked to a specific element. For example, the liver is linked to the wood element, while the heart is linked to the element of fire. In this system, the organs are linked energetically to one another through the life energy (or chi) that flows from one organ to another in what is called the Five Element Creation and Control Cycle.

In this cycle, one organ—the "Mother Organ"—feeds and nurtures the next organ by giving it or sharing with it a strengthening flow of energy. For example, if one organ becomes depleted of energy, it will draw too much of the energy from the preceding organ and deplete it. Thus, it won't have enough energy to give to the following organ.

Many TCM healers have created healing exercises that nourish the five elements. I've created my own version of this practice by developing an exercise that utilizes this concept.

I personally use this exercise all the time to help energize and balance my internal organs. This wonderful, nurturing exercise can help to heal and balance your hormones and support the health of your entire body.

In this exercise, all of the organs in the Creation and Control Cycle are supported through a constant flow of healing energy. This will help to strengthen all of the major organs of your body, not only helping to bring you back to a healthy female hormone balance, but also improve the general health and well-being of your entire body, as well as your energy and mood.

- Sit in a relaxed position with your arms resting comfortably at your sides. Visualize the beautiful healing energy of Divine light and love flowing gently into your liver (your liver is located in the right upper abdomen.) This light is golden or white, depending on the color you prefer. It is nurturing, soft, and very feminine. It cleanses, heals, and rejuvenates every cell of your liver. Feel love and appreciation for this wonderful healing energy.
- Now, feel this Divine loving and healing energy flow into your gallbladder (your gallbladder is located next to your liver in your right upper abdomen). Feel its beautiful energy bathe every cell of your gallbladder, healing and restoring it to perfect health. Your gallbladder is so grateful for the healing it is receiving.
- Next, allow the Divine healing light to flow gently into your heart (located in your left upper chest), opening your heart center to love and appreciation for everybody and everything in your life. Feel your heart fill and overflow with love. Every cell of the heart is healed, blessed, and nurtured as this Divine light restores it to perfect health.
- This beautiful, healing light now moves into your small intestine (located in the middle of your abdomen). Give thanks and appreciation to this healing light as its energy deeply heals every cell of your small intestine, restoring them to perfect health as it heals and improves your digestive function.
- The light of Divine healing now moves into your spleen (located in your left upper abdomen), blessing, nurturing, and healing it. To show your appreciation and gratitude for this healing, silently repeat the words "thank you, thank you, thank you" as your spleen becomes full of light, full of love, and totally healed.
- This beautiful, soft healing energy now flows into your stomach (located in the center of your upper abdomen). Your stomach relaxes and feels totally nurtured as this healing energy gently bathes each of its cells. It feels healthier and more rejuvenated than it has in years. Your stomach is so grateful for this blessing as all spiritual, emotional, and physical blockages are cleared from its cells and tissues.

- This loving and compassionate energy of healing now flows into your lungs (located in both sides of your chest), bringing joy and happiness to all of its cells and tissues. This healing is kind and compassionate, cleansing all negativity and blockages, leaving the lungs full of radiant health and fully rejuvenated. Your breath now flows deeply and healthfully into and out of your lungs.
- This golden-white light then moves gently and peacefully into your large intestine (located in your lower abdomen). It cleanses every cell of your large intestine, improving its heath and elimination function. Your large intestine is so appreciative, so blessed by all of this love and light. It is thankful for this great honor and gives thanks to the Divine many times for this blessing of restored heath and well-being.
- The beautiful Divine light and love next moves into your kidneys (located in your mid to lower back). This is an incredibly important healing since your kidneys not only help to regulate your fluid balance, but also are the center of all the reserve energy of your body for all of the other organs. Take a few moments to let this Divine light cleanse, heal, bless, and fill every cell of your kidneys with the most loving energy. Love and appreciate all of the healing that your kidneys are receiving, as they become healthier, stronger, and full of light.
- Lastly, this Divine healing light moves to your bladder (located in the middle of your lower abdominal region, just above your pubic bone), clearing it of all blockages. Any areas of darkness are now cleansed and purified, and it is now full of light. Your bladder is so peaceful, so happy, bathed in this compassionate and kind healing energy of love and light.

You have now completed a wonderful healing of the 10 major organ centers in traditional Chinese medicine. You can also ask this beautiful healing light to come into any other organs that you want to give special attention to like your pancreas, adrenals, ovaries, nervous system, and brain, as well as your hypothalamus, pituitary gland, and pineal gland (all of which can be treated energetically in the third eye area, between your eyebrows). Be sure to end each session by thanking the energy of Divine light and love. Do this exercise as often as possible. Even once a day would be very beneficial as you heal and balance your hormones and body. I also recommend that you share this exercise with your husband or significant other, as well as other members of your family and dear friends, so that everyone can enjoy the benefit of much-improved health.

* * *

Rebalancing yin and yang energy through your body's meridian system can be a powerful way to stimulate hormone production and balance your body. Using acupuncture and acupressure is a great way to clear any blocks you may be experiencing so you can keep the chi flowing in a healthy, balanced way. Add in a daily practice of my Heal the World exercise, and you'll be well on your way to optimal hormonal and whole-body health.

In the next chapter, we'll take a look at how chakras relate to chi and the meridians, and how you can use these specialized energy centers to create great health and well-being.

chakras–
your spinning wheels
of wellness

23

Chakras (Sanskrit for wheel) are specialized energy centers located at seven different points throughout your body. Many centuries ago, the yogic tradition of ancient India described the presence of these specialized spiritual-energy centers in the body. They called the centers *prana*, and believed that the flow of this subtle energy through them was strongly affected by your personality structure and your emotions, as well as by your state of spiritual development.

As we discussed in the earlier chapter, Asian medicine calls this energy chi, which travels throughout your body via the meridians. As I indicated previously, the point on your skin where the energy surfaces is called an acupuncture point. Some of the major acupuncture points also correspond to the seven chakras.

When your chakras are balanced, they are the same size and shape, and spin in a clockwise direction. If they are knocked out of balance due to emotional or physical stress or illness, chakras can change both shape and motion. They can appear as elliptical or closed, and can spin counterclockwise, back and forth, stop and start, or stop completely. In other words, how a chakra spins and looks directly relates to the energy of the chakra, the health of its corresponding organ system, and the emotional and physical states of the person. The chakras can also greatly affect your hormonal health.

YOUR BEAUTIFUL AURA

Each individual spinning chakra creates its own field and energy, the frequency of which determines the color of a particular chakra. These seven fields then combine to produce an auric field—or your aura. The amount or intensity of energy produced by a particular chakra or group of chakras determines the color of your aura.

A Western Take on an Eastern Practice

Asian and Hindu medicine have recognized the existence of prana or chakras for centuries. However, this knowledge didn't make its way West until quite recently. The first modern description of auras was made in 1729 by Sir Isaac Newton. He wrote about an "electro-magnetic light, a subtle, vibrating, electric and elastic medium that was excitable and exhib-ited phenomena such as repulsion, attraction, sensation, and motion."

Nearly 200 years later, Dr. Harold Saxton Burr defined this electrical nature of the body as life-fields. He was able to detect these "L-fields" in humans, animals, plant life, seeds, and even slime molds.

In recent years, orthopedic surgeon Dr. Robert O. Becker and his colleagues have estab-lished with certainty the relationship between regeneration and electrical currents in living things. For more than 30 years, Dr. Becker and his research team have shown that elec-trons flow through the cells of the nervous system, creating a magnetic field that can affect an organism's ability to sense and evaluate damage occurring anywhere in the body. This electromagnetic flow provides cells with ability to either maintain a healthy cell or stimulate healing within an injured cell. Many claim that this electromagnetic field is, in fact, chakra energies of the auric field.

Not surprisingly, all seven chakras are individually linked to neurological synapses (ganglia), small nerve bundles that operate like little brain centers. Each chakra then pro-cesses and remembers different emotional events and traumas that have occurred to you throughout your life. In fact, you can even store specific types of emotional memories in these centers.

This might explain why different types of emotional distress seem to affect one part of the body more than another. Often, when you have trouble dealing with the emotions and feelings associated with a particular chakra, the resulting constriction of energy flowing into the gland or body part also connected with that chakra can result in disease or a negative health concern.

Reading the Chakras

Each chakra has a color, emotion, gland, and body part associated with it. The first three chakras represent the earthly world, while the last three represent the spiritual realm. The middle one, or fourth chakra, connects these two worlds.

The first chakra is located at the base of your spine. It corresponds with large intestines, hips, and thighs, and is connected to the concept of survival and security. When out of balance, it can lead to instability, grief, and self-centeredness, as well as hemorrhoids, con-stipation, and sciatica.

The second chakra is located midway between your pubic bone and navel. It corresponds with your ovaries, kidneys, and bladder. It is also the center of your sexual relationships with others. When out of balance, it can cause you to be either over- or undersexed. It can also lead to fertility difficulties, menstruation problems, or kidney and bladder conditions.

DARLENE'S STORY

"Darlene" was a passionate woman who had enjoyed many sexual relationships, but few emotionally satisfying ones. At the age of 24, she married a classmate from graduate school. After four years of constant fighting, they divorced, leaving her alone with their child.

From that time on, she continued to have many sexual relationships, but she still could not become emotionally involved, feeling she could neither trust nor depend on the men she dated. During this time, Darlene also began to notice changes in her body. Her breasts became smaller and smaller (a sign her fourth chakra was shutting down), while her lower abdominal and pelvic area began to get larger and accumulate weight, a reflection of her expanding second chakra.

By the time she reached her 50's, Darlene suffered from ovarian cysts and fibroid tumors, reflecting, in part, the energy imbalance between her second and fourth chakras. She was also very unhappy about the excess weight that had developed in her second chakra area. However, neither dieting nor working out regularly at the gym corrected this imbalance in her figure. Until Darlene learns to open up emotionally and take it a bit slower sexually, she will continue to have difficulty correcting her figure issues.

KRISTINE'S STORY

"Kristine," an incredible, loving, selfless 60-year-old woman, is moderately overweight, with most of the weight in her upper body, especially in her breasts. This is likely due to the fact that she relates to those around her so strongly through her fourth chakra, the chakra that is associated with love and nurturing. But while she cares for others selflessly, she keeps her own problems, cares, and concerns to herself, not wanting to be a burden to others.

In addition to causing feelings of increased self-consciousness, her large breasts also cause a great deal of discomfort in her upper back, neck, and shoulders. After using a successful weight loss program, Kristine was able to lose 20 pounds, but she still hasn't been able to drop down a bra size or two, as she had hoped, because of the blockages in her fourth chakra.

Your third chakra is located between your navel and the base of your sternum. It corresponds with your adrenal glands, liver, stomach, pancreas, and small intestine. This chakra is responsible for feelings of personal power, as well as strong emotions like anger and greed.

When out of balance, it can lead to powerlessness, doubt, and aggression, as well as hypoglycemia, diabetes, poor digestion, and hepatitis.

The fourth chakra is located in the center of your heart. It corresponds with the thymus, your master immunity-regulating gland, as well as your heart, lungs, and breasts. How you give and receive love and nurturance resides in this chakra. When out of balance, it can lead to loneliness, passivity, insensitivity, or a state of over-selflessness, as well as breast diseases, stroke, high blood pressure, colds and flu, lung disease, and immune-related diseases.

The fifth chakra is located at your throat. It corresponds to your thyroid and vocal cords. It is associated with communication, self-expression, inspiration, and creativity. When out of balance, it can lead to obsession and lack of expression/communication, as well as laryngitis, stutter, and thyroid problems.

NANCY'S STORY

"Nancy" learned that it was unsafe to express her feelings with her family at a very young age. If she became angry or upset, she was severely reprimanded or punished by her parents. As a result, she learned to stuff her feelings with food. By the age of 11, she was one of the heaviest girls in her class.

Nancy's habit of shutting down her fifth chakra continued into her adult life. By suppressing her upsets, frustrations, and even sadness through overeating, she caused a ricochet effect on the organs associated with her third chakra—the chakra associated with the digestive organs and how personal issues are handled on an emotional level.

By the time she was in her mid 40's, Nancy was not only overweight, especially around her midsection, but she also suffered from heartburn and gall bladder disease, as well as hypothyroidism. While she has tried a number of dietary programs over the years, nothing will take hold permanently until she can change her pattern of stuffing her feelings with food, rather than unburdening her fifth (and third) chakra and expressing her emotions.

The sixth chakra, known as your "third eye," is located at the point where your eyebrows meet the bridge of your nose. It corresponds with your hypothalamus and pituitary gland, as well as your eyes, ears, and sinuses. It is associated with intuition, imagination, psychic abilities, and clarity of thought. When out of balance, it can lead to fuzzy thinking and intellectual stagnation, as well as eye disease, hearing loss, and sinus conditions.

Finally, the seventh chakra is located at the top of your head. It corresponds with the pineal gland and brain, and is associated with spirituality and your connection with God. When out of balance, it can lead to confinement and close-mindedness, as well as depression, insanity, epilepsy, and cranial pressure.

Reading the Chakras' Mind

Every chakra has an organ system, emotion, and specific health condition(s) associated with it. Use this chart to discover which of your chakras may be out of balance.

	First	Second	Third	Fourth	Fifth	Sixth	Seventh
Location	Base of spine	Midway between pubic bone and navel	Midway between base of sternum and navel	Center of your heart	Throat	"Third eye" between your eyebrows, where bottom of forehead meets top of nose	Top of your head
Emotion	Stability, security	Sexuality, creativity	Self-esteem	Love, nurturing	Self-expression	Intuition, inspiration	Spirituality
Organ System	Large intestines, hips, thighs	Ovaries, kidneys, bladder	Adrenals, liver, pancreas, stomach, small intestines	Thymus, heart, lung, breasts	Thyroid, vocal cords	Hypothalamus, pituitary gland, eyes, ears, sinuses	Pineal gland, brain
Health Concern	Sciatica, intestinal concerns	Fertility, menstrual issues, menopause, kidney or bladder problems	Ulcers, diabetes, digestion issues, low blood sugar, gallstones	Breast and lung disease, high blood pressure, stroke, heart disease	Thyroid concerns, laryngitis	Eye disease, headache, hearing loss	Insanity, epilepsy, depression

Promote Healthy, Balanced Chakras

I've found that the regular practice of affirmation and meditation are great tools for restoring health and balance to all of your chakras. Use each of these exercises daily to keep your "spinning wheels of health" moving in the right direction.

Healing Chakra Affirmation

I have developed the following affirmation to help heal and balance all seven chakras. These can be easily used and repeated for a few minutes each day.

First Chakra: I feel safe and secure in the world around me. All of my needs are satisfied.

Second Chakra: I have plentiful reserves of energy that nourish my femininity and my creativity.

Third Chakra: I handle my life with calm and self-confidence.

Fourth Chakra: I am a vehicle for love. I give and receive love and joy in all of my relationships.

Fifth Chakra: I express my thoughts, needs, and desires honestly, freely, openly, and completely.

Sixth Chakra: I see the world around me with perfect clarity. I trust my intuition as well as my intellect to guide the choices I make.

Seventh Chakra: I live every day of my life according to the spiritual beliefs I hold and cherish.

Balancing Chakra Meditation

This meditation is designed to soothe and reenergize your chakras, while also helping to enhance the flow of chi throughout your body.

1. Sit comfortably in a chair, with your arms placed gently at your side. Keep your feet firmly on the ground.
2. Close your eyes and breathe slowly and deeply—inhaling and exhaling slowly and fully.
3. Visualize a ball of golden light at the base of your pelvis, in the area of your first chakra. Feel the deep, healing energy the light emits.
4. Picture the ball unraveling into a long, thick cord with a golden weight on the end. This is your grounding cord.
5. Let this golden weight sink deeply into the earth until it reaches a spot where you feel grounded, safe, and secure.
6. Continue to breathe deeply, enjoying the feeling of your grounding cord establishing itself in this place of safety. Stay there for a few minutes.
7. When you feel relaxed, calm, and reenergized, open your eyes. Remember that your cord is in place and grounding you.
8. In this place of safety, allow your own negative energy (anger, frustration, judgments, and upsets), as well as those of others to be released from your body,

down your grounding cord, and back into the earth, where they are neutralized back into non-harmful energy.

9. Now picture this golden light and energy flowing up from the center of the earth, through your legs and into each of your chakras. Allow the energy to cleanse, nourish, and fill the chakras, helping them to spin in the proper direction as they become fully energized with loving, nurturing, healing energy.

10. When each chakra has been filled with the golden light, release the energy back down into the earth. Continue to breathe deeply, enjoying the feeling of healthy, balanced chakras and a strong, powerful grounding cord planted deep in a place of safety. Stay there for a few minutes.

11. When you feel relaxed, calm, and reenergized, open your eyes.

⋆ ⋆ ⋆

Discovering the relationship between your chakras, body, mind, and emotions gives you yet another step in your journey to great hormone health. In the next chapter, we'll take a look at how specific colors can give your chakras another boost, and how you can use those colors to generate health and happiness.

24 a rainbow of healing

Color can have a profound effect on physical and emotional health. Color therapy is based on the theory that every color has a different energetic pattern. When a particular color enters your eyes and hits your retinas, it is converted into its specific energy frequency. The energy then travels to your brain, which processes the color and triggers reactions that can affect your physical and emotional health. Color therapy has been used to heal conditions as diverse as menstrual disorders, insomnia, depression, anxiety, migraines, vision disorders, skin problems, digestive illnesses, asthma, dyslexia, and epilepsy.

The most convincing theory of how color affects your physical and emotional well-being is due to its effect on your body's chakras. Each chakra acts as a relay station, absorbing energy from the environment and distributing it to the specific organs associated with each of these energy centers. Your chakras also play an important role in translating emotional states into physical conditions and concerns.

As I indicated in the previous chapter, every spinning chakra creates its own energy field, the frequency of which determines the color of a particular chakra. As such, using the specific color associated with a chakra can help to alleviate specific emotional and physical conditions. For instance, the heart chakra's corresponding color is green and the emotion is inner harmony. Therefore, the color green, which resonates harmony and balance, can be useful in treating heart disease and hypertension. Similarly, the root chakra is associated with the color red, and regulates your body's strength and vitality. Disorders that can cause fatigue and lack of vitality, such as anemia, can be treated with the color red.

Make Color Work for You

Color therapy is a very easy technique—which is why I not only recommend it to others, but also do it myself! I've found that many women have a well-developed sense of intuition and will find that they instinctively choose or are drawn to colors that provide them with the energy that is deficient in their bodies. For example, women who are estrogen dominant and are suffering from the expansive effects of too much estrogen—or postmenopausal women who have retained many of the yin characteristics like excellent fluid reserves and a peaceful and calm mood, but are yang deficient and may lack libido, low energy, poor mental acuity, or have difficult losing weight—will find they are best with colors like red and orange, or even yellow. These colors are heating and help to dry up or contract the over-expansiveness that these women are suffering from.

Conversely, women who are estrogen deficient-fast processor will feel best with cooler, more energizing and expansive colors like blue, lavender, and green. These colors can reduce heat in your body, and promote more peace and calm, as well as more yin qualities in your body.

In addition, if you are anxious, you may decide to wear more cooling and relaxing colors like blue and green, which can help bring your emotions back into balance. Conversely, if you are feeling depressed, a bright red or orange outfit may be just the thing you need to perk you up! In short, choose colors that support what you are trying to accomplish. Wearing the "wrong" colors can literally worsen your hormone imbalance and possibly even your general health, even if the effect is subtle for some women.

And speaking of clothing, I also recommend that you organize your closet according to the chakra system—going from the cool, relaxing colors to the hotter, more energizing ones. This will help you match your wardrobe and jewelry to your mood and energy level each day.

You may also want to take inventory of the color palettes in your home. Are they working to enhance the mood that you are trying to set for your greatest health and well-being? For example, do you want your bedroom to be a room for peaceful, deep sleep and relaxation, or do you want it to create passion and enhanced sexual activity? If the colors of your home aren't helping you reach your goal of optimal health, it may be time to invest in a can of paint and repaint your walls!

The Chakra-Color Connection

Use the following chart below to can determine which color you should works best for your particular emotional or physical need.

	First	Second	Third	Fourth	Fifth	Sixth	Seventh
Color	Red	Orange	Yellow	Green	Blue	Violet	White
Mood	Stimulating	Revitalizing	Energizing	Balancing	Restful	Relaxing	Soothing
Health Condition	Nervousness, constipation	Appetite, breathing, reproduction	Digestion, nervous and liver function	Stabilize emotions	Blood pressure	Sleep, heart rate	

"Sarah" was an amazing 88-year-old woman who was a busy professional in the health-care and complementary medical field. When I spoke with her about her choice of colors in her wardrobe, she gave me a spirited and fun account of why she liked to wear warm colors like red and orange.

Sarah was an incredible and wise woman who had been active, strong, and healthy most of her life. She attributed her health, in part, to her understanding of the importance of balance. She would pick her clothes and jewelry each day by tuning into her body to determine what colors would best promote a healthy balance in her mind, body, and spirit.

Because she tended toward accumulating excess weight, a slower metabolism, and a more sluggish disposition, as well as large, sturdy bones, Sarah usually favored the hotter colors like read and orange, which picked up her mood, gave her energy, and even stimulated her metabolism.

A Colorful Exercise

Some of the more well-known ways to use color therapy include colored lights (more on this in the next chapter), visualizing with certain colors, using colored oils for a massage, wearing certain colors, painting your bedroom or living room a specific color, or even eating certain colored foods.

One of *my* favorite color therapy techniques involves using colored construction paper during my daily meditation practice. Follow these steps to take full advantage of the healing effects of color.

- Purchase 11x17 sheets of construction paper in the color you want. Use your intuition to pick the color you are most drawn to or those that stir up the emotion you desire or ease your particular physical ailment. If you are estrogen dominant (too yin), use hot colors like red, scarlet, and hot orange to dry out, shrink, contract. Conversely, if you are estrogen deficient-fast processor (too yang), use cooler colors like violet, lavender, and blue. Be sure you buy various shades of the color—such as hot pink, salmon, rose, etc.
- Place the sheets of paper up on a white wall or other white background.
- Sit in front of the color in a calm, relaxed manner. Make sure you are breathing slowly and deeply.
- Set your intention. Ask your body to use this color to balance your hormones and heal your tissues, organs, and/or mind. Visualize your body healing.
- Stay calm and relaxed as you look at the color for several minutes.

You can keep the sheets of paper up for several hours or even days after your session. Glancing at the colors every so often will provide a subliminal reminder of the healing you're trying to achieve.

A Colorful Meditation

As you perform this exercise, concentrate on the flow of chi as it transports the various colors throughout your body. At the end of this exercise, you should feel more vital, with your chakras freshly recharged and balanced.

1. Sit comfortably in a chair with your arms resting gently at your side.
2. Pay attention for a minute or two to your breathing as you begin to inhale and exhale slowly and deeply.
3. Visualize a pool of bright red energy below you, running deep beneath the earth.
4. As you take a deep breath, begin to feel that bright red energy slowly flowing into your feet and rising up your legs. As this energy fills your legs, you may feel a slight weight or fullness. You also may see with your inner eye the blocked areas or areas that are dark or muddied energy in your legs begin to melt away and disappear.
5. Next, let this bright red energy flow into your first chakra, filling your thighs, hips, and lower pelvic region.
6. As the first chakra becomes full, allow the excess energy to flow out of the chakra and back down into the earth like the cycle of life itself.
7. With the pool of radiant energy beneath your feet, change the color to bright orange, then yellow, green, blue, violet, and eventually white. Feel this energy as it moves up through your body, feeding and nourishing each chakra and its associated organs and tissues.
8. Let it flow out of each chakra, back into the earth.
9. When the color white reaches your 7th chakra, it should flow out of the energy center on top of your head.

* * *

Now that you understand how color can be used to balance your chakras, and therefore, your yin-yang duality, let's explore take color therapy one step further and discuss the amazing benefits of light therapy.

25

light your way to hormonal health

One of the most powerful ways to use color to optimize hormone health is colored light therapy. I love this type of therapy because it is so gentle, yet very effective in helping to bring women back into hormonal balance, especially when used in conjunction with my nutritional, diet, and other hormone-balancing programs that I discuss in this book.

Much like color therapy, the energy that your body takes in through light-emitting devices has a warming, contracting, drying, yangizing, and energizing effect when the red and orange part of the visible light spectrum is utilized. This can be very helpful for women with estrogen dominance. In contrast, the blue and violet part of the visible light spectrum is cooling, calming, relaxing, yin, and expansive to the body. This can be very useful for estrogen deficient-fast processors. Green is best to help promote balance between the two polarities.

I first became aware of the existence of colored light therapy as a third year medical student. At that time, I was doing my pediatric rotation, and I learned that colored light, specifically blue light therapy, was being used to treat jaundice in premature infants in order to protect them from brain damage.

The idea that such a gentle and non-invasive therapy could help save the lives of newborns was very intriguing to me. I decided to delve into the research and discover what other health conditions this amazing therapy could treat. I began to intensively study the medical research on colored light, along with a very good friend of mine who was a biophysicist at NASA and had a similar interest in this area. During the early 1980's, I purchased one of the first colored light lasers available in the United States, and he and I performed research studies on plant growth and laser therapy. My interest developed into a passion for the healing benefits of colored light, which continues to this day.

I personally experienced the tremendous benefits of red light more than 25 years ago. At that time, I was going through a period of intense fatigue, very likely triggered by too much stress and hard work. (I had a thriving and very busy medical practice, was teaching at Stanford University Medical School, and was taking care of my newborn daughter). Luckily, I pulled out of it pretty quickly and was able to regain my normal state of high energy and vitality.

Besides putting myself on a very strong nutritional supplement program, I started to take red light "baths." This not only restored my energy, but also helped me maintain hormonal balance, as I was more of an estrogen dominant type during this period of time.

Over the years, I have continued to take colored light treatments—especially bright energizing colors like scarlet, red, and orange—to support my mood and energy, and to balance my female hormones. I also used some of the more calming green and green-yellow lights. And, as I entered my late 50's, I found that my body really seemed to crave the deep, sustained energy that blue and violet light produces for balance. These calming colors also provided me with a wonderful quality of relaxation.

Even more wonderful is the fact that colored light therapy, when used properly, does not have any of the negative consequences and side effects that are often seen with conventional medical therapies, such as surgery and most medications.

The Early Research

Light therapy, particularly sunlight, has been in use since ancient times. In fact, in the early 1800's, physicians throughout the world believed that sunlight could cure a wide range of conditions, including inflammation, tuberculosis, and even paralysis. During this time, some studies even found that colored light produced dramatic effects on the brain and the nervous system. However, it wasn't until the 1870's that researchers began to look in earnest at the possible therapeutic benefits of colored light.

One of the pioneers in colored light therapy was General Augustus J. Pleasanton. In 1876, General Pleasanton reported that the use of blue light—from the sun or from an artificial source—was effective in stimulating the endocrine glands and nervous systems, both of which have significant effects on your mood, level of energy, and sleep patterns.

One year later, prominent physician Dr. Seth Pancoast filtered sunlight through panes of red or blue glass and found that this could either increase or decrease the activity of the nervous system, and that by these opposing colors, he could create emotional as well as physical balance in the body. More than a decade later, Dr. Neils Finsen took the treatment one step further and used red light to treat smallpox lesions.

The Twentieth Century

All of these early pioneers paved the way for more intense research on colored light during the 20th century. In the early 1900's, Dr. Harry Spitler began researching this type of therapy to treat patients. By the 1920's, his research revealed that certain portions of the brain that directly control both the autonomic nervous system and the endocrine system are regulated, at least in part, by light. He also discovered that light may play a very significant role in altering behavior and physiological function. In other words, simply altering the color of light entering the eyes could disturb or restore balance within the autonomic nervous system. In this way, light can not only affect your emotional makeup (mood, energy, etc.), but it can also have an impact on several physical functions, including sleep.

This research focus progressed significantly in the 1950's, when Russian scientist, S.V. Krakov discovered that the color red stimulated the sympathetic portion of the autonomic nervous system, while the color blue stimulated the parasympathetic portion. In 1958, Dr. Robert Gerard confirmed this finding.

In Gerard's study, blue, red, and white lights of equal brightness were each projected separately for 10 minutes on a screen in front of 24 normal adult males. He found that red light stimulated the sympathetic nervous system, increasing the level of alertness, excitement, and tension in the subject, while the blue and white lights stimulated the parasympathetic nervous system and generated a sense of calm and relaxation.

Research Today

One of the best-known and widely respected modern-day researchers of colored light is Dr. Norman Shealy, a neurosurgeon by training and a prominent practitioner of complementary medicine. He has taken the research on colored light therapy's effect on the brain one step further by actually incorporating light therapy into his practice, using flashing bright light and colored light to treat depression and pain. Dr. Shealy has found that stimulating colors like red and relaxing colors like blue and violet has an effect on many neurochemicals, neurotransmitters, and even hormones, including sex hormones.

In one research study that he conducted, he found colored light therapy had dramatic effects on female sex hormones, the precursor hormones such as DHEA, and the neurochemicals and neurotransmitters that regulate hormones. In this study, he found that red light increased the level of 14 out of the 40 neurochemicals and hormones measured, while green light affected 20, and violet light affected 15. This study and others like it have led to a fascinating field of research called syntonic optometry. One of the key areas of research in this field includes the effect of colored light on neurochemicals that regulate female hormone production.

Thanks to all of this research, color therapy is currently used by practitioners such as psychologists and acupuncturists to help restore and enhance healthy hormone function, as well as emotional and physical well-being. On the "hot" end of the visible light spectrum, deep and bright red and orange lights have been shown to create energy, stimulate sex drive, regulate menstruation, ease migraines, and alleviate depression. Conversely, the "cool" end of the visible light spectrum (namely blue and violet) is very relaxing. In addition to improving sleep quality, these colors can help to lower blood pressure, heal tissue damage, alleviate seasonal affect disorder (SAD), and even treat acne! Green is the color in the middle of the visible light spectrum, and is often used to provide balance to the body.

How Colored Light Works

Colored light is absorbed into your body through your eyes or skin. When taken in through the eyes, colored light is converted into electrical impulses through the action of millions of cells that are sensitive to light and color. The electrical impulses move along the optical nerve to the hypothalamus gland in the brain, which regulates a variety of body functions including breathing, digestion, temperature, blood pressure, mood, and sexual function. The resultant stimulatory effect that light has on the hypothalamus can affect the hypothalamus's action on the pituitary gland. The pituitary controls the secretion of many hormones, including luteinizing hormone (LH) and follicle-stimulating hormone (FSH), both involved with the menstrual cycle. The pineal gland, located in the brain, also receives light waves through the eye, which are then transformed into nerve impulses capable of affecting hormones. The hypothalamus, through the pineal gland, also controls the body's internal clock, the circadian rhythms that pace and synchronize biological events.

When taken in through the skin, colored light can penetrate up to one inch in the soft tissue. By traveling energetic pathways, light therapy has a therapeutic effect on the endocrine glands and other organ systems.

Now, let's take a more detailed look at the two types of therapeutic light therapy colors that are the most helpful for female hormonal balance and overall health and well-being.

Healing Benefits of Red Light

As I mentioned at the beginning of this chapter, red light greatly boosts energy, and is very useful for estrogen dominance, due to its heating and contracting effects on the body. Russian biophysicist Tiina Karu, Ph.D., of the Laser Technology Center in Moscow, studied these and other effects of red light therapy. She is one of the most renowned researchers on red light in the world, and I first learned of her impressive and tremendously compelling body of research on red light back in the mid-1980's.

Dr. Karu and other researchers made a landmark discovery in the way red light affects our bodies at the cellular level. Various wavelengths of red light easily penetrate the skin and stimulate energy production within the mitochondria, the energy-producing powerhouses of the cells. They enable the energy from food to be released and trapped as high-energy bonds called adenosine triphosphate (ATP). ATP is found in all of our cells and releases energy needed to fuel nearly all chemical reactions in our bodies. Thus, red light therapy helps your body create energy, vitality, and stamina, so every tissue and organ system can run more efficiently.

In general, red light is profoundly anti-aging and promotes health, strength, and vitality for virtually every organ in the body. It helps ease hormone-related conditions such as PMS, irregular menstrual cycles, menstrual cramps, bloating, lack of libido, energy, stamina, and poor mental acuity in postmenopausal women with excellent yin reserves, but who suffer from symptoms of yang deficiency. Since these women tend to have slower metabolisms, red light therapy helps them to lose weight by speeding up their metabolism through the sympathetic nervous system. It has also been found to have a stimulatory effect on the pituitary and immune systems.

More specifically, red light has been used to heal bone conditions such as osteoarthritis and fractures. It also helps to relieve pain and inflammation in joints, muscles, and tendons, and stimulates the healthy circulation of blood to tissues. Red light also helps to heal repetitive stress syndrome such as carpal tunnel syndrome, and skin conditions such as varicose vein ulcers and diabetic wounds. Plus, it improves blood flow to the heart in individuals with coronary artery disease, eases migraine headaches, improves energy levels in women with chronic fatigue, and helps reduce chronic lymph-related edema in women who have undergone mastectomy for breast cancer.

A number of studies have also found that when certain photosensitive chemicals are injected into cancerous tissue, the chemicals selectively accumulate in cancer cells. The tissue is then exposed to red light, which activates the chemicals and destroys the cancerous tissue.

ROSE'S STORY

"Rose" had suffered from a terrible pain in her neck for several years. It was so bad that she had to hold the back of her neck just to look up.

She had seen every type of health practitioner under the sun—conventional doctors, chiropractor, massage therapist, acupuncturist, and on and on. Nothing worked. In time, they all told her the same thing—she would have to learn to live with the pain.

During this time, Rose attended a conference on natural and alternative health therapies. One of the exhibitors had a red light laser device and gave Rose a demonstration. He used the laser on her neck for three minutes and the pain went away. More miraculous was that the pain never came back!

Rose borrowed one of these lasers for 30 days. She used it every day and felt amazing. All of her aches and pains disappeared and her mood was great. However, within a week of sending the laser back to the manufacturer, she began to feel terrible. She was depressed and found herself crying all the time for no reason.

When Rose told me about her experience, it was obvious to me that she had a very significant red light deficiency that would require on-going light exposure. Rose and I discussed this, and she immediately purchased an LED red light blanket for home use. She started using it every other day for 15 minutes at a time. She now enjoys a pain-free life, fantastic mood, and very positive outlook on life.

Red Light and Hormone Health

Red light triggers sympathetic nervous system function, which causes your heart and pulse rate to speed up, your muscles to tense, and your body to get rid of excess fluids through increased urination. Plus, more calories are burned up and utilized for energy.

You may benefit from red light therapy if you are estrogen dominant or an estrogen deficient-slow processor. Many women with excess estrogen suffer from a slower, more sluggish metabolism, excess weight that can be difficult to lose, constipation, fluid retention, PMS, fluid-filled cysts in the breasts and ovaries, fibroid tumors, and irregular periods. If this sounds like you, red light can be helpful.

Red Light and Migraines

I've been aware of the use of red light therapy to treat migraines for years, and have even seen my own mother benefit from using it for her headaches (see sidebar for her story). Unfortunately, this information has never been reported by the mainstream media, until a study conducted at San Jacinto Methodist Hospital in Baytown, TX, was reported a few years ago in *Family Practice News*.

In the study, researchers gave dark red contacts to 33 patients, predominantly female, with a history of light-sensitive headaches. They found that 31 patients enjoyed pain relief within 90 minutes, and 26 reported a complete absence of pain. Of those who had total pain relief, most patients experienced relief within five minutes, and approximately 50 percent relief was obtained within 20 minutes. And five lucky participants felt relief within 10 seconds after putting in the second lens. Researchers concluded that "red-tinted contact lenses provided rapid, safe relief to most patients with acute migraine pain."

I believe that one of the reasons red light works so well to treat migraines is that it reduces inflammation and stimulates the healthy circulation of blood to tissues—both of which are critical factors when treating migraine headaches.

If you are interested in trying red contact lenses, work with an ophthalmologist or optometrist to ensure the proper fit. For an ophthalmologist in your area, log on to *www. aao.org*; to find an optometrist, visit *www.aoa.org*.

MY FAMILY HISTORY

My grandmother, my mother, and my daughter (at puberty when she was entering her teenage years) all suffered with migraines. I can still remember my Grandma Rose hiding in her darkened bedroom until her migraine pain and sensitivity to light went away.

continued on next page

My mother, also a physician, suffered terribly from migraines. I can remember my father, a doctor himself, throwing up his arms in frustration since no known medication effectively prevented or stopped her painful and debilitating chronic migraines. Even my daughter Rebecca wasn't free from this family legacy, enduring the pain of migraines when she reached puberty. Don't ask me why, but my sister and I are the fortunate ones: in the last four generations of women in my family, we're the only ones who have never had a migraine. And believe me, I appreciate that blessing!

Fortunately, my mother and daughter were able to overcome their migraines with a program that included a diet that eliminated headache triggers, a regimen of nutritional supplements that corrects underlying imbalances, and light therapy. In fact, my mother completely prevented any recurrence of her migraines for many years by using red light therapy.

Red Light and Pain

Red light has been used to treat pain and stiffness for several decades with great results. In one study, 100 patients with chronic neck and shoulder pain due to osteoarthritis, muscle spasms, or a sprain were divided into two groups. In the first group, participants were exposed to a red light laser for up to 90 seconds, while the second group was exposed to a "fake" laser. Sixty-five percent of the group who received the red light therapy enjoyed a 30 percent reduction in their pain, while less than 12 percent of the people in the "fake" laser group saw this level of relief.

A separate study, also with 100 participants, had similar results. In this study, people who received red light laser therapy noticed significant pain reduction after just one treatment, and the pain continued to be eased or even diminished after 24 hours.

Red Light and Lymphodema

Several years ago, a report on the use of red light therapy in the treatment of post-mastectomy secondary lymphodema was published in the journal *Lymphology*, and the results were promising. Women treated with red light therapy once or twice a week for 10 weeks showed measurably less arm swelling, edema volume, and tissue pressure, and marked improvement in subjective complaints, including "aches/pains, tightness, heaviness, cramps, pins/needles, and mobility of the arm," with even greater improvement in the hand and forearm.

The women in the study also showed gradual softening of the skin and tissues, as well as improved skin integrity. Over a three-year period, some of the improvement in their symptoms gradually decreased, but their arm swelling, pressure, and hardness all continued to show improvement.

In a more recent, double-blind, placebo-controlled Australian study published in *Cancer*, 61 women with post-mastectomy lymphodema received 16 red light treatments twice a week for six weeks, then once a week for four weeks, for approximately 10 minutes each session. At the end of the 10 weeks, 31 percent of the women enjoyed a measurable decrease in swelling, volume of edema, and hardening of the upper arm. Plus, they enjoyed these benefits for an amazing six months after the red light treatments were discontinued.

Red light has also been shown to help activate the local immune system by stimulating the specific types of white blood cells that kill, consume, and/or carry away pathogens. This creates a more sanitary cellular environment, thereby reducing the risk of skin infections—a significant problem for women with lymphodema.

Finally, red light is reported to enhance the activity of *phagocytes*, cells that are thought to help reduce tissue swelling by breaking down protein-based debris in the damaged area, including excess scar tissue. The overall effect in the treatment of secondary lymphodema appears to be the creation of a healthier tissue environment, with faster regeneration of damaged vessels and enhanced circulation.

Red Light and Circulation

Several studies have shown that red light therapy enhances circulation. One study in particular illustrates this point in the case of peripheral neuropathy (PN). In a double-blind study from the *Journal of Diabetes Complications*, 2,239 patients with PN found that infrared light therapy relieved numbness and neuropathic pain by 66 and 67 percent, respectively.

In a separate study from *Acta Diabetologica*, an eight-week course of infrared therapy in 22 patients with long-standing, profound PN brought reversal of symptoms. Scientists believe the therapy stimulates nitric oxide production, which improves circulation and nerve function.

JACKIE'S STORY

"Jackie" is a dear friend and colleague of mine. Early in May 2003, her husband "John" developed flu-like symptoms. While they rarely sought conventional medical help, he felt so awful that they made an appointment with a doctor.

After a brief examination, the doctor told John that he had "swimmer's ear." However, after a few days, John's condition became even worse. Jackie noticed that the right side of his mouth was drooping and his eye looked strange. They went back to the doctor, who acknowledged that he had misdiagnosed John. This time, he said that John had Bell's palsy.

continued on next page

JACKIE'S STORY   *continued*

Jackie was skeptical of this new diagnosis, and rightly so. Within a couple of days, John's health deteriorated quite rapidly. He could no longer eat, drink water, or eliminate. Eventually, he became so ill that at about 2:00 in the morning, John fell and Jackie couldn't get him up. Still unclear where she found the strength, she was able to get him down the stairs and to the emergency room.

Once there, the doctors tried to tell her that he was simply constipated. It took her 15 hours, but she was eventually able to convince them that they needed to admit him. At that point, the doctors went into high gear. They did an MRI and discovered that John had suffered a stroke.

While John was recuperating in the hospital, Jackie was scheduled to host a personal empowerment conference. Nearly 80 percent of the attendees also happened to be in the healing arts. During the conference, Jackie told the participants about John's condition. Afterwards, a woman named Sandy approached her about a cold, red light laser that she used. She told Jackie that her aunt had also had a stroke and that the doctors had written her off. Sandy used the laser on her aunt, and soon after the treatment, the aunt was up and walking around, asking for something to eat. Sandy offered to treat John with the laser.

Jackie told John about the device, but he declined. Seeing as he was still in the hospital, he didn't think it would be appropriate. However, a week later, once John had been released and was resting at home, he agreed to let Sandy treat him.

Jackie watched as Sandy used the device on John. Sandy placed the laser on the base of his neck, where the stroke had occurred. Jackie watched in amazement as the distortion in his face completely disappeared and his face returned to normal. Afterwards, John regained his speech, his balance, and most everything.

While John still has some diminished range of motion in his right shoulder, he and Jackie are both convinced that the red light laser was responsible for giving him back his life and dignity.

Red Light and Cancer

With the use of a technique known as photodynamic therapy, researchers have been able to use red light to selectively kill cancer cells for more than 30 years. In photodynamic therapy, a physician injects the patient with a dye that is selectively taken up by cancer cells. When activated by ultraviolet light, the cells actually show up as bright red. This not only allows the physician to make a diagnosis of cancer, but she can also use the UV light to mark where the cancer is located.

Once the cancer is identified, the physician uses a red light laser to target the cancer cells. Within hours of the treatment, the cancer cells begin to die, leaving the surrounding, healthy tissue unharmed.

Photodynamic therapy has been used successfully to treat more than 3,000 cancer patients with a wide variety of malignant tumors all over the world. In fact, when used in combination with surgery, chemotherapy, radiation, and/or immunotherapy, photodynamic therapy successfully reduces the size and occurrence of tumors 70–80 percent of the time. Photodynamic therapy is most commonly used to treat gynecological, colorectal, and metastatic breast cancers, as well as cancers of the bladder, lung, and esophagus. In addition to photodynamic therapy, protocols are available to treat a variety of cancers with red light laser therapy alone.

EXCITING NEW DEVICE

There is an exciting product gaining interest in the realm of light therapy and cancer—a hand-held imaging device called iFind. This machine is about the size of a deck of cards and uses infrared light, which is just outside of the range of visible light, right next to the red side of the spectrum. The device is primarily used to detect breast cancer by monitoring the differences in blood oxygen ratios in normal tissues versus growing cancers. Plus, the infrared light measures blood flow in different areas of the breasts. Since tumors require large amounts of blood to grow, those areas of your breasts that indicate greater blood flow may indicate an abnormality.

Early research studies have found that iFind has an extremely high success rate in detecting cancerous growths. It takes just five minutes to use, and if atypical blood flow is detected, the device beeps out a warning.

Red Light for Macular Degeneration

Red light is currently being used in a revolutionary new way—to treat age-related macular degeneration (AMD). Charles McGee, M.D., an innovative researcher in the field of colored light therapy and the developer of the "X Light," shared several case histories with me regarding individuals who used red light therapy to successfully treat AMD, including one 80-year-old woman with intermediate AMD. After using a red LED (light emitting diode) in each eye for 10 minutes each day for several months, her vision improved perceptibly.

While the exact mechanism of why red light therapy may specifically benefit AMD is not yet known, I suspect that red light works, in part, by improving the production of ATP within the cells of the eyes, thereby promoting the healing process. Still, I would love to see more research done in the area of colored light therapy for eye disease, since it holds so much promise.

In the meantime, if you are interested in the use of red light therapy to treat AMD, I suggest you seek a physician who has experience with colored light therapies, rather than try to treat AMD with colored light on your own.

AMERICA IS BEHIND THE TIMES

While red light therapy has been widely used throughout the world, it is only in limited use here in the U.S. Why? The FDA does not recognize it as a viable treatment, even though NASA has used it to treat astronauts for years, particularly for wound healing. As a result, most conventional physicians don't offer it.

This is unfortunate, as many well-designed, double-blind, placebo-controlled studies have been conducted with red light therapy in Canada, England, Australia, Norway, Turkey, Austria, Greece, Brazil, and Ireland. They have looked at red light's ability to treat a variety of conditions, including osteoarthritis, infected wounds, burn scars, ankle sprains, bone implants, bone defects, and surgical incisions—all with significantly positive results.

Hopefully, with more education and patient demand, the U.S. will catch up with the rest of the world.

Healing Benefits of Blue Light

Researchers have only recently begun to delve into the rich, healing benefits of blue light. And they are finding some pretty amazing results. As I indicated earlier, blue light is highly successful for treating infants with jaundice. But other studies have shown it has more far-reaching potential.

Blue light can be helpful for women with estrogen deficiency. It has also been shown to be effective in healing injured tissue and preventing scar tissue, treating several types of cancers and non-malignant tumors, skin and lung conditions, jet lag, and insomnia, as well as raising serotonin levels. Additionally, research from the American Association for the Advancement of Science has found that blue light is helpful for a myriad of psychological issues, including depression (particularly seasonal affect disorder), anxiety, anorexia, bulimia, and alcohol and drug addictions.

Blue Light and Hormonal Health

Cooling, calming, and relaxing blue and violet light therapy can be beneficial for women suffering from estrogen deficiency. As you know, women with this imbalance are more like to suffer from the uncomfortable symptoms of excess heat, hot flashes, insomnia, mood swings, anxiety, arthritis, muscle aches and pains, and vaginal and skin dryness.

Blue and violet light therapy can help to cool down, calm, and relax estrogen deficient-fast processors who are feeling too anxious and overstressed. Calming down the brain, nervous system, and metabolism can help to bring these types of estrogen deficient women back into better hormonal balance and restore their yin.

Blue Light Increases Serotonin Levels

Several very recent studies, most notably from the Thomas Jefferson Medical College in Philadelphia, have found that blue light is critical for the suppression of melatonin production. One study looked at the way nine different colors of light, ranging from indigo to orange, affected 72 healthy volunteers. The participants were examined at midnight, when melatonin levels are usually the highest. The volunteers' pupils were artificially dilated. They were then blindfolded for two hours. Researchers took blood samples, exposed the participants to a randomly selected hue of colored light for 90 minutes, and then took another blood sample from the volunteers. They found that those participants who were exposed to blue light had the greatest changes in melatonin levels.

As we discussed back in chapter 11, melatonin is produced from serotonin. Therefore, the researchers concluded that when melatonin production is suppressed, the level of serotonin in your brain increases. This can have a whole range of physical and emotional benefits, including easing PMS symptoms, depression, and anxiety.

Blue Light and Rheumatoid Arthritis

A study from Dr. Sharon McDonald found that when rheumatoid arthritis (RA) sufferers were exposed to blue light, the majority enjoyed a significant degree of pain relief. Dr. McDonald had 60 women with RA place their hands into a specially-designed box while she shined blue light onto their hands for up to 15 minutes. Even with such a short exposure time, most of the participants experienced a significant amount of pain relief.

McDonald concluded that the reduction in pain was specifically due to the blue light, as well as the length of time participants were exposed to it. She found that the longer a patient was exposed to blue light, the greater their chance of reduced pain.

Blue Light and Acne

Researchers conducted studies at two different sites in the U.S., where they exposed more than 50 patients to blue light on one side of their face for 15 minutes twice a week. At the end of one month, half of the participants experienced a significant reduction in acne. This improvement continued for another month, and was maintained for three more months following the treatment.

A second study was performed on nearly 300 men and women in Mexico and Europe. In this study, researchers exposed the patients' whole face to the light. They found that 74 percent of the participants had significant improvement, with only seven percent exhibiting no response. They also found that the blue light treatment had no negative side effects. I believe this because isolating only the blue portion of the visible light spectrum eliminates the potentially more dangerous invisible bands of ultraviolet light that have been linked to sun burns, skin aging, cataracts, and increased risk of skin cancer.

Based on these and other similar studies, the Food and Drug Administration (FDA) has approved a new, physician-administered, high-intensity, narrow-band blue light device to treat moderate acne. The treatment works to destroy the bacteria that cause acne, thereby helping to heal the skin.

USING COLORED LIGHT

The goal of colored light therapy is to help create a balance within your body. If you are estrogen dominant, you need red light to help you contract and heat up. Conversely, if you are an estrogen deficient-fast processor, you'll want to veer more towards blue light to soften and cool down.

Whichever color makes the most sense for you, I suggest that you start with the light of that color, and as your emotions and level of energy come back into balance, you can begin to work with both types of colored lights. Once you are in good emotional and energetic balance, you'll want to use both colors to support and strengthen your brain, nervous, and hormonal systems.

Use Red Light if You Have...
- Estrogen dominance
- Estrogen deficiency–slow processor
- PMS
- Fluid retention
- Cysts in breasts or ovaries
- Irregular menstruation
- Depression
- Lack of zest for life
- Mental confusion/sluggishness
- Severe obesity
- Difficulty losing weight
- Edema, false fat
- Chronic fatigue
- Low energy
- Low libido

Use Blue Light if You Have...
- Estrogen deficiency–fast processor
- Anxiety
- High blood pressure
- Hyperthyroidism
- Stress
- Insomnia
- Impatience
- Dry skin/tissues
- Acne
- Diarrhea

Applying Colored Light to the Body

In addition to regular exposure to natural sunlight, you can use colored light in three different ways: lasers (which are mainly used for red light therapy), light-emitting diodes (LEDs), or a colored glass or gel filter. Unlike the light bulbs we use in our homes and offices that radiate light throughout the room and are made of many colors, lasers travel as a single beam in one direction and are made up of a single color. Traditionally, there have been red light lasers, though new lasers are now becoming available that utilize other parts of the color spectrum. For example, blue lasers are effective for mood and brain function, while violet is great for treating infection, including dental-related infectious issues such as gum infections, cavities, and root canal infections, as well as infectious diseases in general.

Lasers comprise one of the fastest growing areas of energy medicine. They offer amazing versatility, and can be extremely beneficial for a wide range of conditions, including menstrual and hormonal issues, cancer, soft tissue injury, brain and neurological diseases, emotional imbalances, and macular degeneration.

Don't confuse these types of lasers with the "hot" lasers used by surgeons to cut, cauterize, and destroy tissue. Light-therapy lasers have a powerful regenerative and healing effect upon many different types of sick or injured tissues. They use coherent energy, which is the same energy used by the cells in your body to communicate to one another. This is one of the reasons lasers are the most efficient energy your body can use to regenerate tissue and increase blood flow. Plus, research is showing that the coherent energy of lasers helps to stimulate the nervous system. This is an exciting area that we are learning more and more about every day.

While these types of lasers are generally safe, they have traditionally been used by health care professionals (although wonderful red lasers have now become available for self-care use at home and are tremendously helpful).

Specific wavelengths of light can also be transmitted through LEDs, which is an excellent method for women who want to use colored light therapy on a self-care basis. Each diode is very small; in fact, the red LEDs currently being used by NASA to promote wound healing of astronauts are no larger than a pinhead. But when linked together, these diodes form a flat panel of colored light that produces a beam that is broader than that of a laser. Unlike a laser, specific wavelengths of LEDs can be used simultaneously with other colored light bands to expand their therapeutic benefits.

The great thing about LEDs is that the light they emit is completely safe and can be used on such sensitive areas as the eyes. Plus, they are much safer to use than lasers, can be bought by anyone, and are readily available for purchase.

The third way colored light is transmitted is through a simple, filtered light. This form of light therapy was practiced in ancient times, and today involves placing a red glass or theatrical gel filter over a common light bulb or a full-spectrum fluorescent bulb, or even in glasses or a contact lens!

LIGHT CREATES COHERENCE

Several years ago, I was doing a research project and looking at tissue samples under a microscope. What impressed me the most were the visible differences between the tissues of children and the elderly.

The cells of healthy children were beautifully organized and neatly lined up in rows, with clear and clean-looking margins. These cells were such a pleasure to look at because they were so orderly and coherent.

In contrast, the cells and tissues of elderly people who suffered from a variety of health-related conditions were not nearly so lovely to look at. Their cells looked like they had truly suffered from the ravages of time. The cells were often irregular in shape, with overlapping and even messy-looking margins. Like a messy desk or closet, they had lost their sharp, clean edges and looked disorganized and incoherent.

One amazing benefit of colored light therapy is that its energizing and balancing effect on tissue helps to restore its coherence and structural and functional integrity, thereby helping to restore its health.

Self-Treating With Colored Light

Colored light can be placed on many different parts of your body. I prefer the area three finger-widths below the navel. You can also use your "third eye"—the point directly between your eyebrows, where the bridge of your nose meets your eyebrows—or the area in the center of your breastbone, at the level of your heart. However, you should avoid this area if you have a pacemaker or known heart disease.

Treatment sessions can last anywhere from just a few minutes to as long as 15 minutes (or even longer if appropriate), depending on what feels most comfortable to you. Not all women need or should use prolonged light therapy. Start out by using any light therapy device for shorter amounts of time (just a minute or two) in the beginning until you know how your body will respond.

If you find that you enjoy colored light therapy and want to use it as part of your regular health program, it is important to be aware that your emotions and level of energy will likely change as you move through different life stages. As this occurs, you may find that you need to modify your colored light program.

Choosing a Light Device

I have reviewed a wide variety of colored light therapy devices. If you are interested in using colored light at home, I recommend the following companies that produce high-quality light devices. (I've also included these companies in the Resource Guide.)

- For an excellent red light laser that can be used on a self-care basis or for professional use, I recommend the Lazr Pulsar 4 from Next Generation Therapeutics (*www.ngtlasers.com* or 866-918-0399). This is the laser I personally use myself.
- For a superb laser that uses probes with different wavelengths of colored light, including red, green, blue, and violet, as well as infrared, I highly recommend (and personally use) the new NGT I, also from Next Generation Therapeutics (*www.ngtlasers.com* or 866-918-0399). While the NGT I is targeted for the professional market, this versatile device can also be bought for home self-care.
- For a very high quality LED device, I recommend the X Light from the Chee Energy Company (*www.cheeenergy.com* or 888-263-9214).
- For a red light only device, I recommend the Red Light Shaker from the Light Energy Company (*www.lightenergycompany.com* or 800-544-4826).
- For an excellent filtered, colored light device, I recommend the Photon Stimulator from LifeForms (*www.photonstimulator.com* or 800-233-1754).
- If you are interested in using light to treat stress, I highly recommend Dr. Shealy's RelaxMate II (*www.soundstrue.com* or 800-333-9185).
- Another great device to treating stress is the emWave Personal Stress Reliever from the Institute of HeartMath (*www.heartmath.org* or 831-338-8500). This amazing device uses colorful LED displays and audio feedback to help you reduce stress by showing you how to create heart-centric, positive emotions.
- If you are interested in trying light therapy for your skin, I recommend the Verilux Happy Skin light unit (*www.verilux.net* or 800-786-6850). I find this device to be particularly exciting because it uses both blue and red light to reduce the bacterial count of acne, as well as the inflammation of the skin's pores.
- To help stimulate your scalp and promote hair growth, I recommend the Viatek HairPRO Laser Hair Treatment Brush (*www.drlark.com* or 800-941-1997).

Note: Colored light therapy is extremely safe; however, I suggest that you consult the manufacturer of the light unit you purchase to see if there are any contra-indications between your condition and their particular product.

Benefits of Sunlight

Sunlight consists of *all* wavelengths of light, those that are visible, and those we cannot see, such as the ultraviolet light associated with tanning and the infrared light associated with heating. The full range of frequencies is necessary to insure physical, mental, and emotional well-being, as the different wavelengths act on the body in specific ways.

As I said earlier in this chapter, the health benefits of light have been appreciated since ancient times. More recent research has proven that various types of light therapy, especially natural sunlight, can enhance hormone production and balance.

Daily exposure to natural sunlight is essential for maintaining robust health. Sunlight is necessary for the timely development of secondary sexual characteristics. Boys who are blind have been observed to have delayed spermatogenesis and onset of ejaculation, and blind girls have delayed onset of menstruation. One theory of how this occurs, based on studies on hibernating animals that remain in darkness for long periods, is that the absence of light suppresses the excretion of gonadotropins (gonad-stimulating hormones) from the pituitary gland.

Everyone needs around one-half to one hour of sunlight each day, taking care, of course, to shield sensitive areas of your body with a good sunscreen to prevent skin damage. However, most people, unless they have jobs that involve outdoor work, spend the majority of the day shielded from sunlight. Window glass, windshields on cars, sunglasses, clothing, and suntan lotion all block sunlight. Smoggy air can also reduce our exposure. Even the coveted corner office, which can have windows on two walls, is not bright enough to be truly life-supporting. Outdoor light is about 100 times more intense than the normal lighting inside a building.

Worse yet, most people in the workforce spend much of their time indoors working under artificial light, much of which is fluorescent. Fluorescent light is not full spectrum, as the wavelengths are not equivalent to those of sunlight. This distribution of wavelengths is particularly noticeable when you purchase clothing in a store under fluorescent lighting, only to find that the color is different in sunlight. You get the same effect of distorted wavelengths from fluorescent street lights: The colors of cars do not appear the same as they do in daylight. When you work under fluorescent light, you are in essence being undernourished light-wise, because the amount of the various color wavelengths differs from that of sunlight and may even be deficient in certain parts of the light spectrum.

Fluorescent lights also emit three types of harmful radiation—X-rays, radio frequencies, and extremely low frequency radiation. Working too close to or working for a long time under fluorescent lighting can reduce the activity of the immune system due to the effects of these radiations. Finally, older fluorescent lighting fixtures were underpowered, causing the lights to flicker. This flickering can cause extreme eye fatigue and affect mental and physical performance in the workplace.

Sun's Absence Can be SAD

The short, dark days of winter can also limit your access to sunlight. Some individuals are sensitive to this seasonal change. Light deprivation can cause them to feel depressed and tired as well as suffer from a reduction in mental clarity. This condition is known as seasonal affective disorder (SAD). While levels of several neurotransmitters in the brain—including melatonin, serotonin, and dopamine—have been implicated in the origin of SAD, the underlying culprit seems to be decreased exposure to sunlight.

Individuals with SAD may have difficulty getting out of bed in the morning and may tend to isolate themselves socially. They may show less interest in sex. Symptoms of PMS, such as irritability and moodiness, may also worsen. The darker winter days are also associated with decreased fertility. It is thought that these changes occur because the lack of sunlight disrupts the natural pacing of hormone production. Such changes in personality, due to hormonal alterations, can stress personal relationships and even affect job performance.

If you doubt the power of decreased sunlight to produce such a constellation of symptoms, consider these points. We know that sunlight triggers cycles and seasonal behavior in animals, including reproduction, hibernation, migration, and molting. Also, a mere 1.4 percent of Floridians suffer from SAD, but almost 10 percent of the population of New Hampshire is plagued by the condition. Moreover, the symptoms of SAD begin earlier for people who live farther north, and abate when they visit sunnier southern climes in the winter.

If you or someone you love is prone to SAD, you should, if possible, spend one to two hours in the sun every day during the winter months, when the sun's radiant energy is at its weakest. Indoor lighting from incandescent or halogen bulbs should also be kept bright.

Additionally, many people have had great success with light boxes. One study, published in *ACTA Psychiatrica Scandinavica*, found that subjects with SAD experienced significant reductions in their depression scores after two weeks of daily exposure to 2,500 lux cool-white fluorescent light between 6 A.M and 8 A.M. Another study from the National Institutes of Mental Health investigated the ability of light boxes to nudge subjects with SAD into their sunnier summer state of emotional well-being. Short winter days were stretched by six extra hours of light—three before sunrise and three after dusk. Each subject was exposed to fluorescent light approximately 20 times the intensity of normal indoor lighting, kept at eye level. Symptoms eased and energy levels rose within days.

Many other investigators have reported similar success stories, making light boxes a widely accepted treatment for SAD. The typical light box available today provides 10,000 lux of bright indoor lighting. (In contrast, sunshine produces 100,000 lux.) The light spectrum used in this product provides minimal exposure to the more harmful ultraviolet and blue rays and tends to emphasize the red rays, which have a mood-elevating effect. The box is positioned one to three feet away from the user, who is free to exercise, read, or work. My patients generally find that 30 minutes of exposure each day, preferably in the morning, is all that's needed to improve mood and reduce SAD symptoms. Certain individuals require longer exposure, up to two hours.

JANE'S STORY

By the time "Jane" came to me for help, she was 49 years old and had spent two perfectly miserable winters suffering from SAD. During her initial consultation, she told me that she had always had a tendency towards feeling mildly depressed, particularly during the week or so before her menstrual periods (when she suffered from PMS). She reported that when she entered menopause at age 47, she began to notice a worsening fatigue during the winter months.

As the days grew shorter, she had trouble just getting out of bed. She felt "blue" and less sociable. She didn't feel "up" for anything, including her normal exercise routine. Come spring, she observed, the symptoms reversed, only to have the cycle repeat the next winter.

Jane had read about the connection between light deprivation and mood before coming to see me. She wondered if she might be suffering from SAD—and was determined not to spend another winter feeling blue.

I suggested that she buy a light unit designed to treat SAD. The results exceeded Jane's expectations. The way she described it, the light treatments were like a "cushion" that prevented her from sinking into depression.

That first winter with the light unit was the best Jane had experienced in years. Using the light unit didn't just relieve her symptoms, it put her back in control of her life.

---

* * *

Colored light therapy and full-spectrum light are both great ways to further support hormone production and health. In addition to getting regular doses of natural sunshine, you can use different hues to bring your hormones back into balance, depending on if you are estrogen dominant, estrogen deficient-slow processor, or estrogen deficient-fast processor. Once your hormones are balanced, you can use a wide spectrum of color to stay in harmony.

Now, let's turn our attention to frequency medicine. We'll discuss how vibrations can help a wide variety of hormone-related health conditions, and what you can do benefit from this type of therapy.

feel the vibration of great health

26

Frequency medicine is by far my favorite form of energy medicine, due in large part to its critical, fundamental benefits to health and well-being. It can be a terrific therapy for women who are estrogen dominant, estrogen deficient-fast processor, or estrogen deficient-slow processor and trying to regain the healthy middle ground of hormonal balance. It is also a fantastic treatment for virtually all other health-related issues.

In the same way that every living thing has an aura or energetic field, all life forms also have a unique energy and frequency. Every cell of your body vibrates at its own specific frequency. The collection of these cells (organs and tissues) vibrates at a different frequency rate than everything else. Not only do organs have their own vibrational rate, but everything else on the planet does as well, including neurotransmitters, vitamins, food, and even emotions.

Similarly, healthy organs and tissues, and even positive thoughts and emotions vibrate at a different rate than unhealthy ones. For example, a healthy liver vibrates differently than a diseased one. The same goes for healthy emotions such as joy, happiness, peace, and calm as compared to negative, emotional vibrations such as anger, resentment, jealousy, and fear, which can literally make you sick. In fact, frequency is completely tied to the concept of life itself because when your cells are moving constantly and pulsing, you are alive. When your cells stop moving and vibrating, you will die.

Moreover, every human being on the planet has the ability to detect the individual vibrations of the people around them. This is the reason that you can tell when someone is looking at you or has entered a room, even if you don't hear or see them. You just *know* they are there.

This model of vibration and frequency underlying the health of all your tissues and organs, and even the existence of life itself, has been supported by many, many research studies. Let me begin to explain it by starting with a more commonplace example—the healing benefits of sound, which is also based on vibration.

The Sound Frequency

Sound therapy can dramatically help to enhance your energy, balance, and mood, and even greatly improve your health, primarily through the therapeutic use of music. While sound therapy is just now coming into more prominence as an effective health-enhancing therapy, this practice has been around for thousands of years. In fact, the earliest record of its use dates back to 600 B.C. when Pythagoras of Samos first lured animals out of the forest by playing his dulcimer.

In more recent times, Dr. Manfred Clynes from Vienna has shown that music does indeed deeply affect emotions, creating a brand new field of science known as sentics to highlight his research. In a nutshell, he found that certain classical music pieces can trigger very specific emotions, regardless of the listener. He tested this by creating a special "finger transducer" that measured the unconscious, downward pressure patterns in a person's fingertip—a technique to detect a person's emotional state. (The technique is so reliable that a similar device is often used by criminal investigators to determine a suspect's level of guilt.) Dr. Clynes found that different pieces of classical music created different patterns of pressure that were consistently associated with a range of emotions.

Medical researcher Sharry Edwards built on this and set out to determine how sound affected a person's physical health, but she took a slightly different approach. Ms. Edwards discovered that she had the ability to "hear" different sound frequencies that were being emitted by different people. She went on to actually record these frequencies, then played those frequencies back for the individuals.

What she learned was that when the person heard their own unique frequency, it had a healing effect on them. The sounds Ms. Edwards was hearing were actually missing frequencies in the person's energy fields. When the missing frequency was replaced (by playing back the person's unique sound for them), healing was able to occur.

Ms. Edwards tested her theory on a number of people, two of whom I'd like to discuss. In the first case, a man was suffering from severe zinc poisoning. He was in critical condition, plagued with several strokes and major organ system failure. Ms. Edwards then played his "key sound frequency" for him, and within 15 minutes, his vital signs had stabilized. Skeptical, the doctors turned off the tape and the patient reverted back to critical condition within minutes. Once the tape resumed, the patient stabilized once again. After continued exposure to the tape, the man was eventually able to get rid of all of the excess zinc in his system.

In the second case, a man who had been involved in a serious motorcycle accident had shattered his kneecap, lost his entire tibia (outside bone below the kneecap), and severed a major artery. Although doctors were able to save his life, they declared that he'd never walk again. Using frequencies based on the atomic weights of calcium and magnesium (the main minerals in bone), Ms. Edwards was able to help the man not only significantly reduce his pain, but also begin walking within 10 weeks. Amazingly, his x-rays also showed that he had actually grown a new kneecap!

The Science of Sound

In their book *Creative Healing*, Dr. Michael Samuels and Mary Rockwood Lane explain, "Sound is what our ears pick up from vibrations moving through air. There are actually air molecules moving in space. There is a motion with a rhythm and a frequency moving in space and time. Our bodies pick up the sound with our ears, and the rest of our body picks up the vibrations in every molecule of every cell."

This may explain the visceral reaction people have to classical music versus heavy metal or other, harsher forms of music. And plants are no exception. Fascinating studies on the healing effects of music have also been done in the field of agriculture. Researchers have found that when plants were exposed to music—Bach, 1920's jazz, or the sitar music of the famous Indian musician Ravi Shankar—the plants demonstrated greater growth activity. When these plants were exposed to hard rock music, they were all dead within two weeks.

Music or sound therapy has been used to treat emotional disorders such as stress, anxiety, and depression, as well as physical conditions like hormone imbalance, heart disease and high blood pressure, diabetes, insomnia, excess weight, arthritis, and even cancer.

Stress and Anxiety

Ralph Spintge, MD, executive director of the German-based International Society for Music in Medicine, looked at the effects of soft, tonal music such as slow Baroque or classical on nearly 97,000 patients before, during, and after surgery. Ninety-seven percent of the patients said that the music helped them relax during their recovery.

Heart Disease

A different study from a hospital affiliated with the University of South Carolina looked at the effect of slow, calming music such as Bach, Vivaldi, Bizet, and Debussy on 20 coronary patients. The researcher found that the music did indeed lower blood pressure.

Similarly, a study from *Applied Research* found that calm, soothing music reduced systolic blood pressure (from 124.3 to 118.6 on average), diastolic blood pressure (78.8 to 75.7 on average), heart rate (91.2 to 89.6 on average), and mean arterial pressure (94.3 to 75.7). Anxiety also decreased, as did pain. One patient even commented, "It was the only 30 minutes of peace I've known in days."

Insomnia

Another study from the *Journal of Holistic Nursing* found that Baroque and New Age music helped 24 out of 25 patients improve their quality of sleep. Several were even able to stop taking their sleep medication.

Excess Weight

Dr. Chen, a physician from China, tested the effects of music on herself. She had been steadily gaining weight over the last four years and was developing many of the symptoms of obesity. She started a holistic weight loss program that consisted of music therapy, exercise, and diet. She listened to a specially-designed weight loss CD three times a day before meals, did a few moderate exercises before eating, and drank some traditional Chinese herbs. Within a month, she had dropped nearly eight pounds. After four months, she had lost 40 pounds.

Rheumatoid Arthritis

A study performed at Lutheran General Hospital in Chicago looked at the effects of classical music on the physical and psychological symptoms of rheumatoid arthritis patients. At the end of 18 weeks, researchers found that patients enjoyed significant improvement in both pain and psychological stressors.

Cancer

Finally, professional jazz musician Fabien Maman teamed up with Hélène Grimal, a senior researcher at the National Center for Scientific Research in Paris. Together, they looked at how a wide variety and frequencies of sound could affect blood cells, hemoglobin, and specific uterine cancer cells. They discovered that even the lower volume of 30–40 decibels caused noticeable changes within the cells. Best of all, as the sounds moved up the scale, the cancer cells would "explode," while the healthy tissues and cells surrounding them remained stable and intact.

Clearly, sound can be a powerful, healing therapy. When it comes to using sound therapy, be sure to choose music that fits your particular hormonal profile. If you have estrogen dominance or are an estrogen deficient-slow processor, you'll want to choose music that is faster-paced and revs you up. The best music would be jazz, tango, and Russian symphony music. If you are an estrogen deficient-fast processor, then slower-paced music that calms and quiets you is more in order. I recommend classical music, waltzes, etc. You can also benefit from nature sounds, such as ocean waves and rainfall, both of which have been shown to bring about a sense of peace and relaxation.

PLAY IT AGAIN, SAM

There is a plethora of research heralding the healing benefits of classical music. These studies have found that classical music can help to heal a variety of health conditions, including:

- AIDS
- Arthritis
- Cancer
- Depression
- Heart disease
- Obesity
- Schizophrenia
- Alzheimer's disease
- Back pain
- Chronic fatigue
- Diabetes
- Menopause symptoms
- Parkinson's disease

Exceptional Healers

Like Chinese medicine, sound therapy also has its share of truly exceptional healers. I'd like to highlight three for you—Paul Scheele, Luanne Oakes, and Robert Aviles.

Paul Scheele

Paul Scheele is the co-founder and creative program designer for the Learning Strategies Corporation, a globally successful, premier developer of self-improvement, education, and health programs. Paul has designed and delivered over 50 different programs relating to professional and personal development.

What makes Paul so unique and exceptional is his ability to teach people how to tap the other 90 percent of the mind that most people never use. He does this by combining his education in biology and human development with a diverse, experiential background in neuro-linguistic programming (NLP), accelerated learning, preconscious processing, and universal energy.

This unique blend has led to several innovative techniques, namely paraliminals. Paraliminals use neuro-linguistic programming—a combination of original music and multiple voices—to guide you into a state of relaxed alertness. The voices deliver messages to different parts of your brain through both the right ear (which feeds the left brain) and the left ear (which feeds the right brain).

The content of Paul's messages differ depending on how each part of the brain best accesses information. Paul uses more logical, linear messages for the left brain, which is more analytical. He then uses softer, more metaphorical and allegorical images and messages for the right brain, which is more intuitive. This allows the listener to more readily make the major shifts in his or her state of physical and emotional health and spiritual evolution, as well as improve the quality of their life.

I am a huge fan of Paul Scheele's music and techniques, particularly his new Sonic Access program, as well as his paraliminal CDs, which use powerful, vibrational sound frequencies to help align your body's own energy systems and bring about amazing, long-lasting changes. If you'd like to learn more about paraliminals, Sonic Access, and any of Paul's techniques, visit *www.learningstrategies.com/SonicAccess* or call 866-292-1861.

Luanne Oakes

Luanne Oakes, Ph.D., has studied both Western and Eastern philosophies for nearly 30 years, focusing primarily on sound, light, and color therapies. She does an amazing job of blending soothing music with verbal, energetic, and vibrational qualities in nearly all of her work.

Medical doctors, psychiatrists, energetic healers, and business people the world over have used Dr. Oakes' teachings and expertise to bring about amazing changes in their own lives. I am particularly fond of her *Spiritual Alchemy* and *Sound Health, Sound Wealth* CDs, both of which are available from Nightingale Conant (*www.nightingale.com* or 800-323-3938).

Robert Aviles

I have recently been using the therapeutic music of world-class musician and composer Robert Aviles, based on the recommendation of a dear friend. The first night I listened to his relaxation CD entitled "Lullaby," I had a distinct improvement in my sleep quality. I slept deeper and more soundly than I normally do, and woke up feeling delightfully refreshed. I have been using it every night since then, with the same results. (See Tammie's story for how Robert's music also helped correct her very serious sleep imbalance.)

One of the most interesting things about Robert is that, other than the basic group classes in grade school, Robert is a self-taught violinist. He played all four years in his high school orchestra, as well as his community orchestra for two years. But music wasn't the only thing Robert excelled at. He was also a bit of a chemistry whiz. He was selected as one of the

TAMMIE'S STORY

Over the last several months, Tammie had become increasingly sensitive to electromagnetic frequencies (EMFs). She became so sensitive, she could "detect" the three cellphone towers' radiation within about a half-mile radius from her home.

This sensitivity caused several serious challenges. She had pain in her hands, short term memory loss, lethargy, difficulty sleeping, and she couldn't use the computer for more than five minutes at a time. She even had to wear silver gloves, a silver hat, and a silver apron to shield her body just to check email. Tammie's problems became so debilitating, she was planning to sell her home.

Of all her difficulties, her sleep issue was the worst. She searched everywhere and tried everything that she thought would help, including products that marketed EMF protection. In many cases, the products didn't work at all, worked for a short time, or even made matters worse.

Then Tammie heard about Robert Aviles' wonderful healing music, as well as the Intention Energy Nanovibe pendant. By gently balancing the left and right sides of her brain, the music and pendant were able to reduce and even eliminate her symptoms. Within five days, Tammie didn't have pain in her hands, could work easily on the computer, and was calm all the time. She could think clearly and was no longer having short term memory problems. She now feels like a new person. She has even decided that she didn't need to move after all, and took her house off the market.

top 50 students of Chemistry in a national competition, and went on to major in pre-med at California State University of Long Beach.

After four years of medical courses, Robert turned his focus away from biology and pre-med and back to music. After two additional years of college study in Composition and Common Practice Theory, Robert went on to receive private study, with an emphasis on counter point and fugal composition. This earned him the equivalent of a Master's degree in Composition.

During his college years, Robert began performing with local groups and working to evolve his sound, instrument, and message. He quickly moved from being a featured musician in a band to forming a group of his own, creating a sound that was innovative and uniquely Robert's.

But Robert never entirely let go of his desire to heal. In 1992, he became a certified Reiki healer and apprenticed under a Native American medicine man from 1993 to 1994, where he discovered the power and intricacies of healing energies. He rounded out his learning in 1994, when he began to study astrology.

Through all of this experience, learning, and practice, Robert began to see the deep and powerful connection between music, energy, and healing of the mind and body. Based on these insights, he developed "Star Songs", in which Robert would translate your own, personal astrological chart into a musical composition. He also teaches and leads seminars in Spiritual Awareness, Healing, and Meditation classes.

Robert founded Music Research Technologies, which is dedicated to the research of music, healing, and spirituality. Additionally, he holds workshops in Cymatics, the study of the relationship between sound and form, as well as in music, healing, and spirituality.

For more information about world-class performer, composer and musician Robert Aviles or to purchase his innovative and inspiring music, visit *www.healinglullabies.com* or *lifeisgood@iegroupusa.com*.

AN EXCEPTIONAL HEALING EXPERIENCE WITH LIGHT AND SOUND

As you likely know by now, I am a passionate advocate of light and sound therapy, and I want to introduce you to one of the newest, most innovative treatment modalities currently in use. It's called The Life Vessel, and it will change your life.

The Life Vessel is a large, enclosed, cutting-edge unit in which the clients lay down for the session. The Life Vessel combines light, sound, vibration, and frequency to assist your body's own natural healing abilities through detoxification, removal of stress, and rebalancing your autonomic nervous system, which regulates every unconscious function within your body and is vitally important for a balanced and properly functioning immune system.

Developed by Barry McNew in 1998, The Life Vessel uses patented technology that is safe and non-invasive. The Life Vessel has gone through nine years of clinical evaluation and testing to substantiate its effectiveness. Positive feedback and testimonials are being collected through the parent facility in Arizona, as well as clinical data in Pittsburgh, PA, where there is a Life Vessel center under the supervision of Valerie Donaldson, M.D.

Dr. Donaldson is the first Medical Doctor to open a Life Vessel center. She first contacted me more than five years ago to share with me the exciting results she had been finding with her patients using the Life Vessel, and the research findings continue to be extremely positive. She currently has on-going clinical studies involving heavy metal detoxification and anti-aging effects in patients using The Life Vessel.

continued on next page

The Benefits of Biofeedback

Next, I want to introduce you to the concept of biofeedback (if you are not already familiar with it). The most beneficial energy-medicine devices are based on this concept. Biofeedback operates on the idea that you have an innate ability to control physical functions in your body. In essence, you can train your body to respond to different stimuli, therefore warding off pain. It's been used to successfully treat migraines, fibromyalgia, arthritis, and back pain.

Biofeedback techniques vary, but they all require the use of devices that measure particular bodily functions—muscle tension, skin temperature, sweat gland activity, brain waves, or heart rate. Once you know the rate of these functions in your body, you can train yourself to manipulate them to achieve the result you want.

For instance, if you suffer from migraines, you can learn to raise the temperature of another body part, such as your hands. This increase in temperature redirects blood flow from the painful, swollen blood vessels in your head, eventually making your migraine subside.

Biofeedback can also help to bring your entire hormonal system back into balance. It is particularly useful for hormone-related issues such as menstrual cramps and endometriosis.

I love biofeedback because you can do it on your own at home with the use of a variety of devices. But for best results, have a few sessions with a trained practitioner. Once you've learned how to control your body's responses, you can practice biofeedback on your own much more effectively.

The Body of Research

There is an enormous amount of research supporting the use of biofeedback for a wide variety of health conditions, including menstrual cramps, migraines, vaginal dryness and pain, high blood pressure, loss of bladder control, and even constipation.

Biofeedback is particularly useful for estrogen dominant women who suffer from menstrual cramps. Because biofeedback helps you determine when your muscles are tense and when they are relaxed, you can learn to move them from a cramped state to one of relaxation. In a study from *Applied Psychophysiology and Biofeedback*, researchers tested nine women with severe menstrual cramps to determine if thermal biofeedback would provide any relief. They tested the women for six months and found that the women did, indeed, enjoy a reduction in their symptoms. Moreover, the benefits lasted for at least two additional months following treatment.

According to a study published in the *Journal of Pediatric Psychology*, researchers at the Children's Hospital in Boston and the University of Pittsburgh tested the effectiveness of biofeedback on children with migraines. Researchers divided 34 children (average age: 12.8 years) into three groups. The first group practiced hand-warming biofeedback, as well as stress management training. The second group practiced hand-cooling biofeedback, and the last group was told they were on a "wait list." Both treatment groups received four biofeedback training sessions, as well as a portable biofeedback machine they could use at home. Researchers found that the children who used hand-warming biofeedback not only achieved a greater improvement in alleviating their migraines, but were able to maintain the improvements for up to six months after the treatment.

Numerous studies have supported this finding for children and adults alike. In fact, even the *Journal of the American Medical Association's* Migraine Information Center lists biofeedback as a successful tool for treating migraines and other tension-related headaches.

Cornell University Medical College has particularly exciting news for women suffering from vaginal dryness and pain, particularly during sexual contact and tenderness to the touch at the entrance to the vagina. Researchers tested 33 women who suffered from vulvar pain for two to six years. Using a portable biofeedback instrument in their homes, all 33 women practiced stabilizing their pelvic floor muscle tone over a 16-week period—strengthening their voluntary contractions, while decreasing the at-rest pelvic muscle tone. By the end of the study, their pain decreased an average of 83 percent. Before the study started, 28 of the women had not had intercourse for an average of 13 months because of discomfort, but by the end of the study, 22 had resumed intercourse. At the six-month follow-up, the benefits were still present.

Similarly, biofeedback has been used successfully to treat menstrual cramps. To do this, you will insert a thermometer-like device into your vagina, much like a tampon. The device is connected to a digital readout machine that monitors your internal temperature. By using the data recorded on the readout machine, you can consciously work to increase your temperature. This will lead to better blood flow and muscle relaxation in your pelvic area, which translates to less severe cramps.

Another study, this one from *Obstetrics and Gynecology*, found that biofeedback is a wonderful treatment option for stress incontinence. Researchers found that 69 percent of women who used biofeedback-enhanced Kegeling saw relief, versus 50 percent for Kegeling alone. A similar study published in the *American Journal of Physical and Medical Rehabilitation* found that 62 percent of women using biofeedback were cured versus only 28 percent with Kegeling alone.

A study published in *Biofeedback and Self-Regulation* found that 26 out of 40 patients with high blood pressure were able to successfully complete one year of biofeedback-assisted relaxation. Researchers measured the patients one, two, and three years after treatment. They found that 31 percent, 38 percent, and 72 percent, respectively, continued to meet the criteria for success. Some of the patients were also able to maintain lower levels of anxiety, cortisol, blood pressure, and muscle tension over a long period.

According to research presented at the annual meeting of the American College of Gastroenterology, biofeedback is also effective as a long-term therapy for the most common cause of chronic constipation. Dr. Satish S.C. Rao and colleagues at the University of Iowa tested 52 patients, 47 of whom were women, on the effectiveness of a three-month biofeedback program versus standard therapy (diet, exercise, and laxatives). Twelve months later, those using biofeedback had significant improvement in bowel movements and reported greater satisfaction with bowel function than those using the standard therapy.

Using Biofeedback

In addition to its effectiveness, one the best things about biofeedback is that you can use it at home.

If you are looking for a general biofeedback machine to balance hormone function and overall health, I recommend the Healing Rhythms System from Sounds True (*www.soundstrue.com* or 800-333-9185).

If you are looking for a biofeedback machine to ease vulvar pain and reduce the pain from menstrual cramps, try the Pathway STM-10 Vaginal and Rectal Intracavity Stimulator from the Prometheus Group (*www.theprogrp.com* or 800-442-2325).

If you are interested in trying biofeedback to help reduce leaks caused by stress incontinence, I suggest using "Myself" (available at many drugstore chains or at *www.dependonmyself.com*) and "PMTx" (available at *www.biolifedynamics.com*). Both are easy to use and come with detailed instruction manuals for first-time users.

Finally, if you would like to find a qualified biofeedback therapist in your area, contact the Biofeedback Certification Institute of America (*www.bcia.org* or 303-420-2902). You may also be able to get a referral through your doctor.

Measure Energetic Frequencies With EPFX-SCIO

The EPFX-SCIO is my very favorite and, I feel, the most powerful and effective biofeedback-based device currently available. This device blends biofeedback with the ability to send therapeutic, corrective frequencies to parts of the body that are either under stress or ill.

The result is a machine that can make energetic adjustments and help restore the "energetic blueprint" or vibrational pattern of many substances and processes—including hormone levels, neurotransmitter levels, blood pressure, coronary artery circulation, neuromuscular reactivity, and mitochondrial function. Likewise, EPFX-SCIO has many powerful frequency programs available to treat pain associated with arthritis, rheumatism, fibromyalgia, muscle inflammation, traumatic injury, and even emotional and spiritual imbalances to help the user evolve on all levels of the body, mind, and spirit. The body then takes this "energetic blueprint" and utilizes it to make changes in its own frequencies toward greater health optimization. As a result, your body can better create greatly improved health and well-being.

The Pioneering Spirit of Energetic Healing

I was first exposed to frequency therapies almost 30 years ago by my friend, Dr. Hazel Parcells, a holistic health practitioner who founded two healing centers in New Mexico. She utilized this type of therapy extensively, using a Rae machine from England, where most of the research in this field has been done. She used the machine on herself as well as others, and she credited it with being one of the reasons she lived to be 106 years old, enjoying great health and a productive life all the while.

Frequency therapy works by neutralizing negative frequencies and helping to restore your body's normal, healthy frequencies, thereby providing you with the energetic blueprint of your own body. Your body can then use this blueprint to help restore the structure and function of your organs, tissues, cells, and even emotions. It helps to energetically regenerate your cells, so your body regains the ability to produce healthy chemicals at healthy levels, as well as to literally regenerate the structure of your body, such as your bones and joints.

Today's Modern Take

Like everything involving technology, the EPFX-SCIO takes the concept and functionality of correcting and normalizing the frequencies of your body, mind, and spirit to a whole new level.

This device was developed by Bill Nelson, a brilliant mathematician. He developed computer software that combines the widely-accepted concept of biofeedback with the groundbreaking abilities of energetic healing. The result is the EPFX-SCIO. In fact, the machine is so exceptional that even the FDA has recognized it as a biofeedback device!

However, it differs from both biofeedback and energetic machines in several critical ways. First, biofeedback teaches you to control your physical conditions with your mind. The EPFX-SCIO uses the biofeedback principle to detect abnormal and aberrant frequencies within your body, and sends you the normal, healthy frequency for your body to utilize and readapt.

Second, the EPFX-SCIO is a software system that is run by a computer. Although the computer and software are electric, the interface between you and the machine is purely energetic.

Lastly, and most interestingly, the EPFX-SCIO also has superb analytic capabilities, far beyond that of any other current biofeedback device. By interfacing with your unique energy field, the machine can test you for thousands of different electrical and chemical indicators. And with speeds of 1/100th to 1/1,000th of a second, the machine can analyze you for more than 10,000 parameters of health, including physical, chemical, emotional, mental, and even spiritual.

Then, in a matter of three minutes, the machine organizes these parameters and ranks them in order from those that are most urgently needing treatment to those that are in the healthy range (anything between 80 and 100 is normal). It also distributes this information to over 200 different programs (biofeedback, acupuncture, chakras, enzymes, adrenal, hormonal, etc.) so you can begin treatment.

RAE'S STORY

Rae started getting ill back in 1995. She was suffering from panic attacks that became so overwhelming she couldn't go more than two miles away from her house. Her mental function also began to severely deteriorate—at times she didn't even know who or where she was.

Seven years later, her hands began shaking so badly she couldn't function. She couldn't get the key in her door, couldn't eat soup, and couldn't type on the computer. It was soon discovered that she suffered from Parkinson's disease, as well as lupus-like symptoms.

While Rae was not in pain, the mental anguish was excruciating. She used to love to dance and socialize with friends, but now was reduced to living like a recluse. Eventually, she stopped leaving her house altogether, and had to rely on friends and neighbors to bring her food and tend to her yard.

After exhausting all my suggestions for treatment, and seeing a tribe of homeopathic physicians, chiropractors, and herbalists to no avail, she began to consider suicide. During what she thought was her final visit to see her son in California, she regained hope.

She met her son's girlfriend, Chandra, who was an EPFX-SCIO practitioner. She told Rae she could help her. Chandra told her about an amazing, cutting-edge technology that generates healing frequencies to reverse the energetic patterns of disease. She immediately began treating Rae, and after just eight treatments, Rae began to consciously notice some profound physical changes.

The shaking went away, the mental clarity started coming back, and most importantly, Rae began to feel like herself again. Today, Rae doesn't shake at all anymore. She is now able to drive and her windows are always wide open, letting in the sunshine where before she lived in darkness. She embraces each day, thanking God that she is not just living, she is alive and thriving!

JOY'S STORY

"Joy," a 47-year-old physical therapist, came down with a terrible case of the flu. She had vertigo, nausea, diarrhea, and headache. It was almost as if she had motion sickness. She felt totally ungrounded and intensely ill, and couldn't imagine how she'd possibly recover.

Joy knew she should get herself on her EPFX-SCIO machine, but was too ill to work it herself. She called a close friend and asked her to come over and help her. Joy hooked herself up to the machine and told her friend what buttons to push.

After three or so hours, Joy felt significantly better. She firmly believes that the machine saved her and allowed her to resume her normal, busy schedule much more quickly than she had expected.

My Personal Experience

I was first exposed to this technology three years ago and began using it a year ago to deal with a very old stress pattern that I was having difficulty getting at any other way. I found it to be tremendously effective in helping me balance my mood, energy, and even hormonal health.

Some Words of Advice

While an Internet search on EPFX-SCIO will likely turn up lots of Web sites and practitioners, there is only one Web site that I recommend—*www.QuantumEducation.com.*

QuantumEducation.com has been developed to provide comprehensive educational programs and training to EPFX-SCIO practitioners, based on my own extensive research with this device.

The reason I am so comfortable recommending Quantum Education is because I know all about it from the ground up. A colleague and I have collaborated for the last four years to design and implement an innovative treatment approach that greatly enhances and expands the power and capability of this device to help restore one's physical health and well-being. In addition, emotional and spiritual blockages that are so disruptive to one's health, including a woman's hormonal health, can be eliminated much more rapidly and in a much more gentle and non-traumatic fashion with my programs.

All levels of EPFX-SCIO training from beginner to advanced are available. Quantum Education will also be offering a variety of training programs for other energy medicine devices such as cold laser therapy. The company also provides a wide variety of educational materials, products and services to the public. For more information, call Quantum Education at 888-674-8227.

To find the name and number of a well-trained, careful practitioner, call Quantum Source for Life at 877-488-4359. Once you find a practitioner in your area, be sure to ask them about their experience and training background, as I've found that getting the most out of your treatment depends largely on the skill of the practitioner. Also, tell them absolutely everything you can think of regarding your health history—your emotional and spiritual as well as physical health. Remember, the EPFX-SCIO is a holistic treatment device.

Next, don't use the machine for testing more than once or twice a week. If you want to do treatments in between your testing session, you need to wait at least 72 hours, as after you do a test and treatment session, your body will be in flux for 1–4 days.

During this transitional period, your body is literally evolving and transforming itself to a higher and healthier state. As a result, you may experience symptoms of detoxification (such as old memories or emotions, fatigue, a mild headache, or a stuffy nose), for a day or two as your body gets rid of whatever caused it to be ill in the first place. Also, don't allow the practitioner to go too heavily into programs that break you down (such as the detox programs), as excessive use can throw you into a severe and prolonged detox. Instead, when doing the detox program, ask them to also concentrate on programs that build you up at the same time.

Finally, be realistic about the time it takes to make these changes. While you may see dramatic changes after your first session, it can take weeks and even months to heal completely, depending on the chronicity and severity of the problem.

Another Fascinating Option

Another fascinating application of therapeutic frequencies is NRG cards. The cards look like a credit card, including a strip on the back. Each card has been imprinted with a wide variety of very beneficial, therapeutic frequencies, depending on the issue that it is helping to resolve. Like the EPFX-SCIO, these frequencies help to create new "energetic blueprints" that your body can then utilize to create a state of greatly improved health in many areas of your life. This helps to promote a much higher level of physical, emotional, and spiritual health and well-being. The range of issues that the specific cards help to deal with is quite varied. They include:

- abundance
- acne
- allergies and asthma
- anti-aging
- anxiety and stress
- arthritis
- autoimmune disease, including lupus, rheumatoid arthritis, and Crohn's disease
- bladder health
- high blood pressure
- blood sugar imbalances
- chronic fatigue
- dental health
- depression
- digestive concerns
- estrogen deficiency issues, such as hot flashes and vaginal and tissue dryness
- estrogen dominance issues, such as PMS, fibroids, endometriosis, and edema
- fibromyalgia
- heart health
- immunity
- infection
- improved libido
- love and joy expander
- respiratory diseases
- optimal nutrition
- acute and chronic pain
- positive life enhancing emotions
- positive relationships
- skin health and appearance
- sleep, calm, and relaxation
- thyroid disorders

When used in conjunction with a good, nutritional and lifestyle-based program, these cards can help to promote healthy hormone balance in women of all ages. Some women reportedly noticed the benefits immediately, while others enjoyed a slower, gentler therapeutic benefit.

NRG cards are produced by a device called the Quantum NRG Bioimprinter. These devices are also available for purchase so that you can make your own cards. Once you purchase an NRG card, it is impregnated with your own particular vibrational pattern by placing your thumbprint on the card. You can then carry the cards with you in your bra, pocket, or placed under your pillow at night while you sleep. I love using my own NRG cards, and use them frequently for promoting better overall health.

You can purchase cards for a very reasonable cost from *www.nrgcards.com* or 888-674-8227.

DIANE'S STORY

"Diane" worked as a night nurse for six to seven years. She went into work about 9:00 or 10:00 P.M. and worked until 7:00 A.M. She had to rearrange her schedule, as well as her internal clock, so she could sleep during the day.

When Diane left her job and returned to a more normal schedule, she found that she had a very difficult time sleeping at night. She had so conditioned herself to work in the evenings that her mind wouldn't slow down and shut off. She'd just lay there thinking about her "to do" list, what she had accomplished during the day, and what she needed to do the next day.

As a result, she had a difficult time falling asleep or staying asleep. When she did sleep, even her dreams were "busy," and when she woke, she was drained, as if she had indeed worked through the night.

Diane heard about the NRG cards and decided to try a "night calm" energy card. She did and it worked! She could relax at night and sleep well. Her dreams returned to a more peaceful, calming nature, and she awoke refreshed and recharged. And because she keeps the card under her sheets, it seems to have had a beneficial effect on her boyfriend. He has even stopped snoring!

FREQUENCIES IN WATER

In his book *The Hidden Messages in Water*, Japanese scientist Masaru Emoto has discovered an amazing, yet simple fact—words, emotions, and even music have a profound effect on water. Specifically, he found that when he exposed the water to different words or different kinds of music, different types of crystals form, and in some cases, no crystals form at all.

The short version of his research is that he would write a word or phrase on a piece of paper, then wrap the paper around the jars of water, with the words facing in towards the water. In other cases, he would play a variety of music in the presence of the water. He would then place the water in a Petri dish and freeze the dish at -20ºC (-4ºF) for three hours in the freezer. According to Dr. Emoto, "The result is that surface tension forms drops of ice in the Petri dishes about one millimeter across. The crystal appears when you shine a light on the crown of the drop of ice." Finally, using high-speed photography, he took a picture of the crystal. To ensure that there were no confounding factors involved, he used different types of water, usually distilled water.

The resultant images are nothing short of amazing. It is difficult to put into writing how deeply the feelings behind the words affected the water. But more importantly, it may provide one explanation of how and why emotions have such a profound effect on your health.

Dr. Emoto found that the word "wisdom" created beautifully-formed crystals, regardless of the language the word was written in. Similarly, when exposed to the words "thank you," the water always formed stunning and complete crystals. And like the word "wisdom," the types of crystals that resulted were always similar, even when the word was written in seven different languages.

Interestingly, when water was exposed to words that create emotional distress, such as "You fool" and "You make me sick," no crystals formed at all. But far and away, the most beautiful crystal was the one formed by the words "love and gratitude."

You may be asking, "How can this be possible? Water reading words or listening to music?" The answer is simple—vibrations.

As I said earlier, every living thing has a vibration and a frequency…including water. According to Dr. Emoto, water is the "transporter of energy throughout the body." He maintains that this is due to vibration and resonance. I couldn't agree more.

Think about a time when your husband, partner, co-worker, or child simply walked into the room, and you immediately knew what kind of mood they were in, even before you saw their face or they said a word. You can't explain it, you "just knew." That is emotional vibration.

Electromagnetic Frequencies

Electrical frequencies are involved in all the chemical reactions of your body. Everything that takes place within your body—whether normal or abnormal—creates a change in your body's electrical field. When you are healthy, these frequencies are very stable. When you are ill or have a disease, the cells misstep and lose their healthy frequency.

By using electromagnetic therapy (EMT), you can enhance overall cellular function and boost your body's ability to heal itself. Research and treatment with EMT began back in the 1930's, but until recently, the world just wasn't ready for it. The brilliant and pioneering scientist and orthopedic surgeon Robert O. Becker did pivotal research in the 1960's, showing that an electrical current could stimulate the healing of broken bones. His books—*The Body Electric: Electromagnetism and the Foundation of Life, and Cross Currents: The Promise of Electromedicine, the Perils of Electropollution*—are classics if you want to delve deeper into the details of EMT.

The underlying premise of Becker's work is that the structure and function of living organisms are based on electromagnetic fields of many sizes, "shapes," and frequencies, ranging from the atomic level to those that surround the entire body. The potentially revolutionary part of this premise is that these fields interact with your biochemistry, and when this bioelectrical conversation is interrupted, your chemical, physical, and hormonal health suffers too. Although Becker started out using simple electric currents directly on bone and looking for the right frequencies to heal, more productive research is being done today with fields that combine electricity and magnetics.

The Father of Bioelectrical Medicine

The early research on the therapeutic benefits of bioelectric medicine go back even further than Dr. Becker's work to that of Raymond Royal Rife. In a nutshell, the late Raymond Royal Rife was a medical visionary. Considered by some to be the "father of bioelectric medicine," Rife developed technology that is used even today in the fields of biochemistry, ballistics, optics, electronics, radiochemistry, and aviation. He built and designed several medical instruments, including the heterodyning ultraviolet microscope, the microdissector, and the micromanipulator.

But Rife is best known for creating a microscope that could see virus-sized organisms, and a radio frequency-emitting ray tube that could target and kill specific microorganisms. Thus, he could treat many conditions, allowing patients to become free of whatever disease was ailing them, including cancer.

Rife's "Universal Microscope" had close to 6,000 parts and could magnify an object to 60,000 times its size. More importantly, it allowed him to view a living virus. Even today's most sophisticated electron microscopes cannot do this.

Because 75 percent of the organisms Rife viewed were visible only with ultraviolet (UV) light, and thereby invisible to the human eye, he needed to develop a means of seeing them. This led him to develop heterodyning—a technique by which he illuminated the virus or bacteria by using two different wavelengths of the same UV light frequency that resonated with that specific organism. When these two wavelengths merged, they produced a third, longer wave that fell into the visible portion of the electromagnetic spectrum. This allowed the organisms to become visible without destroying them.

Using this microscope, Rife was able to see and identify the human cancer virus. Upon closer observation, he noticed that its vibrations caused it to take on a purplish-red color.

He questioned if the microbe causing this frequency could be destroyed by another frequency that resonated at the same vibratory rate as the microbe. In an effort to answer his query, Rife spent hours on end sitting at his microscope, adjusting his frequency device, until one day he reached a certain frequency that caused the virus to glow brighter then go out. Immediately thereafter, the microbe itself disintegrated. He repeated this process several times, always getting the same result.

Rife had unwittingly discovered the mortal oscillatory rate (MOR)—the electromagnetic frequency at which a specific organism is destroyed. Because every cell vibrates at a specific and unique frequency, identifying that frequency, then increasing its amplitude causes structural stresses that distort and eventually destroy the organism. Using this technique, Rife could destroy a virus without disturbing or harming surrounding tissue.

Frequencies Destroy Cancer

It was one thing to identify viruses under a microscope and destroy them on a Petri dish, but would it work in humans? To find out, Rife first injected mice with the BX virus. After they developed cancer, he exposed them to his predetermined frequency. The cancer was destroyed. Every time.

With the safety of his treatment assured, he was eventually pressured to test his theory on humans. In 1934, he exposed 16 terminal cancer patients to frequencies appropriate for their cancers. Treatments usually lasted 3–5 minutes and were administered every three days. At the end of 90 days, 15 of the 16 patients were completely cured. The final person was cured after an additional 30 days of treatment.

Word of Rife's microscope and frequency instruments quickly spread, and soon he was working with many of the top doctors and researchers of the time. The demand grew so much that in 1937, Rife formed Beam Ray, a company to manufacture his frequency instruments.

In 1950, Rife and new employee John Crane began to build more frequency instruments. They soon took on traveling salesman John Marsh. In 1957, Marsh was visiting his parents in Dayton, Ohio when a sore throat sent him to family physician Dr. Robert Stafford.

Marsh told him about the benefits of the Rife machine, and said that if Dr. Stafford ever had a terminally ill cancer patient, he should call him.

Six months later, Stafford had an 82-year-old female patient named Mrs. Byess with end-stage cancer and a life expectancy of 2 to 3 weeks. He called Marsh and Marsh brought him a machine. Dr. Stafford treated her for 3–5 minutes every other day. Within two weeks she began to recover. She eventually got out of bed, was walking around, and made plans to go home. Unfortunately, she never made it home, as she fell and broke her hip while climbing a flight of stairs and died a week later. However, an autopsy found no cancer in her body at the time of her death.

Rife's Work Today

While no original microscope or frequency machine of Rife's exists in its original state, more and more researchers are looking to the past in their efforts to heal in the future. Specifically, researchers published in the *Townsend Letter for Doctors and Patients* mentioned the use of energy-based frequency at clinics throughout the world. They believe that electromagnetic frequencies are at the source of all chemical and mechanical reactions in the body, and that by finding and applying a frequency that resonates with particular tissues and organs, you can help those tissues and organs heal. For example, they found that nerves regenerate at 2 Hz, bone grows at 7 Hz, ligaments heal at 10 Hz, capillaries are stimulated at 15, 20 and 72 Hz.

Their explanations of how electromagnetic therapy works is an echo of Rife's research nearly 80 years ago. "An assembly of cells, as in a tissue or organ, will have certain collective frequencies that regulate important processes, such as cell division. Normally, these frequencies will be very stable. If, for some reason, a cell shifts its frequency, entraining signals from neighboring cells will tend to reinstall the correct frequency. However, if a sufficient number of cells get out-of-step, the strength of the system's collective vibrations can decrease to a point where stability is lost."

Using Rife

I wish I could direct you toward medical professionals currently using this form of treatment. Unfortunately, this technology is considered "taboo" by conventional medicine, and finding a physician using a machine in an office setting is very difficult.

Fortunately, it is completely legal for you to own an EMT device and treat yourself at home. I have shared this information with family and friends, and they have subsequently used these devices to treat conditions as varied as herpes, insomnia, colds, flu, and digestive complaints.

Machines can differ in price (ranging from $700 to $4,000), in the method of energy output, and how the frequency is induced into your body.

1. **Radio Frequencies.** This is the delivery system that Rife used. While some machines still use radio frequencies, they cannot be used at the incredibly high frequencies used by Rife, as they would disrupt modern AM radio. With this system, frequencies are introduced to your body through radio frequencies that are transmitted through inert gas-filled tubes.

2. **Electrical frequencies (TENS).** These are more readily available, and usually involve either a hand-held or attachable electrodes. While you can vary the intensity, more sensitive people may prefer a remote-controlled device. With this system, the electric current is introduced via small contact pads that are placed on your body.

I am particularly fond of the following EMT device companies:

- Resonant Light Technology (*www.resonantlight.com* or 250-338-4949). This Canadian firm sells a programmable frequency generator that induces frequencies into your body through hand-held electrodes. They also have a radio frequency device for non-contact frequency induction.

- Alternative Technologies (336-885-6625). This company sells a pre-programmed frequency generator that contains over 500 programs for various health conditions. This device uses hand-held electrodes or foot pads for frequency induction.

- Bruce Stenulson (*www.stenulson.net/althealth.com* or 719-836-2489). Bruce sells a very sophisticated, custom-made device that uses argon gas-filled tubes that vibrate at whatever frequency you set.

The Research Continues

Thankfully, many researchers continue to look at how EMT can heal the injured and diseased. Let's take a closer look at the areas where EMT is the most promising: hormone balance, stress and mood, osteoporosis, pain management, and cancer.

EMT and Hormone Health

Research has shown that specific frequencies can be used to strengthen and support brain neurotransmitters and neuropeptides, as well as adrenal, ovarian, pituitary, and hypothalamus function by helping to restore their "energetic blueprint" or vibrational pattern. As we've discussed in previous chapters, these variables are crucial to the production of all hormones, especially the five sex hormones. I personally feel that the EPFX-SCIO that I discussed earlier is the most powerful and effective frequency device you can use for treatment with these types of therapeutic frequencies in your body.

WHAT'S YOUR PULSE?
EMT is a great way to bring your brain chemistry, neurotransmitters, hormones, and chi back into balance. Women who are estrogen deficient-fast processors should use very slow treatments with a very slow pulse (cool and slow down with a low frequency). Conversely, estrogen dominant women or estrogen deficient-slow processors are more expansive and need to speed up with a higher, faster pulse in order to receive a contractive and heating effect.

EMT and Stress/Mood

During any 24-hour period, you experience many different states of consciousness, from heightened awareness and activity to deep sleep. Each of these states has a particular brain wave pattern associated with it, and these waves can be detected by using a very sensitive amplifier called an electroencephalograph (EEG). These brain wave frequencies change depending on the neural activity within the brain.

While British researcher Maxwell Cade found 15 different wave patterns associated with human activity, we tend to group these patterns into four major categories:

1. **Beta:** Consists of rapid pulsations of between 14 and 30 cycles per second (measured as hertz, or Hz). This is your normal waking-state pattern and is used for problem solving and reacting to external stimulation. This pattern range allows you to respond quickly to events, do calculations, and process and create complex functions. Beta is increased under stress and anxiety in order to deal with immediate problems.

2. **Alpha:** This is the feel-good brain wave frequency that occurs in focused imagery, meditation, daydreaming, or in rhythmic athletic activity such as yoga or Tai Chi. Its frequency range is 9 to 13 Hz.

3. **Theta:** The theta pattern is from 4 to 8 Hz and tends to be produced during deep meditation and as you become drowsy and near sleep. It allows for deep unconscious imagery, and often great creativity is experienced in this state. Theta patterns are evident during rapid eye movement (REM) sleep, when most dreaming occurs.

4. **Delta:** This is the slowest of the brain wave frequencies and is the rhythm of deep, dreamless sleep, during which your body accomplishes its physical restoration. The waves vary between 1 and 3 Hz in this state.

Controlled external-stimuli pulsed light, sound, or electromagnetic waves are able to dictate the level of activity of the brain through the process of entrainment. Entrainment occurs when the brain's activity level synchronizes with and tracks the pattern of an external source such as pulsed light or sound. The brain literally gets in lockstep with the external frequency pattern. Entrainment to sound is often accomplished by feeding signals of different Hz into each ear, such as 90 Hz in the left ear and 100 Hz in the right ear. The two brain hemispheres then work together to produce a brain wave pattern in the 10 Hz range (the difference between the two frequencies), which is the feel-good alpha state.

Since the brain is unable to resist getting into lockstep with the external stimulus, if you are highly stressed, you can force your brain and nervous system into any relaxed state that you desire and for any length of time. The opposite is also true, of course: The brain can entrain to high-frequency beta states with highly stimulating music and disruptive sounds. If you are in stress overload or fatigue, be very careful of the external stimulation you are exposed to so you do not unwittingly add to your stress level.

Besides stress reduction and relaxation, mind "software" has been developed to use brain wave entrainment for incredible advances in optimal learning, treating insomnia and sleep disorders, enhancing creativity and performance states, dealing with panic disorders and anxiety, controlling anger, augmenting self-esteem and confidence, and controlling psychophysiological disorders such as migraine headaches and chronic pain.

One of the best devices for stress reduction is the Total Relaxation from Binaural-Beats (*www.binaural-beats.com*).

EMT and Osteoporosis

Research has clearly demonstrated that electromagnetic therapy can speed up the healing of broken bones. The racehorse industry was the first to successfully apply and demonstrate the principles of EMT on healing bone fractures. This provided some basis for the FDA to approve pulsed electromagnetic frequency/field (EMF) generators for human use on bone fractures that are unable to heal or mend, as well as to fuse spinal vertebrae in people with chronic, severe back pain.

However, the mechanisms for creating better bone density in someone with osteoporosis are different. There are two primary types of cells that affect bone density. Osteoclasts resorb (or take away old) worn out bone, while osteoblasts build new bone.

Research indicates that electromagnetic currents slow bone resorption, but don't reliably build bone. This may have to do with a feedback system in which the osteoblasts are stimulated by activity from the osteoclasts. If osteoclast activity is suppressed, osteoblast activity is also suppressed.

Even so, I strongly encourage women with osteoporosis to consider the use of electromagnetic therapy to help significantly slow bone loss. Once you've started using an EMF device for osteoporosis, keep using it along with your exercise, diet, supplement, and hormone balance program until a bone density test shows that your bone density is increasing.

It is important to use a very low frequency EMF device that generates a negative field, or a pulsed field, rather than a positive field. In the 1970's, researchers found that while exposure to the negative field of a magnet produced beneficial effects on living organisms, exposure to a positive field created stress. Prolonged exposure to a positive magnetic pole has been shown to increase acidity, reduce the oxygenation of cells, slow metabolism, and increase pain.

There are a variety of these devices available, starting at about $399 for the EarthPulse (*www.earthpulse.net* or 772-485-9724). Devices can go as high as $2,650 for the Bemer 3000 (*www.bemt.net/products.php* or 877-362-3637).

EMT and Pain Reduction

While most of the research on EMT has centered around mood and insomnia, there is a bevy of studies showing that it is highly beneficial for reducing back pain, arthritis, fibromyalgia, and migraine headaches.

According to a study from the *Journal of International Medical Research*, researchers divided 36 people with chronic lower back pain into two groups. The first group (17 people) received pulsed EMT three times a week for three weeks. The second group (19 people) received a placebo treatment. Those participants in the EMT group enjoyed significantly greater pain relief than those in the placebo group.

EMT is also highly beneficial for treating arthritis. One study tested the effectiveness of EMT on 114 people with osteoarthritis. Researchers divided the participants into two groups. The first group received conventional medication (NSAIDs and chondroprotective agents), while the second group received the same medication, plus EMT treatments. The treatments lasted 20 minutes and there was a total of 10 sessions. Those patients who received the EMT treatments saw reduced pain, less stiffness, and lower levels of inflammation than the medication-only group. Additionally, the pain relief and anti-inflammatory effects took place the by second or third treatments.

EMT is also effective in treating rheumatoid arthritis (RA). I am personally thankful for the therapeutic benefits of EMT for this disease after working with precious and adorable children suffering from RA during my earlier years in clinical practice. Anything that can help relieve the symptoms in these children and improve their overall quality of life is much appreciated. One study in particular highlights these benefits.

Researchers tested 138 children with RA. The children were divided into three groups. The first group received EMT treatments on five acupuncture points for 30 minutes a day for 10 days. The second group received EMT treatments on the same five acupuncture points for 30 minutes a day for six days. The third group received EMT on just two acupuncture points, located near the thymus and most severely affected joint. All three groups enjoyed a 50 percent reduction in pain, 80–90 percent improvement in joint function, and reduced morning stiffness. Interestingly, the relief in joint symptoms was most significant in patients in the third group, where the acupuncture points were specifically selected for thymus and affected joints.

Finally, EMT has been found to be fantastic for headache and migraine relief. A study of 56 patients with severe headaches found that EMT was more effective than intravascular laser application. Patients in the EMT group received seven treatments to three acupuncture points for a total of 40 minutes each treatment. They reported complete pain relief from their headaches after just one treatment.

EMT and Cancer

Clinics in other parts of the world are using EMT to treat cancer patients with great success. The findings from these and other studies indicate that EMT can bring about cell death in cancer cell cultures and animal tumors. EMT has even been found to increase key cellular activity that enhances immunity and strengthens the immune system.

* * *

Frequency medicine has a long and varied history. Whether you use sound to soothe your mood, biofeedback to retrain your body, vibrational medicine to bring your cells back into balance, or EMT to treat a specific condition, there is no denying that frequencies can work wonders to restore optimal health.

Since we've covered quite a bit of material in this section, I thought it would be best to give you a quick, easy-to-read reference guide of the different types of energy medicine available.

Acupuncture	Chakras	Color Therapy	Light Therapy	Frequency Medicine
Electro-acupuncture Acupressure	Affirmations Meditation	Chakra exercise Visualization Colored-paper exercise Clothing/jewelry Home décor	Sunlight Red light Blue light Lasers LEDs Filtered glass Tinted contacts	Sound therapy Biofeedback Vibrational medicine (EPFX-SCIO) Electromagnetic therapy (EMT)

Section Four: Summary

In this section, we looked at the myriad of ways you can use energy medicine to restore hormone function. We discussed the fascinating concept of restoring chi and yin-yang balance with acupuncture and acupressure, as well as realigning your chakras.

We then delved into the rainbow of treatment options with color therapy. We took this concept to the next level with light therapy, and looked at how different ends of the spectrum can help to restore and strengthen hormone function.

Finally, we explored the fascinating world of frequency medicine. We examined the history and therapeutic benefits of sound therapy and the work Raymond Royal Rife did with electromagnetic therapy. We also took a peek into the future and discussed the advances in vibrational medicine with the EPFX-SCIO, as well as biofeedback.

Regardless of where you are in your hormonal cycle, the many and varied types of energy medicine can *all* help to bring your hormones back into optimal balance and health.

In Section Five of *Hormone Revolution*, we'll take a look at how your lifestyle can affect hormone production and balance. Specifically, we'll discuss the foods that can help or hinder your hormonal balance, the role stress plays in hormone function, and how regular exercise can keep you on track with great hormonal health.

the optimum lifestyle for healthy hormones

As we've seen throughout this book, there are many ways you can work to balance your hormones. You can use nutritional supplements, bioidentical hormones, and the vast array of energy medicine techniques available to you.

In this section, let's take a look at how you can support healthy hormone production by making good lifestyle choices. You'll learn how the proper diet for your hormonal type can help or hinder your health. You'll discover how damaging stress can be to hormone production, as well as your overall well-being, and how beneficial a healthy attitude and positive emotions can be to your hormones and entire body. Feeling loving and joyful can literally make your cells and tissues sing! Finally, I'll show you how to choose the best exercise programs and routines for your particular hormonal makeup.

By making these key changes to your lifestyle, you can help to ensure the health and support of your hormones throughout your life. Let's get started!

your perfect diet

27

Over the course of more than 30 years in medical practice, the one thing I know for sure is that how and what you eat has a profound effect on your health, well-being, and hormonal make up. But, contrary to what the latest fad diet may profess, there is no perfect diet for women that works for everyone.

Instead, you need to eat a high-nutrient diet that complements your particular body and hormonal type. To start, every woman needs to eat the way our ancestors ate—close to the earth, consuming lots of high-quality, nourishing, whole fresh foods. Where women eat closer to the earth, such as Asians and Pacific Islanders, and consume more plant-based foods, they have fewer menopause symptoms and a lower incidence of breast cancer.

Everyone should also aim for a Mediterranean-style diet. According to a study from the *Journal of the American Medical Association*, people who eat a Mediterranean-type diet are less likely to die of coronary heart disease, cardiovascular diseases, and cancer. This diet is rich in fruits, vegetables, fish, nuts, whole grains, and fats such as olive oil. It is also low in white flour, sugar, and the saturated fats found in dairy products.

However, not every woman should eat the same types of foods, even under the Mediterranean diet umbrella. Instead, you should choose foods that support your particular hormonal profile. And the easiest, most effective way to do this is to look at the pH of the foods you eat.

Understanding pH

All substances in nature can be classified according to their relative acidity or alkalinity. The origin of the word *acid* is the Latin word "acidus," which means sour or tart. These qualities characterize many of the common acidic substances that we come in contact with, such as the vinegar used in salad dressings, which contain acetic acid; soft drinks, which contain phosphoric acid and carbon dioxide; and black tea, which contains tannic acid. Citric acid is found in grapefruits, oranges, lemons, and limes; and tartaric acid comes from grapes.

In contrast, alkaline substances have a bitter taste and feel slippery or smooth on the tongue. A good example is sodium bicarbonate, also known as baking soda, which is used as an antacid.

The acidity and alkalinity of all substances are expressed in terms of pH, which measures the concentration of hydrogen ions. A pH ranking above 7.00 indicates that a substance is alkaline, and below 7.00 is acidic. Pure water has a pH close to neutral, or 7.00.

The pH measurement is an extremely sensitive calibration, with an increase or decrease from one whole number to another indicating a tenfold increase or decrease in hydrogen ion concentration. Thus, seemingly small shifts in the pH value of a substance can reflect significant changes in its relative acidity or alkalinity.

How pH Functions Within Your Body

Your body contains trillions of cells, fluid-filled structures that contain many alkaline substances: minerals such as calcium, magnesium, potassium, and sodium, as well as oxygen and bicarbonate. The combination of all of these substances within the cell produces a slightly alkaline intracellular pH of just above 7.00. The cells are also surrounded by fluids that contain alkaline minerals.

Not only are the cells of the body alkaline, but the blood that circulates throughout your body must maintain a very narrow range of slightly alkaline pH, 7.35 to 7.45. The constancy of the blood pH is fundamental to the body's ability to maintain a relatively unchanging internal environment. The blood is constantly exposed to a variety of mostly acidic substances. Various things, from the foods you eat and the stresses in your life to the pollutants you are exposed to—as well as your own metabolic processes—produce chemicals within the body that are often more acidic than your own slightly alkaline pH.

All of these substances are carried within the blood, which transports them to the cells for use as nutrients or carries them away from the cells as waste products. All of these substances potentially disrupt the healthy pH of the blood. As a result, your body has to have a mechanism to both neutralize and eliminate these substances in order to keep the pH of the blood constant. This is the pH-regulating system. Its importance is illustrated by the fact that a person cannot live more than a few hours if the blood's pH goes below 7.00 or above 8.00. For example, blood with a pH of 6.95, which is only slightly acidic, can lead to coma and even death.

A few compartments of the body, primarily those of the digestive tract, have a pH range that differs from that of the blood. For example, the pH of saliva is 6.0 to 7.5, which is needed to begin the digestion of starches in the mouth. Proteins are much harder to break down than carbohydrates and require an acid environment for their digestion—found in the stomach, which secretes hydrochloric acid. This brings the pH of the stomach down to a highly acidic 1.0 to 3.5.

Once the food leaves your stomach, it must be brought up to an alkaline pH so that the enzymes necessary for further digestion can be activated within the small intestine. The breakdown of nutrients into small particles as well as their absorption occurs in the small intestine. These processes also require an alkaline environment to proceed efficiently.

Digestive juices containing sodium and potassium bicarbonate that are secreted by the pancreas into the small intestine have an alkaline pH varying from 8.0 to 9.0. Bile produced by the liver and secreted into the upper part of the small intestine also helps in the process of digestion by breaking down fats. Bile has a pH of 7.8, which is also slightly alkaline. Finally, the intestinal glands, which are located over virtually the entire surface of the small intestine, produce intestinal secretions that have a pH of 7.5 to 8.0.

Regulating pH Within Your Body

The pH-regulating system of your body is very complex and is made up of many parts. Within the body, the various parts of your pH-regulating system are carefully orchestrated to work well together. The system includes the alkaline minerals contained both inside and outside the cells, as well as the mineral reserves stored within your bones. You also have three buffer systems in your blood that help to keep its pH constant.

In addition, your lungs help to regulate pH by breathing in alkaline oxygen and eliminating acidic waste products in the form of carbon dioxide. Finally, your kidneys eliminate excessive amounts of either acid or alkaline substances from the body through the urine.

The pH-regulating system tends to be healthy and to work efficiently in children and young adults. The healthy buffering capability of most young people is due to the robust mineral reserves stored in their bones, robust buffer systems, and strong lung and kidney function. However, as people age and experience the mostly acidifying stresses of modern life, the pH-regulating system begins to decline in its efficiency.

This decline is a part of the normal aging process and can be accelerated by years of acidifying stress or eating a standard American diet. As a result, with age, more and more individuals who formerly had good pH balance tend to become overly acidic.

The pH–Estrogen Imbalance Connection

As I've told you throughout this book, there are three different and very distinct hormonal types—women who are estrogen dominant, women who are estrogen deficient-fast processor, and women who are estrogen deficient-slow processor. (If you feel you need a review of this concept, see Chapter 13 for more details.)

Let me give you a quick summary of the three concepts here. I'll discuss each type of diet as it relates to your hormonal type in much more detail further on in the chapter.

If you are estrogen dominant (see Chapter 10), you tend to produce excess estrogen during your reproductive years. Because estrogen is a major growth promoter, you can enjoy some great benefits of lots of estrogen, including beautiful, moist, dewy-looking skin and strong bones and muscles. However, there can also be a grave downside as well, such as the tendency towards problems like PMS, uterine fibroid tumors, ovarian and breast cysts, excess weight, and breast cancer. Therefore, you would want to avoid foods that will make you expand and reinforce the growth-expansive effects of your abundant estrogen production. When choosing foods, you need to avoid the highly alkaline ones. They are more typically seen in a primarily vegetarian diet with lots of whole grains and legumes and higher pH fruits and vegetables. These foods tend to have a more expansive effect on the body. Instead, you need to opt for more contractive, drying, and acidic types of foods, such as condiments like vinegar and lemon juice, as well as more acid-forming meats, fruits, and vegetables.

Conversely, if you are estrogen deficient-fast processor you are producing too little estrogen. Unlike your estrogen dominant sisters, you need to retain more fluid in your body, and build more moisture content back into the structural elements of your body, like your bones and connective tissues. Therefore, you need a much more alkaline, vegetarian-centered diet that helps you expand and build, and should avoid anything drying, contractive, or highly acidic.

Then there's the third hormonal type—estrogen deficient-slow processor. If you are postmenopausal, but tend to retain fluid and gain weight and have a bigger, denser body, you have yin excess. You don't have enough of the yang qualities that limit, dry, and contract this expansiveness naturally from within your own body. While you can still benefit from estrogen supplements if you have vaginal dryness or depression, you need to carefully build up and support your contractive and energizing yang components. This will support your energy, vital life force, libido, and mental acuity, and help to drain off excess fluids and weight. Because you tend toward being more yin than yang, you should follow a modified estrogen dominant, more highly acidic diet to help you contract, and become drier and less expansive.

Selecting the Proper Foods

This very helpful chart is my gift to you to help you to learn the relative acidity or alkalinity of the foods that most women eat on a daily basis. It gives the pH of foods prior to being consumed and does not reflect the substantial acid production that some of these foods can trigger within the body.

I put this chart together based on scientific research done at major universities. This information was obtained from technical sources compiled at the University of California Davis, Department of Food Science and Technology; and Cornell University, Department of Food Science. In addition, I obtained the pH value of certain foods from their appropriate professional associations such as the National Coffee Association. You will notice that while most food groups are listed, oils are not. Oils do not have a pH since they cannot be mixed with water, which is necessary for taking pH measurements.

The chart will help you to plan a diet best suited to your hormone profile, depending on whether you are estrogen dominant, estrogen deficient-fast processor, or estrogen deficient-slow processor. As you work to modify and improve your own diet to best support your hormonal and overall health, I strongly recommend that you refer often to this chart when making your food selections.

PH OF COMMON FOODS AND BEVERAGES PRIOR TO BEING CONSUMED

Highly Acidic Foods (pH between 1 and 4.6)	pH Range Prior to Being Consumed
Beverages	
Ginger ale	2.0–4.0
Lime juice	2.2–2.4
Lemon juice	2.2–2.6
Wines	2.3–3.8
Cranberry juice	2.5–2.7
Cider	2.9–3.3
Grapefruit juice	2.9–3.4
Currant juice	3.0
Orange juice	3.0–4.0
Apple juice	3.3–3.5
Pineapple juice	3.4–3.7
Prune juice	3.7–4.3
Tomato juice	3.9–4.3

continued on next page

Highly Acidic Foods (pH between 1 and 4.6)	pH Range Prior to Being Consumed
Fruit	
Lime	1.8–2.0
Lemon	2.2–2.4
Cranberry sauce	2.3
Gooseberries	2.8–3.1
Loquats	2.8–4.0
Orange	2.8–4.2
Plum	2.8–4.6
Rhubarb	2.9–3.4
Apple	2.9–3.5
Raspberries	2.9–3.7
Grapefruit	2.9–4.0
Boysenberries	3.0–3.3
Strawberries	3.0–4.2
Blackberries	3.0–4.2
Kumquat	3.1–3.5
Quince	3.2
Blueberries	3.2–3.6
Pineapple, crushed	3.2–4.0
Crab apples, spiced	3.3–3.7
Kiwi	3.3–3.8
Apple sauce	3.4–3.5
Apricots	3.5–4.0
Pineapple, sliced	3.5–4.1
Fruit cocktail	3.6–4.0
Raisins	3.6–4.2
Vegetables	
Sauerkraut	3.1–3.7
Cucumber	3.1–3.8
Tomatillo	3.9–4.1

Moderately Acidic Foods (pH between 3.1 and 5.6)	pH Range Prior to Being Consumed
Dairy Products	
Yogurt	3.8–4.2
Sweeteners	
Fruit jellies	3.0–3.5
Fruit jams	3.5–4.0
Condiments and Seasonings	
Vinegar	2.4–3.4
Pickles, sweet	2.5–3.0
Pickles, dill	2.6–3.8
Pickles, sour	3.0–3.5
Fermented olives	3.5
Mayonnaise	3.8–4.0
Beverages	
Beer	4.0–5.0
Fruit	
Peach	3.1–4.7
Cherries	3.2–4.7
Pear	3.4–4.7
Mango	3.9–4.6
Asian pear	4.2–4.6
Guava	4.3–4.7
Banana	4.5–5.2
Vegetables	
Tomato	3.7–4.9
Potato salad	3.9–4.6
Eggplant	4.5–4.7
String beans	4.6

continued on next page

Moderately Acidic Foods (pH between 3.1 and 5.6)	pH Range Prior to Being Consumed
Red Meat	
Dry sausage	4.4–5.6
Dairy Products	
Cottage cheese	4.1–5.4
Condiments and Seasonings	
Fermented vegetables	3.9–5.1
Red pimento	4.3–5.2

Low Acid to Alkaline Foods (pH between 4.61 and 9.5)	pH Range Prior to Being Consumed
Beverages	
Coffee	4.9–5.2
Mineral water	6.2–9.4
Distilled water	6.8–7.0
Fruit	
Figs	4.6–5.0
Papaya	5.2–5.7
Persimmon	5.4–5.8
Avocado	5.5–6.0
Dates	6.2–6.4
Cantaloupe	6.2–6.5
Melon	6.3–6.7
Vegetables	
Pumpkin	4.8–5.5
Sweet pepper	4.8–6.0
Spinach	4.8–6.8
Carrot	4.9–6.3
Squash	5.0–5.4
Asparagus	5.0–6.1
Turnip	5.2–5.6

Low Acid to Alkaline Foods (pH between 4.61 and 9.5)	pH Range Prior to Being Consumed
Cabbage	5.2–6.3
Broccoli	5.2–6.5
Parsnip	5.3
Sweet potato	5.3–5.6
Onion	5.3–5.8
Peas	5.3–6.8
Turnip greens	5.4–5.6
White potato	5.4–6.3
Artichoke	5.6
Cauliflower	5.6–6.7
Parsley	5.7–6.0
Celery	5.7–6.1
Alfalfa tops	5.9
Corn	5.9–7.3
Lettuce	6.0–6.4
Mushrooms	6.0–6.5
Brussels sprout	6.3–6.6

Beans

Baked beans	4.8–5.5
Dried beans	4.9–5.5
Kidney	5.2–5.4
Lima	5.4–6.5
Soybeans	6.0–6.6

Nuts and Seeds

Walnuts	5.4–5.5
Almonds	> 6.0
Flax seeds	> 6.0
Hazelnuts	> 6.0
Pecans	> 6.0
Poppy seeds	> 6.0
Pumpkin seeds	> 6.0
Sesame seeds	> 6.0
Sunflower seeds	> 6.0

continued on next page

Low Acid to Alkaline Foods (pH between 4.61 and 9.5)	pH Range Prior to Being Consumed
Fish and Shellfish	
Halibut	5.5–5.8
Sardines	5.7–6.6
Tuna	5.9–6.1
Mackerel	5.9–6.2
Oysters	5.9–6.7
Clams	5.9–7.1
Codfish (canned)	6.0–6.1
Salmon	6.1–6.5
Haddock	6.2–6.7
Whiting	6.2–7.1
Catfish	6.6–7.0
Scallops	6.8–7.1
Crab	6.8–8.0
Shrimp	6.8–8.2
Poultry	
Chicken	5.5–6.4
Duck	6.0–6.1
Egg yolk	6.0–6.3
Egg white	7.9–9.5
Red Meat	
Beef	5.3–6.2
Pork	5.3–6.4
Corned-beef hash	5.5–6.0
Spiced ham	6.0–6.3
Hot dogs	6.2
Dairy Products	
Roquefort cheese	4.7–4.8
Most cheeses	5.0–6.1
Parmesan cheese	5.2–5.3
Evaporated milk	5.9–6.3

Low Acid to Alkaline Foods (pH between 4.61 and 9.5)	pH Range Prior to Being Consumed
Whole cow's milk	6.0–6.8
Butter	6.1–6.4
Camembert	6.1–7.0

Grains

Wheat	> 6.0
Rice	> 6.0
Barley	> 6.0
Oats	> 6.0
Rye	> 6.0
Millet	> 6.0
Quinoa	> 6.0
Amaranth	> 6.0
Hominy	6.9–7.9

Baked Goods

White bread	5.0–6.0
Date-nut bread	5.1–6.0
Soda crackers	6.5–8.5

Sweeteners

Molasses	5.0–5.4
Glucose syrup	5.2
Honey	6.0–6.8
Brown-rice syrup	6.1–6.4
Maple syrup	6.5–7.0

Condiments and Seasonings

Hot peppers	4.8–6.0
Garlic	5.3–6.3
Cocoa	5.5–6.0
Ripe, canned olives	5.9–7.3
Dutch processed chocolate	7.0–8.0

CONDIMENT CONUNDRUM

There is a lot of misinformation about the relative acidity and alkalinity of foods. Many other books have acid/alkaline food charts; however, these charts tend to contradict one another. One chart will list a food as being highly acidic, while another chart will state that the same food is highly alkaline. This can be very confusing to the reader who is trying to use this information to make intelligent choices.

For example, some people claim that lemon juice and apple cider vinegar can be used to alkalinize the body because, once eaten, they turn alkaline in the body. As a result, they can be used to counteract or treat over-acidity. This is not so. Lemon juice and apple cider vinegar are actually very acidic because their alkaline mineral content (such as calcium, magnesium, potassium, and sodium) is extremely low. Thus, these foods have no internal buffering from minerals to bring up their own pH and thereby counteract their naturally high acid content.

When you consume them, they do become much more alkaline in the body. But that's only because all acidic foods have to be buffered by your body's own pH-regulating system to maintain the slightly alkaline pH of your blood. This occurs partially at the expense of your bones, which will release and deplete their own alkaline minerals to keep your blood pH slightly alkaline.

The following chart compares the pH and mineral content of lemon juice and apple cider vinegar with other common flavorings. The more-alkaline choices have a pH of 5 or higher, because they are internally buffered by their own higher content of alkaline minerals.

Food	pH	Calcium	Magnesium	Potassium	Sodium
Lemon juice	2.2–2.6	2 mg	1 mg	15 mg	3 mg
Lime juice	2.2–2.4	1 mg	1 mg	17 mg	0 mg
Cider vinegar	2.4–3.4	0.8 mg	3 mg	14 mg	trace
Blackstrap molasses	5.0–5.4	137 mg	52 mg	585 mg	19 mg
Tahini	>6.0	64 mg	14 mg	110 mg	17 mg
Flax meal	>6.0	35 mg	63 mg	120 mg	7 mg
Kelp	NA	156 mg	104 mg	753 mg	42 mg

Eating for Your Type

Throughout my medical career, women have come to me, telling me that they can't lose weight, even though they are eating what the "experts," health magazines, and latest fad diets are telling them they should eat. And the reality is they are often eating foods that we normally consider to be healthy, but they are not necessarily healthy for their body type.

By following the correct diet based on your own specific hormonal and health needs, you can stay extremely healthy and balanced. However, if you eat foods outside your health zone, you may aggravate any underlying health and hormonal imbalances. I call this diet "eating for your type."

Let's use a common problem—excess weight—to illustrate this concept. What I've learned through extensive research and clinical experience is that if you are overweight, you are very likely eating the wrong foods for your hormonal and body type. Instead, you need to eat the right foods, in the right ratios and proportions, for your hormonal type if you want to lose weight and keep it off.

To help you better understand this concept, let's take a look at each hormonal type and the types of foods they should be eating in more detail.

Diet for Estrogen Dominance and Estrogen Deficient-Slow Processors

If you are in your 30's, 40's, and early 50's and are prone towards estrogen dominance, or are estrogen deficient-slow processor, this is your best diet. Women in both of these scenarios tend to have great reservoirs of alkaline minerals contained within their cells, tissues, and bones that give them ample buffering capability well into old age. Even in their 80's and 90's, they do not tend to develop many of the common diseases related to overacidity, such as osteoporosis, kidney, or lung failure—provided, of course, that their other physiological functions remain strong.

A patient that I saw some years ago exemplified this issue. "Josephine," a 45-year-old woman, was a classic estrogen dominant type. She suffered from PMS and ovarian cysts, and had heavy menstrual periods throughout much of her life.

Josephine was raised on a traditional Polish diet that was high in meat protein and saturated fat. She continued to eat this way throughout her entire adult life. A physically strong and highly energetic individual, she was concerned about her elevated cholesterol level because of a strong family history of heart disease. After reading several books on cardiovascular health, she tried to become a vegetarian. After a week of eating mostly grains, beans, raw salads, and steamed vegetables, she no longer felt like herself and complained of feeling tired and listless. She quickly went back to her old dietary habits.

Months later, Josephine came to see me. I explained that she was sabotaging her health by eating the wrong foods. Based on my dietary recommendations, she began to substitute fish and range-fed poultry, as well as game meat like venison (which is low in saturated fat) for the fatty red meat that was her chief source of protein. She found that she felt surprisingly healthy and energetic after eating these very acidifying and contractive meats. She also began to supplement her diet with various types of fiber to help promote the elimination of estrogen and cholesterol from her body. In time, Josephine lost weight, gained energy, and lowered her cholesterol and estrogen levels.

Similarly, "Ginny" was a 56-year-old estrogen deficient-slow processor. She was 30 pounds overweight, having gained 10 pounds each decade since her 20's. She had a calm, peaceful demeanor, but her libido and "get up and go" were quite low. She was fortunate in that she didn't suffer from hot flashes and had amazing, healthy bone density, but she suffered from low back pain, sore hips, and sore knees. In fact, she had been diagnosed with osteoarthritis.

When Ginny was younger, she dealt with terrible PMS and heavy menstrual bleeding. She had even had surgery to remove fibroid tumors. I asked her what her typical diet consisted of and, sure enough, it was high in grains, sugar, and saturated fats. I suggested that Ginny reduce her whole grain and simple carbohydrate intake and eat more animal-based protein, whole fruits and vegetables, especially more acidic choices such as lemons, oranges, berries, and spinach; liberal amounts of highly acidic condiments like vinegar and lemon juice; and more heating spices such as cinnamon, ginger, and pepper. Once she made these dietary changes, her weight melted off, her libido started to improve, and the discomfort in her joints steadily improved.

As Josephine's and Ginny's stories illustrate, a more acidic and heating diet is critical for estrogen dominant women and estrogen deficient-slow processors to help them become drier, more contracted, and balanced. These high-alkaline producers may actually benefit from the wide variety of valuable nutrients contained within highly acidic and more heating foods. Such individuals can handle these foods' low pH without experiencing negative side effects. For example, certain fruit juices that are high in potassium citrate and alkaline salts of citric acid can be used to maintain energy and stamina while participating in athletic activities. Such drinks are best used by high-alkaline producers who can tolerate their higher content of simple sugar and do not develop tissue reactions such as canker sores, heartburn, and other types of irritation from the use of these drinks.

While alkaline individuals are not prone to these and other diseases related to overacidity, they may have a higher risk of heart attacks, strokes, and cancer of the breast and colon than their peers who follow a more vegetarian-based diet. Since the digestive function of most high-alkaline producers is so strong, they typically eat a diet high in animal protein and saturated fat. This may result in elevated blood lipids and the buildup of plaque within the arteries, thereby increasing their risk of cardiovascular disease. This is a common scenario among hard-driving, typically alkaline CEOs, who run their companies with enormous energy and staying power right up to the time that they have their first heart attack, in their 50's or 60's.

When estrogen dominant women and estrogen deficient-slow processors do try to follow the trends and adopt a low-fat, low-protein, and high-complex carbohydrate diet with a more vegetarian emphasis such as those advocated by Dean Ornish, MD, the Pritikin Institute, and even the American Cancer Society, they feel weak, devitalized, and mentally foggy. Eating this way will cause them to lose their natural robust energy and stamina, and their performance in many areas will begin to suffer.

BEST FOODS FOR ESTROGEN DOMINANT AND ESTROGEN DEFICIENT-SLOW PROCESSORS

Women with estrogen dominance or estrogen deficient-slow processors need to eat a more acidic diet that can help to bring estrogen back into balance in younger women, as well as restore the more yang, drying, and contractive qualities of the body in women who are well into their menopausal years. The best foods for the job include:

- High fiber foods such as buckwheat and flaxseed
- Citrus fruits (oranges, limes, lemons, grapefruit), berries, pineapple
- All vegetables, especially sauerkraut, spinach, cucumber, tomatoes, asparagus, and broccoli
- Free-range poultry and wild fish
- Free-range beef and lamb, as well as game meats like venison
- Soy and soy-based foods
- Vinegar
- Hot, spicy foods
- Nuts like almonds and walnuts

Naturally alkaline people instinctively gravitate to a highly acidic (but very unhealthy) diet of red meats that are high in saturated fat, soft drinks, sugar, white-flour products, beer, wine, caffeinated beverages, and fruit juices in order to maintain their pH at a healthy balance. While you do need to eat a highly acidic diet, you should aim for healthy foods that fall toward the more acidic side of the pH scale.

While these individuals can handle the acidity of this type of standard American diet, this type of diet lacks the essential nutrients that all women—whether estrogen dominant or deficient—need to maintain their health and well-being. High-alkaline producers are better served by following a diet that is both highly acidic and nutrient rich. This type of diet includes seafood, poultry, vegetables, fruits, legumes, whole grains, and condiments like lemon or lime juice and vinegar—basically, a more highly acidic version of the Mediterranean diet, but with a very limited amount of grains.

I've had many of my high-alkaline patients tell me they felt terrible when they tried to eliminate meat from their diet. That's because some women tend to be so alkaline that their bodies actually feel their best and they have the most energy with highly acidic red meats like free-range organic beef, lamb, and game meat like venison and buffalo. Fish is another great source of needed protein, as well as healthy polyunsaturated oils, which lower cholesterol, prevent clotting, and promote cardiovascular health.

However, while naturally alkaline people can eat more of the meat, fruit, and vinegar-doused antipasti, vegetables, and salads, overly acidic people (such as estrogen deficient-fast processors) should emphasize more of the vegetables, whole grains, and legumes of this regimen. In addition, these individuals should significantly decrease their intake of highly acidic foods and beverages that have a deleterious effect on health. This category includes alcohol, coffee, tea, soft drinks, and rich, sugary desserts.

Additionally, the fatty foods that alkaline types tend to eat can also lead to weight gain. This is particularly true if these individuals are older and have begun to lose their oxygenating ability. As oxygen intake begins to decline, women burn calories less efficiently. Since fat has more than twice the number of calories of protein and starch, eating a high-fat diet can easily lead to weight gain. To counteract this tendency, alkaline individuals need to reduce their fat intake by eating leaner cuts of meat, more salads and steamed vegetables, and substituting butter with healthier fats and oils, such as extra-virgin olive oil and flaxseed or flax oil.

Finally, estrogen dominant women should avoid antacids such as baking soda (sodium bicarbonate) and Tums. Although these remedies help tens of millions of Americans counter the ill effects of gastric overacidity, canker sores, and other minor ailments related to overacidity, I have seen them produce toxic effects in my naturally alkaline patients. These people tend to become bloated, gassy, fatigued, and even panicky when using these remedies since they tend to push these individuals' pH even further toward the alkaline side (of course, overly acidic individuals should avoid the overuse of antacids also).

SCENT-SATIONAL SPICES FOR ESTROGEN DOMINANCE

Women with estrogen dominance and estrogen deficient-slow processors can enjoy a wide variety of heating spices. These spices, often found in Mexican and Indian cuisine, stimulate metabolism, create heat and contraction within the body, and "burn up" excess fluid and weight. Among the best spices are:

- Turmeric (curry)
- Ginger
- Cayenne pepper
- Chili powder and chili peppers
- Cumin
- Cloves
- Cinnamon

Eat Your Nutrients

What you eat should also reinforce what you are taking in supplement form, which I discussed in Chapter 11. For estrogen dominant women, this should include key antioxidants, probiotics, fiber, essential fatty acids, and lots of water. These foods not only help to regulate the level of estrogen in your body, which is very important in younger, estrogen dominant women, but also help to bring estrogen deficient-slow processors back into better chemical and energetic balance.

Astounding Antioxidants

As I told you back in Chapter 11, certain antioxidants are critical for women with estrogen dominance and estrogen deficient-slow processors. The best of the best include beta-carotene, lutein, lycopene, flavonoids, and DIM.

Beta-carotene is a plant-based, water-soluble precursor to vitamin A that is abundant in the ovaries, and is found in very high concentrations in the corpus luteum and the adrenal glands—both of which produce progesterone to help balance the estrogen excess in estrogen dominant women, and support progesterone levels, even if greatly reduced after menopause. Research studies have also found carotenoids such as beta carotene are useful in treating or preventing conditions related to estrogen dominance, including ovarian cancer, heavy menstrual bleeding, and benign breast disease. Additionally, studies have shown that high levels of vitamin A can help reverse fibrocystic breast disease.

To ensure that you are getting enough beta-carotene in your diet, be sure to include plenty of the following foods: carrots, kale, spinach, squash, sweet potatoes, mangoes, cantaloupe, apricots, and cabbage.

DIET AND FIBROCYSTIC BREASTS

Nearly 30 percent of American women suffer from fibrocystic breasts. And, it's no surprise that the standard American diet is partly to blame.

Researchers have found that caffeine (coffee, black tea, cola, and chocolate), as well as excessive saturated fat and salt play a large role in the disease. Fortunately, by reducing or eliminating these foods from your diet and eating foods high in fiber, fresh fruits and vegetables, raw seeds and nuts, and wild-caught seafood, you can reduce your risk for fibrocystic breasts.

The carotenoid *lutein* plays a major role in the luteal phase, the time from ovulation to menstruation when the corpus luteum of the ovaries produces progesterone. This is because lutein is abundant in the corpus luteum and provides it with its distinctive yellow color. (For a refresher on the role the corpus luteum plays in ovulation, refer to page 91.)

Make sure you are getting enough lutein by eating yellow and orange foods such as corn, eggs, and sweet potatoes; and green leafy vegetables, especially spinach and collard greens.

Lycopene is one of the most concentrated carotenoids found in the blood, organs, and tissues of the body. One of the most important health benefits of lycopene is its ability to reduce the risk of cancer, particularly cancers of the reproductive tract. One study in particular from the *International Journal of Cancer* found that the 75 percent of women who ate the least amount of tomatoes (a rich source of lycopene) were three to five times more at risk for pre-cancerous lesions of the cervix than those who ate a lycopene-rich diet. Another study found that a diet high in lycopene significantly reduced the risk of ovarian cancer in premenopausal women. Investigators suggested that consumption of fruits, vegetables and food items high in carotene and lycopene, particularly raw carrots and tomato sauce, may reduce the risk of ovarian cancer.

Help reduce your risk for estrogen-dependent cancers by eating foods high in lycopene, including tomatoes and carrots, as well as red peppers, watermelon, apricots, cantaloupe, pumpkin, guava, and sweet potatoes.

DIET AND BREAST CANCER

According to a study from *Nutrition and Cancer*, women with breast cancer who ate higher dietary fiber and more vegetables and fruits that contained folate, vitamin C, and carotenoids had lived longer than those women who ate fewer foods containing these nutrients. Additionally, researchers found that those women who ate a diet higher in fat did not live as long as those who chose a lower fat diet.

To reduce your risk for breast cancer, be sure to eat a high-fiber, low-fat diet rich in vegetables, fruit, and lean protein.

Flavonoids encompass a wide group of antioxidants, including bioflavonoids and flavanols. Bioflavonoids are usually found in the pulp and rind of citrus fruit. They have weak, estrogen-like properties, and have also been shown to interfere with the production of estrogen by binding to estrogen receptor sites. In this way, bioflavonoids work to normalize estrogen balance, bringing excessively high estrogen down to more normal levels. Because bioflavonoids do bind to estrogen receptor sites, they can also act as a supplemental form of estrogen, helping to combat common menopausal symptoms such as hot flashes in women who are in their menopausal years and lack their own natural production of estrogen.

Flavanols, namely polyphenols and catechins, also bind to receptor sites, which is why they have been found to be so beneficial in protecting women from cancer. By binding to breast tissue estrogen receptors sites, polyphenols work to prevent carcinogens (tumor promoters, hormones, and growth factors) from binding to and harming the cells. In essence, the polyphenols "seal off" the tissue from invasion by carcinogens.

The superior antioxidant properties of polyphenols also help in the fight against heart attacks and other forms of cardiovascular disease. Japanese researchers have found that tablets of green tea extract providing 254 mg of catechins raised blood levels of antioxidants and reduced plaque-forming oxidation.

Foods rich in bioflavonoids include citrus fruits (lemons, oranges, tangerines, grapefruits, and limes) and buckwheat (a gluten-free grain that is not botanically related to wheat). Other good sources are apricots, cherries, grapes, plums, blackberries, papayas, green pepper, broccoli, and tomatoes. Foods rich in flavanols include green tea, apples, grapes, and onions.

DIM, or diindolylmethane, is found in *Brassica* veggies. Research has shown that when DIM is ingested, it not only encourages its own metabolism, but also that of estrogen. While it is not an estrogen or even an estrogen-mimic, its metabolic pathway exactly coincides with the metabolic pathway of estrogen. When these pathways intersect, DIM favorably adjusts the estrogen metabolic pathways by simultaneously increasing the good estrogen metabolites and decreasing the bad.

Make sure you are getting plenty of this amazing antioxidant by loading up on broccoli, bok choy, kale, cauliflower, cabbage, and Brussels sprouts.

Potent Probiotics

Women with estrogen dominance and estrogen deficient-slow processors whose diet is high in saturated fats, such as butter and dairy products, especially cheese and ice cream, often stimulate the growth of unhealthy, anaerobic bacteria in their intestinal tract. These bacteria chemically change the breakdown products of estrogen into forms that can be reabsorbed back into the body, thereby elevating your own levels of estrogen. Let me explain this a bit further.

As I mentioned in Chapter 11, these bacteria split estrogen from the binding substances that cause estrogen to be inactivated in your liver, which actually helps regulate your estrogen levels by binding to and detoxifying estrogen as it passes through the liver into your blood circulation. From the liver, estrogen is then secreted into your intestinal tract, where it is normally eliminated from the body. However, when these unhealthy, anaerobic bacteria predominate in the intestinal tract, the splitting process that they initiate on the bound estrogen then causes free estrogen to be reformed within your intestinal tract. Because this free estrogen can then be reabsorbed back into the circulation, it increases free estrogen levels within the blood.

To suppress the growth of these unhealthy bacteria, you should not only reduce your intake of saturated fat (which can lead to the problem in the first place), you also need to increase your intake of probiotic-rich, fermented foods, which recolonize your intestinal tract with healthy bacteria. These include yogurt (preferably soy or goat), kim chee, pickles, and sauerkraut, as well as taking probiotic supplements like lactobacillus and acidophilus.

Essential Fatty Acids

Essential fatty acids (EFAs) are health-promoting nutrients that your body needs to perform a whole range of functions. Estrogen dominant women will find that proper amounts of EFAs will help to reduce the inflammation and pain seen in conditions such as endometriosis and menstrual cramps. Women who are estrogen deficient-slow processors need EFAs to prevent a wide range of health concerns, including heart disease and breast cancer.

There are several different types of EFAs, but the two main categories include omega-3 fatty acids—eicosapentaenoic acid (EPA) and docosahexaenoic acid (DHA)—and omega-6 fatty acids (linoleic acid). Your body converts all EFAs into either series 1 or series 3 prostaglandins, potent hormone-like substances with a wide range of benefits that are essential for good reproductive health, and also help reduce fatigue and boost immune function. However, the production of prostaglandins shifts depending on the level and type of fatty acids in your body.

Omega-3s

Omega-3 EFAs consist primarily of EPA and DHA. EPAs are your heart-healthy fats. They also promote beautiful, healthy skin, hormonal balance, and immune function. EPA also makes serotonin, the "happy" neurotransmitter.

DHA, on the other hand, is a natural brain booster. Your brain needs DHA to create healthy nerve cell membranes. Your brain uses nerve cells for mood, attention, and memory.

Omega-3 fatty acids are converted into anti-inflammatory series 3 prostaglandins. Among other things, these prostaglandins help reduce inflammation that can lead to sore joints and brain fog.

Two of the best sources of omega-3 EFAs are flaxseed and fish. (Other good sources include soybeans, hemp powder, walnuts, canola oil, eggs, organ meats, and some forms of algae.) In the case of flaxseed, both the oil and the ground meal are rich in EFAs.

When it comes to fish, I recommend cold-water choices such as salmon, tuna, and mackerel. The colder the water a fish lives in, the more omega-3 its body requires and possesses, simply to keep it warm enough. Other amazing sources of omega-3–rich fish include sablefish, shad, and oysters.

Sablefish, also known as butterfish, is a white fish from the cold, deep waters of Alaska that contains about 3,000 mg of omega-3 fatty acids in a five-ounce filet. Many people describe the taste of this white fish as a "butter-infused halibut." I eat it frequently and find it to be delicious!

Shad, a member of the herring family, is a bony fish from the northern Atlantic and northern fresh water lakes and rivers. Both the meat and eggs are rich in flavor and omega-3 fats, with a six-ounce filet boasting nearly 5,000 mg of EFAs.

Usually prized for their aphrodisiac properties, oysters are surprisingly rich in EFAs. Just six oysters contain as much as 2,000 mg of omega-3 fatty acids, as well as good amounts of zinc and selenium.

Omega-6s

There are three main types of omega-6 fatty acids: linoleic acid (LA), arachidonic acid (AA), and gamma linolenic acid (GLA). You only need to supplement with GLA, because you get enough of the other omega-6 fatty acids through your regular diet. However, the stress of daily life (as well as poor nutrition, alcohol, chemical carcinogens, cholesterol, saturated fats and low levels of some vitamins) may prevent your body from turning linoleic acid into GLA.

The reason GLA is particularly important for women is that it is converted into series 1 prostaglandins that help ease depression, prevent breast tenderness, balance blood sugar, and may also play a role in preventing certain cancers.

The best food sources of omega-6 fatty acids are whole grains, seeds, and vegetable oils. Other oils such as evening primrose, borage, and black currant are especially rich stores of GLA. If you would prefer to take a supplement, try 3,000–4,000 mg of evening primrose oil per day.

Get Into Balance

Back in cavewoman times, our diets contained between a 4:1 and a 1:1 ratio of omega-6 to omega-3 fatty acids. Today, the ratio is closer to a very unhealthy 20:1 or 30:1.

Our high consumption of vegetable-based oils (containing omega-6), low intake of fish, and focus on decreasing overall fat in our diet has led to inadequate levels of omega-3 fatty acids in the body. Some groups, such as vegetarians, are particularly vulnerable to omega-3 deficiencies because they don't consume any animal foods, including omega-3–rich fish.

Fantastic Fiber

Dietary fiber is a key component to eliminating excess estrogen from your body. According to a study from Tufts University Medical School, vegetarian women excrete two to three times more estrogen in their bowel movements than do other women who eat a diet lower in fiber and higher in fat. This is great news for estrogen dominant women who are trying to reduce the estrogen load in their body.

In addition to regulating estrogen levels, fiber also binds to cholesterol. This helps to keep your bad cholesterol levels in a healthy range, which is great for estrogen deficient-slow processors.

According to a study from the *Journal of the American Neutraceutical Association*, fiber also helps to lower glucose concentration and triglyceride levels. Researchers asked nine women with high blood pressure to eat 40 grams of flaxseed every day for 12 weeks. At the end of the testing period, the women's average glucose levels decreased by 16 percent and their triglyceride levels dropped 25 percent (from 202 mg/dl to 150 mg/dl).

Moreover, fiber has been found to promote feelings of satiety (helps to prevent overeating and food cravings), slows the digestive process, supports weight loss, promotes regular bowel movements and healthy colon function, and works to maintain normal blood sugar and insulin levels. These are all great benefits for both estrogen dominant women and estrogen deficient-slow processors.

There are two types of fiber: soluble and insoluble. Soluble fibers (dissolvable in water) are found in fruits, vegetables, nuts, and beans. Insoluble fibers (not dissolvable in water) are found in oatmeal, oat bran, sesame seeds, and dried beans. To ensure that you are getting adequate amounts of both kinds of fiber (and therefore ensuring the effective elimination of excess estrogen), be sure to eat whole-grain cereals and flours; brown rice; all kinds of bran; fruits such as apricots, prunes, and apples (with skins); nuts and seeds; beans, lentils, and peas; and a wide variety of vegetables. Several of these foods should be included in every meal.

MARY'S STORY

"Mary," a 40-year-old woman with two young children, came to see me because her PMS was causing her to feel moody and irritable every month. She would yell at her children or withdraw from them when her moodiness was at its worst. She also complained that she was constantly snacking on cookies and potato chips during the week before the onset of her period.

By eliminating these foods from her diet and replacing them with lots of fresh fruits and vegetables, plenty of wild-caught, omega-3–rich fish, and high-fiber foods, Mary was able to reduce her PMS symptoms. Her moodiness disappeared, her food cravings diminished, and she was able to relax and enjoy her family.

Wonderful Water

Estrogen dominant women and estrogen deficient-slow processors need to drink lots of water to encourage the healthy detoxification of estrogen and other toxins. A great way to do double duty in this arena is to drink oxygenated water—in particular, a brand called hiOsilver (*www.hiosilver.com* or 713-937-8630).

This water is infused with pure oxygen and bottled in glass, so that the oxygen doesn't leach out. It also contains 10 times the oxygen of ordinary water. On top of that, this water will stimulate your metabolism and allow you to burn even more calories as it oxygenates your body! This can help to reduce excess weight and release fluid from the body.

Diet for Estrogen Deficient-Fast Processor

"Lorraine" came to me complaining of extreme pain, stiffness, and immobility in her fingers, wrists, elbows, knees, lower back, and feet. Every morning, she felt like she could barely move, and was especially concerned by the patches of redness on her hands, elbows, and shoulders that took several hours of activity before finally going away. Lorraine also told me that she was feeling more nervous and agitated than she could ever remember feeling in the past.

She had recently entered menopause and now, at age 53, was really beginning to suffer from menopausal symptoms, which she found to be extremely uncomfortable. These symptoms included dryness of the mouth and extreme thirst, which was worse at night. Her hot flashes and night sweats were unbearable. She was also sleeping very poorly and suffered from vaginal dryness. Moreover, she disliked how dry her skin had become and the wrinkles that were appearing around her eyes and mouth. Even her hair was drier and thinner than it had ever been.

With all of these extreme symptoms, it was obvious to me that she was in the throes of estrogen deficiency, as well as a very severe yin deficiency, which was clearly aggravated by her diet.

The hot, spicy, red meat-based meals full of peppers and chili that Lorraine loved were much too yang for her hormonal and energetic type. When she ate these foods, not only did her arthritis worsen, but she also suffered from excruciating hot flashes and skin and tissue dryness. While her diet would be more tolerable for a woman with estrogen dominance, it was destroying her health, as she was menopausal and was no longer creating the moisture and fluid balance she needed to handle such a yangizing and heating and drying diet. I explained that her diet had to undergo a significant makeover, with the elimination of these very acidic, heating foods; instead, she needed to adopt a much more alkaline, cooling, and calming cuisine.

Lorraine discarded her old ways of eating and switched to yin-enhancing types of foods that were much milder and more cooling, such as cooked grains, beans, salads, and lightly-steamed vegetables. I also recommended that she trade in her hot spices for neutral or cooling spices like peppermint, lemon balm, cilantro, marjoram, basil, chamomile, and saffron.

Almost immediately, she noticed an improvement in her degree of pain and immobility. On a scale of one to 10, her pain rating of 12 dropped to four or five with just nutritional changes alone. With an estrogen- and yin-supportive nutritional program, Lorraine's other symptoms began to resolve, and over the next few months, she was starting to feel much more comfortable.

Like Lorraine, if you are an estrogen deficient-fast processor, you need to avoid acidic, spicy, heating foods and eat a more alkaline and cooling diet that will help to restore you to a naturally healthy state of slight alkalinity. Avoid highly acidic and hot, spicy foods and choose cuisine that is more alkaline in its pH. Foods that are higher in alkaline minerals and have a pH of 5.0 or 6.0 and higher are best. The more alkaline foods are also higher in nutrients and full of the alkaline minerals needed to restore the alkaline reserves in your cells, tissues, and bones. Plus, these foods tend to be less allergenic and less likely to cause inflammatory reactions, which acidify your cells. Equally important, this diet will decrease the wear and tear on your buffer systems and organs of elimination by reducing the acid load of the body. This diet will also cause fewer inflammatory reactions.

The alkaline power diet has enormous variety and includes a tremendous range of flavors. Its major food groups include vegetables, gluten-free grains, legumes (beans and peas), small amounts of raw seeds and nuts, organic eggs, fish, shellfish, sea vegetables, and fruits like papaya and melons. Ground, raw flax meal deserves a special mention as a rich source of both alkaline minerals and anti-inflammatory polyunsaturated oils.

Eating these types of foods will help to lessen the acid load of the body and reduce the wear and tear on your pH-regulating systems, while also increasing your physical energy, stamina, and resistance to disease. Better still, the alkaline power diet provides many health benefits such as reducing the risk of heart attacks and strokes, cancer, and crippling, inflammatory conditions like arthritis.

Avoid Acidic Foods

If you are estrogen deficient-fast processor, the constant consumption of highly acidic food will, over time, rob you of your energy and vitality, reduce your mental clarity, and even dampen your optimism and enthusiasm for life. You may experience a slowdown in your ability to recover from injuries, surgery, and strenuous physical activities. The overconsumption of acidic foods can also cause you to become more prone to infections, runny noses, and allergic reactions. You may also notice an increase in menopausal symptoms, as well as aches and pains. I've had many overly acidic and estrogen deficient-fast processors tell me that drinking a glass of orange juice triggered heartburn, drinking a cup of coffee caused bladder discomfort, and eating dairy products triggered nasal congestion.

In my clinical practice, I have found that the ingestion of more-acidic, low-pH foods such as citrus fruits and juices, different types of vinegars, and highly spicy seasonings like ginger and peppers can be incredibly stressful to overly acidic persons, despite these foods' potential health benefits for the more expansive, alkaline woman. The reason for this is that their highly acidic pH can trigger either immediate or slower-acting stress responses within the body. For example, many of my estrogen deficient-fast processor patients have frequently complained about citrus fruits and vinegar causing unpleasant reactions like canker sores, heartburn, bladder pain, and joint discomfort. Other potentially nutritious, but highly acidic, foods like tomatoes, pineapple, raspberries, and wine can also cause similar symptoms. Repeated consumption of these low-pH foods tends to trigger chronic damage, inflammation, and overacidity in the affected tissues of sensitive people.

Interestingly, these symptoms can occur in some individuals even before the food has left the stomach. This suggests that a non-chemical process may be taking place since the pH-regulating systems of the body cannot work this rapidly. To explain this phenomenon, some researchers have suggested that certain stress factors, like the overacidity of foods, may cause an immediate electrical imbalance within the body, which is then followed by the actual chemical responses to the stressor agent.

If you are estrogen deficient-fast processor, your diet and food selection should concentrate on foods with a very high nutrient (especially alkaline and trace minerals) content that have a pH above 5.0, which is only mildly acidic. This will create a diet that has a vegetarian emphasis, but includes rich sources of proteins like legumes, whole grains, raw seeds and nuts, and fish and shellfish. Fish and shellfish do not have the tougher, harder to chew protein found in red meat. As a result, the stomach generally needs to produce less hydrochloric acid to digest these foods than is necessary for the breakdown of red meat. Fish such as salmon, mackerel, trout, and tuna also contain anti-inflammatory polyunsaturated oils rather than the inflammatory saturated fats found in red meat and dairy products.

MINERAL-DENSE SEA VEGETABLES

An easy and delicious way to get tons of alkaline minerals in your diet is with sea vegetables. If you are not familiar with these exotic and tasty vegetables, I strongly suggest that you acquaint yourself immediately.

Sea vegetables are extremely rich in minerals. For example, one tablespoon of kelp contains 156 mg of calcium, 104 mg of magnesium, and 753 mg of potassium. Talk about a bone blockbuster!

In addition to kelp, other types of sea vegetables include dulce, nori, and wakame. To make sure I am taking advantage of this spectacular mineral profile, I personally try to eat seaweed salad or sushi several times and week. Sea vegetables are also available in a shaker at most health food stores and can be used in place of salt.

Essential Fatty Acids

We discussed the importance of essential fatty acids (EFAs) for estrogen dominant women and estrogen deficient-slow processors, but these incredible healthy fats are also critical for estrogen deficient-fast processors. When estrogen levels decline with menopause, many women begin to experience drier, thinner skin. Fortunately, the moisture can continue to be provided to tissues of the skin, vagina, and bladder, as well as the hair, by increasing the intake of fatty acid–containing foods.

In fact, a study published in the *British Medical Journal* found that women who consumed foods rich in EFAs enjoyed greater vaginal lubrication and tissue thickness. Over a six-week period, researchers took smears from the vaginal wall every two weeks to see if the addition of these types of foods would cause a beneficial hormonal effect on the vagina. Typically, the vaginal mucosa thins out and becomes more prone to trauma and infections as the estrogen level drops with menopause. Interestingly, the vaginal mucosa responded significantly to the additional ingestion of flaxseed oil and soy flour, but returned to previous levels eight weeks after these foods were discontinued and the women went back to their usual diet.

Additionally, adequate amounts of EFAs (namely omega-3 fatty acids) have been found to substantially reduce your risk of heart disease by lowering LDL (bad) cholesterol and triglycerides, preventing blood platelets from becoming sticky, and reducing blood pressure. Plus, GLA, a critical omega-6 fatty acid, has been shown to alleviate depression, balance blood sugar, and ease pain associated with rheumatoid arthritis.

To ensure you are getting adequate amounts of omega-3 EFAs, be sure to stock up on flaxseed and fish (especially salmon, tuna, mackerel, sablefish, shad, and oysters). Other good sources include soybeans, hemp powder, walnuts, canola oil, eggs, organ meats, and some forms of algae.

The best food sources of omega-6 fatty acids are whole grains, seeds, and vegetable oils. Other oils such as evening primrose, borage, and black currant are especially rich stores of GLA.

As I mentioned on page 369, you need to make sure you are eating the right ratio of fatty acids. Ideally, you should aim for a 4:1 and a 1:1 ratio of omega-6 to omega-3 fatty acids. This is especially important for estrogen deficient-fast processors, as too much omega-6 side can increase your risk for certain chronic diseases such as atherosclerosis or clogged arteries. Similarly, too little of the omega-3 fatty acid DHA is associated with depression and memory impairment.

GET NUTTY!

One of the tastiest sources of EFAs is nuts, especially almonds, walnuts, and cashews. While EFAs in general provide a whole host of health benefits, nuts in and of themselves have a lot to brag about.

One study from *Preventive Medicine* found that people who ate nuts more than four times a week had a 37 percent lower risk of coronary heart disease than people who ate nuts rarely, if at all. Another study, this time from *Circulation*, found that people who ate eight to 13 walnuts a day had enhanced dilation of their arteries. This is great news for women with high blood pressure! Lastly, a study from the *British Journal of Nutrition* found that people who ate nut butters up to four times a week enjoyed a significant reduction in death from cardiovascular disease.

I strongly recommend that you make nuts a regular part of your diet, but do so in moderation. Because they can be high in fat and may be difficult for estrogen deficient-fast processors to digest, I recommend eating no more than 10–15 raw nuts per day three or four days a week. (I don't recommend roasted or salted nuts.)

continued on next page

Beneficial Beans and Grains

Legumes (thin beans and peas) are great sources of fiber, and their complex carbohydrates are broken down slowly in the body, benefiting women with blood sugar imbalances or diabetes, both of which are causes of obesity. They are also excellent sources of low-fat protein, particularly when combined with whole grains.

Often referred to as "cereals," whole grains also contain fiber, as well as protein, carbohydrates, fats, vitamins such as B complex and E, and numerous minerals, including calcium, magnesium, potassium, iron, copper, and manganese. They are also excellent sources of lignans, plant chemicals that act like mild estrogens in women, helping to balance estrogen levels.

Once plant lignans are eaten, intestinal bacteria convert them to substances that are weakly estrogenic and can provide additional nutritional support to menopausal women deficient in this hormone. This was confirmed in a study appearing in *Proceedings of the Society for Experimental Biology and Medicine*. Flaxseeds are 100 times richer in lignans than any other plant. Other sources of essential fatty acids include evening primrose oil, borage oil, and black currant oil. Unlike flaxseed oil, these other oils are not used as foods, but as nutritional supplements.

Spectacular Soy

Weak estrogenic activity is found in a variety of plant foods, including grains, vegetables, legumes, nuts, and seeds. However, for therapeutic purposes, only soybeans contain sufficient active compounds to approximate the effects of estrogen produced by the body.

The phytoestrogens in soybeans are two substances called genistein and daidzein, which belong to the class of chemicals called isoflavones. Soy isoflavones were first discovered during the 1930's, but their potency was not assayed until the 1950's. At that time, genistein was found to be 50,000 times weaker than a synthetic form of estrogen more commonly used at that time. Asian women eat much more soy products, and thereby phytoestrogens, in their traditional diet (which provides between 50 and 150 mg of isoflavones per day) than American women, whose isoflavone intake is virtually zero. This was confirmed in a study published in the *Lancet*, which found that Japanese women who regularly eat a range of soy products had 100 to 1,000 times more isoflavone breakdown products in their urine than Western women, who do not commonly eat soy foods.

Menopausal women in Japan who continue to eat their traditional diet tend to be less troubled by symptoms such as hot flashes. Similar studies recently conducted in the United States also monitored soy intake and menopausal symptoms and confirmed these findings. Eating soy-based foods resulted in a reduction in the severity of hot flashes and also promoted the growth of vaginal tissues, counteracting the tendency of this tissue to thin after menopause.

Eating soy-based foods also has several other long-term health benefits. Unlike prescription estrogen, soy does not appear to have a carcinogenic effect on uterine cells or breast tissue. In fact, it appears to be cancer-protective for several reasons. Not only does soy reduce the production of estrogen within the body, but it also directly inhibits the growth of breast cancer cells.

A review article appearing in the *Journal of the American Dietetics Association* confirmed that two compounds in soy, protease inhibitors and phytic acid, both have anticarcinogenic activity. The writers noted that soybean intake is associated with reduced rates of prostate, colon, and breast cancer. Women in Japan who regularly eat large quantities of soy foods have an incidence of breast cancer four to six times lower than that of women who do not include soy in their diet.

Other studies currently in progress suggest that soy can have a beneficial effect on both blood fats and bone metabolism. While estrogen is often prescribed to prevent heart disease and osteoporosis, soy offers a food-based approach to the same health issues.

To receive optimal therapeutic benefits, be sure to read labels to make sure that your total soy intake is at least 30 to 50 g of soy protein per day. For example, one glass of soy milk contains between two and 10 grams of protein, soy burgers typically contain eight grams, and soy cheeses four grams per slice. Soy sauce, however, is of very little benefit as a phytoestrogen. For women who do not like soy foods, soy-based protein powders and capsules now contain pre-measured amounts of isoflavones.

If you find that soy foods cause digestive upset such as gas, bloating, or intestinal discomfort, I suggest that you either take a digestive enzyme specifically formulated for bean and vegetable intake when eating soy or use soy isoflavone capsules (50–100 mg per day). If you are allergic to soy, then avoid consuming it entirely.

Win With Water

Drinking pure, alkaline water helps to dilute the acid in your system. But if you want to up the stakes in your favor, opt for mineral water with an alkaline pH. Stick to non-carbonated varieties, since many sparkling mineral waters lose their natural alkalinity when carbonated with acidifying carbon dioxide.

But the "best in show" for alkaline water has to be mineral water with natural bicarbonate. A study presented at a meeting of the American Society for Bone and Mineral Research found that women who drank 1.5 liters per day of bottled mineral water that contained bicarbonate for four weeks saw less calcium loss than those women who drank water without bicarbonate.

When it comes to alkaline mineral water with natural bicarb, I'm a huge fan of Trinity water from Paradise, Idaho (*www.trinitysprings.com*). It contains 10 mg of bicarbonate, a healthy dose of silica, and an astounding pH of 9.6.

You can also make your own alkaline water with a water ionizer. I am partial to the AlkaZone by Better Health Lab, Inc. (*www.alkazone.com* or 800-810-1888). I also like Micro-water (*www.1microwaterco.com* or 740-758-5707), a highly sophisticated water ionizer that recently became available in the U.S. and Canada.

Better Health Lab also sells Alkaline Booster—tasteless, colorless, liquid mineral drops that you add to your water. Three or four drops can have the same alkalinizing benefits as the entire water ionizing system attached to your kitchen sink. Alkaline Booster is ideal for travel and can easily fit in your purse.

REVERSING ROSACEA

Rosacea is a skin condition characterized by ruddy cheeks and small pimples. Although we don't know why people develop this skin disorder, we know that the redness, bumps, and blemishes that occur are the result of enlarged, dilated blood vessels. We also know that rosacea isn't caused by a virus or a bacterial infection, so it can't be spread from person to person.

According to a report issued by the American Academy of Dermatologists (AAD), nearly 14 million Americans have rosacea, yet nearly 75 percent of them don't know it. The AAD also reports that women are more likely than men to get the condition, and that women often develop rosacea during menopause. Additionally, if you are between ages 30 to 50, have a fair complexion, have ancestors from northern Europe, or have family members with rosacea, you are have a greater chance of getting the condition.

At first, rosacea will present as a flushed appearance on the cheeks, forehead, and nose. If left untreated, symptoms can also develop on the neck, back, ears, scalp, and inside and around the eyes. In an advanced stage, a person may develop a bulbous nose or thickened, distorted patches of skin. Aside from being unsightly, rosacea can be extremely painful. Many women describe it as a stinging or sunburn sensation, due in part from inflammation that occurs during flare-ups.

continued on next page

Adopt a Preemptive Strategy

The best strategy for treating rosacea is a preemptive one. First and foremost, it's important to get an accurate diagnosis before you begin any treatment therapies. So you should see a dermatologist as soon as possible. Since many over-the-counter topical creams and gels can actually exacerbate the condition, I recommend lifestyle changes rather than self-treatment. Here are some recommendations.

- Avoid things that trigger your face to become flushed. These include highly acidic foods, such as spicy and fried foods, sugar, caffeine, dairy products, trans fatty acids, and alcoholic beverages. The National Rosacea Society also identified Mexican food; hot sausage; hot peppers; black, red, and white pepper; paprika; vinegar; and garlic as triggers. Also keep a journal of triggers (foods, activities, medicines, etc.) to share with your doctor.

- Determine whether any of your cosmetic products are aggravating your condition. Ask your dermatologist to recommend skin-care products that are non-irritating.

- Protect your skin with a sunscreen containing SPF 15 or higher. I especially recommend using products that contain zinc oxide (which blocks harmful rays) and wearing a hat.

- You also need to be careful not to scrub or rub your face roughly. You don't want to be the cause of your own redness.

- Finally, you should take a good, high quality multinutrient that contains 25–100 mg of the **B-complex vitamins—especially riboflavin (B$_2$), which has been shown to be effective in treatment of rosacea.**

Treatment Options

There are two treatment options to consider: intense pulse light therapy and cosmetic procedures. These treat blemishes and reduce the appearance of red lines due to broken blood vessels.

Intense Pulse Light Therapy

I am a big fan of light-based therapies, so I was particularly excited to come across a study published in the *Journal of Drugs in Dermatology* on its effectiveness for treating rosacea. Thirty-two patients completed one to seven treatments with intense pulsed light. At the end of the treatment period, 83 percent noticed less redness; 75 percent reported an improvement in their skin texture and a reduction in flushes; and 65 per-

continued on next page

REVERSING ROSACEA   *continued*
cent reported a decrease in their number of pimples. Ask your dermatologist about this safe alternative.

Cosmetic Procedures
In general, I am not a big fan of cosmetic procedures. If you decide to explore either of these options listed below, make sure you go to a licensed dermatologist who specializes in cosmetic procedures.
- Glycolic acid peels have been used effectively to treat rosacea. Known for their ability to reduce fine lines and wrinkles, the fruit acids used in glycolic acid peel treatments will significantly improve your skin's texture, reducing redness and ridding your skin of break-outs.
- Laser therapy can be used to erase the redness at the skin's surface due to broken blood vessels. Although it is safe, laser therapy is quite expensive and requires many visits before true results are seen.

Inflammation and Hormone Health

All traumatic injuries are characterized by an inflammatory response. Similarly, internal injury to tissues due to such stressors as infectious bacteria, viruses, allergens, and toxins can also cause inflammation. Inflammation of an injured area is characterized by swelling, heat, stiffness, a reduced range of motion, and pain on weight bearing or use of the extremity or joint. No matter where the site of the injury, the physical manifestations are the same.

When an area of the body becomes inflamed, the blood vessels and capillaries in the injured area begin to dilate (expand), allowing fluids carrying the body's own healing substances to reach the area quickly. At the same time, the capillary walls become more permeable, and fluids force their way into the surrounding tissue, causing congestion.

Very quickly more fluid and waste accumulate than the area can handle. Helper cells seal off the damaged area, creating fibrin clots made of protein, to prevent the spread of bacteria and toxins to surrounding areas. The result is blockage of the blood and lymph vessels, leading to redness, bloating, swelling, heat, pain, and the formation of excess fluids in the tissue (edema). For example, when injury occurs in the intestinal tract due to an offending food, your abdomen and midriff can swell.

Eating the wrong foods can cause inflammation in three ways—allergic reactions; injury to digestive organs; and production of series 2, inflammation-causing prostaglandins. When your body detects an allergen, it releases histamines and other chemicals to the affected areas, often causing that area to swell.

Your body tries to control and regulate the damage caused by inflammation through the production of the adrenal hormone cortisol. The immediate effect of cortisol is to block most of the factors that are promoting the inflammation, so that the rate of healing is enhanced. Cortisol production, as well as sex hormone production from the adrenals, is regulated by the same mechanism through the hypothalamus and the pituitary. This is done through the secretion of corticotrophin-releasing hormone (CRH) from the hypothalamus and adreno-corticotropic hormone (ACTH) secreted by the anterior pituitary gland.

Foods can also injure your digestive organs, namely the liver. When the liver's function is impaired and it cannot fully detoxify certain compounds of our diet, toxic by-products will accumulate in the body. Alcohol is particularly taxing to the liver, causing inflammatory changes which can diminish its ability to operate at peak performance. Increased alcohol consumption can also cause mild inflammation of the pancreas, abdominal bloating, swelling, and discomfort. Similarly, excess sugar in the liver can impair its function. When the liver stores too much glucose, it must work harder to produce bile and essential digestive enzymes. Over time, this maltreatment takes its toll on the liver, resulting in damage to the liver cells, which, in turn, manifests as inflammation.

Lastly, prostaglandins, the short-lived hormones we talked about in relation to essential fatty acids, can be either inflammatory (primarily series 2) or anti-inflammatory (primarily series 3). Simply increasing your consumption of foods, especially from the series 3 category (omega-3 EFAs found in cold-water fish, flaxseeds, soybeans, walnuts, etc.), versus those high in the inflammatory series 2 prostaglandins (red meat and dairy products), will help to eliminate this source of inflammation.

Different Women, Different Inflammatory Effects

When inflammation in a woman is poorly controlled or chronic, as it is in so many women today, the adrenal glands are significantly weakened by this constant inflammatory stress. This also significantly decreases sex hormone production by the adrenal glands. In estrogen dominant women, this can result in estrogen/progesterone imbalances, with increased levels of both estrogen and inflammation, leading to bloating, fibroids, endometriosis, menstrual cramps, breast lumps, and ovarian cysts.

In women who are estrogen deficient-fast processors, the process of inflammation not only reduces sex hormone production, but also generates heat internally. It causes a woman to become yin deficient and lose her calming, cooling yin fluids and become more yang, dry, hot, and contracted. This can worsen all menopause symptoms, including hot flashes, night sweats, and skin and vaginal dryness. Inflammation can even predispose a woman to health issues such as rheumatoid arthritis, colitis, and heart disease.

You can help to bring inflammation under control and take the stress off of your adrenals by improving your diet. Simply eliminating those foods that trigger false fat in your body and replacing them with common, non-inflammatory Mediterranean-style cuisine will help you restore healthy hormone production.

ESSENTIAL DIGESTIVE ENZYMES

The inflammatory process is also controlled by numerous digestive enzymes, especially the body's own pancreatic protein-digesting (proteolytic) enzymes, which eliminate debris at the injury site and initiate the repair of tissue. These enzymes also break up the fibrin, which is made of protein, so that it can be excreted.

Digestive enzymes keep the pathological process from spreading and considerably reduce the duration of the injury by speeding up the healing process. Thus, abundant production of or supplementation with digestive enzymes can greatly limit the severity and scope of inflammatory diseases or external injuries. This means a reduced risk of serious health conditions, including cancer, heart disease, arthritis, and high cholesterol.

A number of digestive enzymes can be used to help ease the effects of inflammation. **I am especially partial to pancreatic enzymes (300–1,000 mg up to four times a day), bromelain (500–1,000 mg two to four times a day), and papain (200–300 mg two to four times a day).** To combat inflammation, take digestive enzymes between meals, as directed above. You can also take with meals to promote healthy digestion.

Common Saboteurs for All Hormone Types

To reduce your risk for inflammation, there are certain classes of food and drink that all women should work to replace, regardless of whether you are estrogen dominant, estrogen deficient-slow processor, or estrogen deficient-fast processor. That's because they have little (if any) nutritional value, and may even cause you to lose valuable nutrients as your body processes them. In some cases, these foods have been shown to actually lead to dangerous health conditions, including damage to your joints, skin, bladder, reproductive organs, and thyroid. Over time, chronic damage to and injury of the affected cells and tissues can lead to reduced energy production, a decrease in oxygen levels, and a loss of alkaline substances and minerals—all of which can contribute to overacidity and, ultimately, disease.

There are five foods that are particularly unhealthy. They include alcohol, caffeine, dairy, sugar, and wheat. Unfortunately, many women unknowingly overeat many of these foods, which worsens their symptoms of hormonal imbalance. Let's take a look at each one individually and how it affects estrogen dominant women, estrogen deficient-slow processors, and estrogen deficient-fast processors.

Alcohol

Numerous studies show that women are markedly less able to tolerate alcohol than men. Women metabolize alcohol slower than men, thus it takes longer to clear out alcohol's toxic effects.

Alcohol is particularly problematic for **estrogen dominant** women, as it increases your estrogen level, and is associated with fibroids, endometriosis, heavy bleeding, and the development of breast cancer. Plus, it may inhibit ovulation. Moreover, excess alcohol can tax your liver, making it more difficult to detoxify excess estrogen, thus allowing more free estrogen to be circulated in the blood. This can lead to a whole host of issues for **estrogen dominant women** or **estrogen deficient-slow processors** (alcohol can cause bloating in these women).

For **estrogen deficient-fast processors**, alcohol can actually worsen every single menopausal symptom, including hot flashes and mood swings. It is particularly pronounced in women who suffer from night sweats and insomnia. Alcohol is a diuretic. This means that overconsumption can lead to dehydration of your skin and tissues, as well as loss of essential minerals through urination.

Caffeine

If you habitually drink too much coffee or cola (12 ounces or more a day), or indulge in a chocolate bar every afternoon, you're putting undue stress on your adrenal glands, which secrete stress hormones. The caffeine stimulates the release of additional stress hormones, increasing your anxiety, and stealing valuable nutrients from the rest of your body to feed your overcharged, stressed nervous system.

In addition to being addictive, caffeine can also affect estrogen levels, increasing blood levels of this hormone and thus contributing to menstrual problems and certain cancers. It can also deplete you of vital B vitamins, which can interfere with carbohydrate metabolism and healthy liver function. Caffeine has also been linked to a worsening of nodules and tenderness in women with benign breast disease. This is a particular concern for **estrogen dominant women or estrogen deficient-slow processors**.

Caffeine also reduces the absorption of iron and calcium. This is problematic for **estrogen deficient-fast processors** who are at risk for osteoporosis. Caffeine also increases blood levels of cholesterol and triglycerides, as well as blood pressure, all of which are risk factors for heart attack. Plus, caffeine has been shown to worsen the frequency and intensity of hot flashes.

If you are a caffeine drinker, I recommend gently easing yourself off by slowly decreasing your intake at a satisfactory speed in order to avoid triggering these symptoms. Start by cutting your consumption in half. For example, if you drink four cups of coffee a day, try going down to two cups. Once you can comfortably maintain this level, reduce your intake by half again (from two to one). And who knows, by that time, you may be ready to eliminate that final cup!

You can also opt for herbal teas, such as peppermint and chamomile for estrogen deficient-fast processors or ginger or chai tea for estrogen dominant women or estrogen deficient-slow processors. I also highly recommend the delicious, herbal coffee substitute Teeccino (*www.teeccino.com*). Kimberly credits Teeccino with helping her break her two cups a day coffee habit.

Dairy Products

Dairy products are one of the primary sources of food allergies in the standard American diet. Symptoms include fatigue, depression, bloating, intestinal gas, bowel changes, wheezing, nasal congestion, and frequent colds.

If you are **estrogen dominant**, such food allergies can also make your PMS symptoms worse. For these women, as well as **estrogen deficient-slow processors** dairy products weaken your adrenal glands over time, greatly increasing your susceptibility to stress. Also, the high saturated fat content of many dairy products is a risk factor for excess estrogen levels in the body. Unhealthy, anaerobic bacteria in the intestinal tract actually convert metabolites of estrogen into forms of free estrogen that can be reabsorbed from the digestive tract back into the body. This elevates your body's estrogen levels, which can aggravate conditions such as fibroids and endometriosis.

In **estrogen deficient-fast processors**, there may be an immediate or delayed allergic reaction to dairy, which manifests as anxiety, irritability, depression or mood swings, insomnia, fatigue, spaciness, dizziness, confusion and disorientation, headaches, and joint pain.

Even if you are not allergic to dairy products, they can be difficult for many women to digest. Plus, the artificial hormones, as well as the pesticides used in livestock feed, make cow's milk an unhealthy choice.

Sugar

Sugar is one of the most overused foods in the Western world. Present almost universally in desserts and sweet snacks, sugar is also an ingredient in condiments such as salad dressings, ketchup, and relish. In addition, foods such as pasta and bread, when made with white flour, act as simple sugars in the body.

Eating large amounts of sugar, especially in a short period of time, can trigger an episode of hypoglycemia (low blood sugar). The mechanism is as follows: Sugar is rapidly absorbed from the digestive tract into the circulation. In response to these elevated blood sugar levels, the pancreas secretes insulin to enable the sugar to be cleared from the bloodstream and be taken up by the cells, where it is used as a source of energy.

In response to large amounts of ingested sugar, the pancreas often overproduces insulin, which causes the blood sugar to fall too low. As a result, hypoglycemia occurs, causing an individual to feel anxious, tremulous, and jittery; in addition, thinking can become confused because the brain is deprived of necessary fuel. To remedy this situation, the adrenal glands release hormones, which cause the liver to pump stored sugar into the bloodstream. However, while the adrenal hormones boost the blood sugar level, they also increase arousal symptoms and anxiety. Both the initial brain deprivation of glucose and the adrenal glands' attempt to restore the glucose levels can intensify symptoms of anxiety and panic in susceptible people. Studies confirm that people who are anxiety-prone are especially sensitive to the emotional effects of a drop in blood sugar.

Estrogen dominant women with PMS may have hypoglycemia related to their menstrual cycles. It is known that women with PMS crave more simple carbohydrates, such as refined sugar and flour. Research shows that 80 to 90 percent of women who eat this way report stress, anxiety, moodiness, and irritability during the week or two preceding menstruation.

My clinical experience is that many of these symptoms can be reversed with dietary changes. An extensive review article on the role of low blood sugar and personality, reported in *Complementary Therapies in Medicine*, provided evidence that low blood sugar is almost always accompanied by personality disorders and that improvement or complete remission is possible with nutritional therapy.

Excess sugar can worsen anxiety and irritability as women transition into menopause, especially in the case of **estrogen deficient-fast processors,** while **estrogen deficient-slow processors** will experience low energy. With both of these groups, too much sugar intake can also aggravate diabetes, elevate triglycoides, *Candida*, food addiction, tooth decay, and gum disease.

PASS ON THE PINK, BLUE, AND YELLOW

While you should work to avoid sugar, don't be tempted by the artificial sweeteners on the market. Not only do they leave a horrible aftertaste, but they are downright bad for you.

Take saccharin for example. Research from the 1980's showed that, in very high doses, saccharin caused bladder cancer in male rats. However, the pseudo-sugar community argued that the doses were so high, and so specific to older male rats (versus other test animals) that the FDA has allowed saccharin to stay on the market. They did have one caveat—there had to be a warning label stating that saccharin might be a carcinogen.

The next option is aspartame, the lovely sweetener decorating restaurant tables across the country with little blue packets. This controversial sweetener is made by combining two amino acids—aspartic acid and phenylalanine—with 10 percent methanol, an alcohol that breaks down into formaldehyde in your body. Yum! This combination has been found to have potent excitatory effects on brain chemistry, often leading to a whole host of health problems, including headaches, dizziness, anxiety, and depression.

Finally, there's sucralose (Splenda), the seemingly miraculous sweetener that "tastes like sugar because it's made from sugar." Well, sort of. Sucralose is made by replacing two of the molecules from table sugar with chlorine, creating a substance 600 times sweeter than sugar. From a health standpoint, those two chlorine molecules are problematic. Rodent research has shown that sucralose causes shrinkage of the thymus gland—up to 40 percent—as well as some enlargement of the liver and kidneys. Considering that a properly-functioning thymus gland is essential for a healthy immune system, this is not great news. But, once again, the manufacturer dismissed these problems as due to high doses, and the FDA has approved sucralose without any long term human studies or formal follow-up.

Wheat and Gluten

Like dairy, many women find they're intolerant to or allergic to wheat products. That's because wheat contains a protein called gluten, which is difficult for your body to break down, absorb and assimilate.

According to a study from the *Archives of Internal Medicine*, more than 1.5 million Americans have celiac disease, a digestive condition that is triggered by gluten—a protein found in wheat, rye, and barley. While celiac disease can represent the extreme end of a gluten disorder, even those women with a mild to moderate case of wheat or gluten intolerance can be putting their health at risk.

Women with wheat intolerance are prone to chronic fatigue, depression, bloating, intestinal gas, bowel changes, post-nasal drip and nasal congestion, and frequent colds. They can also suffer from mood disorder, migraine headaches, and fibromyalgia.

Spectacular Substitutions

One of the most difficult things to do as a physician is to tell someone that they would have to give up something they enjoy. In fact, I'll never forget one female patient in particular who burst into tears when I suggested that she avoid wheat and dairy. She reminded me that she was a homemaker on a limited budget. The list scared her as she felt she had to replace everything in her pantry and refrigerator. That would cost quite a bit, she sobbed. Plus, she worried she'd have to learn a completely new way of eating before she felt better.

Since then, I never tell a woman to avoid a food or food category without giving her several great alternatives that she will love.

- **Alcohol Substitutes:** non-alcoholic wine or beer; sparkling water and lime twist; mineral water with a few drops of flavored, sweetened stevia (Sweet Leaf has the best)
- **Caffeine Substitutes:** Teeccino herbal coffee, green tea, herbal tea, carob bars
- **Dairy Substitutes:** soy, rice, or almond milk; goat, rice, or soy cheese; rice or soy ice creams. Great brands include Good Karma Organic Rice Cream and Soy Delight
- **Sugar Substitutes:** xylitol, erythritol, maple syrup, honey, agave nectar
- **Wheat Substitutes:** oat, soy, corn, rice, millet, quinoa, and buckwheat breads, crackers, pizza crusts, bagels, and pasta. Great brands include Pamela's, Gluten-Free Pantry, Namaste Foods, Foods by George, Glutino, and Bionaturae

* * *

I know the scope of changing your dietary habits can be overwhelming. Don't expect to change your diet overnight; instead, phase your changes in one week at a time. Keep in mind the time-tested fable about the tortoise and the hare. The tortoise won because slow and steady always wins the race! The same lesson applies to all of these principles—give them time to work.

And remember, the mile-long journey of restoring your health starts with a few small steps. So, when you look back over a year, you'll be astonished at the amount of health and well being you've regained if you just keep at it and stay with your own healing program.

healing foods for hormonal health

28

As you've learned, all women should be eating a close-to-the-earth, Mediterranean-style diet modified to their particular hormonal profile, based on the pH of food. If you are estrogen dominant or an estrogen deficient-slow processor, you need to choose foods that are more acidic, energizing, and spicier. Conversely, estrogen deficient-fast processors should be choosing more cooling, calming, and expansive foods from the alkaline side of the scale.

But, regardless of where you are on the hormonal scale, there are three amazing nutritional regimes that can benefit all women. Not only do they help to restore and balance hormone levels, but they have amazing health benefits for your overall well-being.

The High Enzyme Diet

Foods that are rich in their own natural enzymes provide you with natural digestants and anti-inflammatory chemicals. In this way, the foods themselves aid in the process of digestion, helping to keep your hormones in the proper balance.

The best foods for an enzyme-rich diet are fresh fruits (particularly ones with low acid content like melons and papayas, if you tend to be an estrogen deficient-fast processor) and vegetables, along with sprouted beans and seeds. These foods are easy to digest because they contain natural enzymes. Aim to include them with many of your meals.

Various plant enzymes assist in the ripening and maturation process as well as the eventual breakdown and decay of the plant. When raw plant foods are consumed, their enzymes assist in the breakdown of food, beginning in the upper digestive tract. As the food passes through the digestive tract, these plant enzymes ease the workload of the digestive system and reduce the demand on the body's store of enzymes. Over time, this assistance can have a restorative effect on the body's digestive capability.

Fresh Fruits and Vegetables

All fresh fruits and vegetables contain natural digestive enzymes. Two fruits in particular, pineapple and papaya, contain some of the most potent protein-digesting enzymes. The proteolytic enzyme in pineapple is bromelain, and in papaya, papain. Of these two, papain is most useful as a digestive enzyme because of its soothing effect on the stomach. Bromelain is used as a potent anti-inflammatory.

However, many individuals with low enzyme production are also highly acidic, and pineapple and its juice are highly acidic and may cause canker sores and digestive upset in overly acidic individuals. Therefore, I often recommend to patients that they include papaya in their diet, and suggest eating pineapple on an infrequent basis. (Women with estrogen dominance and estrogen deficient-slow processors can better handle pineapple.) Luckily, the best delivery system for bromelain and papain is in supplemental form, which allows one to benefit from the enzymatic properties of both pineapple and papaya, without the acidic concerns.

Sprouted Seeds, Grains, and Legumes

All sprouted seeds are exceptionally rich sources of natural enzymes. A seed that is in the process of sprouting is in a very active state of maturation, rich in enzymes and nutrients. When a seed sprouts, its nutrient value multiplies many times.

As sprouts germinate, they generate increased levels of calcium, potassium, sodium, iron, phosphorous, and vitamins A, B_1, B_2, B_3, and C. Germination also converts a significant portion of the carbohydrates in sprouts into easily digestible protein, and it reduces the oligosaccharides (gas-forming compounds in beans), making sprouts less likely to produce that uncomfortable effect. But that's not all. Sprouts are also incredibly easy to digest. As such, it is much easier for their nutrients to reach your blood and cells.

Alfalfa sprouts contain as much beta-carotene as carrots, as well as high levels of calcium, iron, magnesium, potassium, phosphorus, sodium, sulfur, silicon, chlorine, cobalt, and zinc. Green peas, lentils, garbanzo beans, sunflower seeds, adzuki beans, and mung beans can all be sprouted.

To significantly increase the level of nutrients and natural enzymes in your diet, add sprouted seeds and beans to your salads or sandwiches. You may enjoy the taste of some sprouts more than others—so experiment. Try sprouted sunflower seeds, flax seeds, radish, broccoli, onions, adzuki beans, garbanzo beans, and lentils.

A wide variety of sprouts are available in local supermarkets as well as natural-food stores and farmers' markets—but be sure to choose sprouts carefully. Several years ago, the sprout industry came under attack because crops of alfalfa sprouts were found to be contaminated with *E. coli* and Salmonella. It turned out that the seeds involved in these outbreaks had not been disinfected prior to sprouting. In response to this situation, the International Sprout Growers Association (ISGA) identified seed sanitation guidelines and provided a voluntary grower certification for those companies willing to have their processes inspected by a third party. Growers that participated in that program have an ISGA seal on their products, so make sure to purchase brands with this seal. Also inspect the sprouts before you buy them to ensure that they look fresh and crisp, not slimy or dark.

You can also grow your own sprouts. I personally buy my sprout seeds from the Sproutman (*www.sproutman.com*), a well-known grower in the field. Sprouting seeds are different from traditional planting seeds in that they are specifically packaged and tested for their ability to germinate into sprouts. Sproutman has sprouting bags and larger automatic sprouters available, but you can also sprout seeds and beans by simply using a large glass jar and some water.

To sprout seeds at home, follow these simple instructions. Once you have the sprouting seeds, wash them thoroughly and place them in a jar of filtered or distilled water. Let them soak for about 24 hours, rinsing them off once or twice and putting them back in the jar with fresh water. Then, pour the water out of the jar, and set the seeds away from the sunlight until they begin to sprout. Make sure to rinse them off two or three times each day while they are germinating. Once they have sprouted, place the jar in sunlight and let the seeds sit there for one or two more days, rinsing them two or three times a day. After one or two days in sunlight, they will be ready to eat, but it's very important to keep them in the refrigerator

Fermented Foods

Fermented foods are staples in the traditional cuisines of Europe, throughout the Mediterranean and Middle East, and in Asia, where the fermented tea *kombucha* is a common drink and fermented soy products such as soy sauce, shoyu, tamari, and tempeh are eaten every day. These cultured foods all contain living microorganisms that enhance the food's flavor, digestibility, and nutritional value, as well as acting as a preservative. Many fermented foods are also rich sources of enzymes that enhance digestive function.

As you know, cruciferous vegetables such as cabbage already contain many compounds that protect against cancer. When they are lacto-fermented, they provide even more anti-cancer compounds.

A recent study found that Polish women who traditionally ate real sauerkraut on a regular basis had a significant increase in the incidence of breast cancer when they moved to America and abandoned their traditional diets. Their relatives in Poland suffered no such increase, and continued to enjoy greater protection from breast cancer. In addition to the anti-cancer compounds, researchers found that extracts from real sauerkraut contained anti-estrogenic agents that were different from any they had seen before.

In another study, fermented soy products had anti-tumor and anti-metastatic effects on laboratory mice, and these effects increased with longer fermentation time. Additionally, a German study found that precancerous colon polyps disappeared after four to six weeks of a diet that included generous amounts of lacto-fermented vegetables. Even more interesting, the polyps stayed away as long as the vegetables remained in the diet.

To get these and other benefits, increase your consumption of fermented foods such as yogurt, sauerkraut, olives, pickles, beer, wine, vinegar, as well as a wide variety of vegetables. Whenever possible, buy these foods fresh, as commercial processing can destroy the beneficial enzymes. You can usually find these in natural-food stores, which sometimes carry items such as freshly made sauerkraut, cured olives, and natural yogurt.

Raw Foods

While all raw foods including fish, meat, and poultry contain enzymes, eating raw flesh foods can be very hazardous due to bacteria and parasites. This is especially true when you do not personally know how the meat, fish, or poultry has been handled since it was slaughtered or caught. Therefore, the eating of raw flesh foods, even though they retain their natural enzymes, is not encouraged.

It is important to know that cooked foods do *not* contain active enzymes. When food is heated above 140°F, all its valuable enzymes are destroyed. All common cooking techniques such as sautéing, frying, boiling, and baking occur at temperatures that are well in excess of this threshold. Even such reputedly healthy cooking techniques as steaming and slow cooking in a Crock-Pot are commonly done at temperatures well above 140°F. All food that is canned or otherwise heat-processed has also lost all of its living enzymes and must rely on the enzymes created by the body for its digestion. The cooking process also destroys certain amounts of vitamins, minerals, and other phytonutrients.

While such food may still have many healthy vitamins and minerals, all of its natural enzymes have been inactivated. Frozen foods, usually considered healthier than canned foods, also retain virtually none of their active enzymes. Almost all frozen foods have been blanched (placed in boiling water for two to six minutes, depending on the fruit or vegetable) prior to freezing with the express purpose of arresting the enzyme activity so as to not bring about other nutritional losses or create off flavors through the activity of the natural enzymes. Commercial fruit juices have been pasteurized, which also inactivates their enzymes. However, fresh juices made at home using a juicer retain the active enzymes found in the raw fruits and vegetables they are made from.

A CAUTION ON EATING RAW SEEDS

All raw seeds, beans, and grains are rich in natural enzymes. However, these plants also contain enzyme inhibitors that prevent self-digestion. Without these inhibitors, the seeds, beans, and grains would ripen and decay before they could find the right location in which to germinate and grow. These foods have naturally extended shelf lives due to these inhibitors, but they can cause digestive difficulties when consumed in large quantities because these inhibitors affect not only the enzymes contained in the plants, but also the enzymes produced by the digestive organs, thereby placing an extra burden on the pancreas. So if you eat raw seeds as snacks, be sure to take supplemental enzymes to reduce the stress on your digestive tract.

When seeds, beans and grains germinate, the inhibitors are deactivated. Cooking also deactivates many of the inhibitors, but experts differ as to whether it completely removes all of them.

Combining Raw and Cooked Foods

It is not necessary to eat only raw foods to receive the digestive benefits of plant enzymes. Raw and cooked foods can be eaten in combination. A bowl of lentil soup and a carrot slaw provide legumes that are cooked (the lentils), coupled with living enzymes in the raw carrots. Poached salmon salad made with sliced onions and served on romaine lettuce is also a mix of both cooked and enzyme-rich raw ingredients.

People with weak digestive function may find that eating mostly raw foods can cause digestion symptoms like gas and bloating. Raw vegetables are made up of nonnutritive cellulose, which is tough, fibrous, and difficult for some individuals to digest. To make fibrous foods more easily digestible, it is important to chew them thoroughly. For patients with sensitive digestive systems, I recommend lightly steamed foods, easy-to-digest dishes like soups, and well-cooked grains along with side dishes of raw foods like salads. (As digestive function improves, my patients are usually able to tolerate more raw foods in their diets.)

If you do enjoy salads and raw vegetables, it is fine to include these more and more in your meals as you restore your digestive function with enzyme-rich foods. However, I recommend making the transition slowly so that your body can adapt.

Healing Sugars

For many years, I have been telling millions of health-conscious women just like you that sugar contributes to countless health problems, particularly table sugar and cane sugar. It increases fatigue, worsens PMS symptoms, aggravates inflammation, contributes to (if not causes) type-2 diabetes, weakens tooth enamel, promotes obesity, worsens hypoglycemia, and feeds *Candida*.

However, there are several health-enhancing, therapeutic sugars that are rarely discussed. These eight amazing sugars—collectively called glyconutrients—have incredible healing powers for a wide variety of conditions that commonly affect women. These include galactose, glucose, fucose, mannose, N-acetylgalactosamine, N-acetylglucosamine, N-acetylneuraminic acid, and xylose. Simply adding these glyconutrients to your diet is helpful for women with all three hormonal profiles.

What are Glyconutrients?

Glyconutrients are an essential component of a special coating that surrounds each and every cell in your body. They serve as the building blocks for the creation of glycoproteins and glycolipids—together, these molecules are called *glycoconjugates*. Glycoconjugates cover the surface of your cells with a sugary coating. This coating plays a crucial role in your body—it ensures that your cells are interacting and communicating properly with each other. Since all body functions start at the cellular level, and cell miscommunication is a leading cause of countless conditions and diseases (including autoimmune disease and cancer), it's obvious that this coating is so critical for good health.

Your body gets glyconutrients in two ways: First, it can make them itself. However, the process of making glyconutrients can be long and difficult—especially if your body is missing certain vitamins, enzymes, or other nutrients involved in the process. Unfortunately, this is all too common in most people. Second, your body can get glyconutrients through the foods you eat, but only two of them—galactose and glucose—are commonly found in the human diet. Galactose is found in many fruits and vegetables, as well as in the lactose of dairy products; glucose is readily available in simple carbohydrate, unhealthy foods like white flour products, but it can also be made from the more complex and healthier carbohydrate foods, like whole grains.

Since all of these foods are staples in the American diet (though I certainly suggest limiting both dairy products and simple carbohydrates), let's focus on the other six glyconutrients and learn how you can get more of them in your body, and how they can benefit your health.

Fucose

Unlike fructose, which has no nutritional value, fucose is key to healthy brain development, brain function, and memory. Numerous animal studies, including one published in *Brain Research*, which found that fucose and compounds containing fucose improve memory formation. In addition, fucose inhibits cancer tumor growth and spread, and it guards against respiratory infections, diabetes, and shingles.

Fucose is found in human breast milk, certain medicinal mushrooms, kelp, wakame seaweed, and marine algae. Since the first two are hard to come by, I advise adding green foods to your diet, including cereal grasses, chlorella, spirulina, and wild blue-green algae.

Mannose

Mannose has antibacterial, antiviral, and antifungal properties. It plays a key role in the formation of cytokines—the chemicals that make you feel achy when you're sick. Cytokines, in turn, stimulate the immune system to fight the parasitic invader. In addition, mannose helps prevent urinary tract infections and stomach ulcers, and research suggests that it stimulates collagen production, which helps to ease the inflammation of rheumatoid arthritis.

Mannose can be found in berries, including blueberries, cranberries, currants, and gooseberries. It's also in green beans, soy beans, eggplant, cabbage, turnips, kelp, and *Aloe vera*.

N-Acetylgalactosamine

This glyconutrient inhibits the spread of tumors, and lower-than-normal levels of it have been observed in people with heart disease. It also appears to prevent inflammation associated with arthritis.

N-acetylgalactosamine is not readily available in the human diet, though it is found in human breast milk, and it is an element of chondroitin sulfate.

N-Acetylglucosamine

N-acetylglucosamine is also difficult to find in the diet. It's most abundant in glucosamine—a metabolic product of this glyconutrient—and in human breast milk. Many studies confirm that N-acetylglucosamine helps repair cartilage and decreases the pain and inflammation of arthritis. In addition, it can help with Crohn's disease and ulcerative colitis, and it has been found to decrease insulin secretion.

The main food source of N-acetylglucosamine is shiitake mushrooms.

N-Acetylneuraminic Acid

N-acetylneuraminic acid is essential for brain development and learning, as well as for memory and performance. It also inhibits strains of the flu virus and influences cholesterol levels by lowering LDL ("bad" cholesterol). High levels of this glyconutrient are found in the brain, skin, kidneys, and other organs.

Not surprisingly, since it's so important for brain development, N-acetylneuraminic acid is mainly found in human breast milk. Unfortunately, there are no food sources.

Xylose

Also known as xylitol, xylose has antibacterial and antifungal properties, and research even suggests that xylose can help prevent digestive disorders and even cancer of the digestive tract. Xylose also appears to discourage pathogens from binding to mucous membranes, and helps promote healthy teeth and gums.

Xylose can be found in guavas, pears, blackberries, loganberries, raspberries, aloe vera, psyllium seeds, broccoli, spinach, eggplant, peas, green beans, okra, cabbage, and corn.

Get More Glyconutrients

While so many of these amazing nutrients are found predominantly in breast milk, there are still many ways you can incorporate glyconutrients into your diet and reap their amazing health benefits.

First, add the foods I've mentioned above into your diet—specifically, green foods, berries, and vegetables. You also can find glyconutrients in a natural form called arabinogalactans (better known as gum sugars), which are found in corn, carrots, radishes, pears, and the herbs curcumin and echinacea. Next, supplement with glucosamine (up to 1,500 mg a day) and chondroitin sulfate (up to 1,200 mg a day). Lastly, replace all white, refined sugar with xylitol.

You can also take glyconutrients in supplement form. I'm particularly fond of Ambrotose from Mannatech, Inc., which contains all eight glyconutrients. You can order it from Tammie Donnelly online at *www.glycoscience.com* or by calling 831-476-1526, or from Jacquelyn Aldana at *www.mannapages.com/ronaldana*. I also recommend ImmunEnhancer™ from Lonza (*www.larex.com* or 201-316-9200).

Green Foods

I first became interested in green foods over 20 years ago when several of my patients, virtually simultaneously, come to my office raving about the benefits they were finding from adding green foods to their diet. Many of my female patients who are in their late 30's and 40's have reported that taking green foods helped to lessen the fatigue and mood swings associated with PMS and perimenopausal hormone imbalances. While I have not found it to be helpful in reducing physical symptoms such as bloating, breast tenderness, and menstrual irregularity, it does seem to promote more efficient liver function. Since the liver has a crucial role in detoxifying and deactivating estrogen, healthy liver function helps to bring estrogen levels into balance, thereby relieving the fatigue, depression, and moodiness often found in perimenopausal women. My menopausal patients have found green foods to be helpful in improving energy, vitality, and stamina, as well as reducing depression and improving detoxification, thereby supporting their overall health.

Green foods are important ingredients in herbal cleansing programs because chlorophyll, which imparts the green color to these foods, helps to neutralize and remove toxins. The greener the plant, the greater the amount of chlorophyll. Foods high in chlorophyll also help heal digestive disorders, provide energy, boost immunity, and prevent deficiency diseases such as anemia. Certain grasses and algae, which are described below, are especially high in chlorophyll.

As cited in an article published in *Mutation Research*, the National Institute for Occupational Safety and Health estimated that millions of workers in the manufacturing sector have been exposed to potentially hazardous chemicals, many of which cause genetic mutation and promote cancer. This same article reports on a study that shows the effectiveness of chlorophyll in counteracting the mutagenic effect of pollutants such as cigarette smoke, coal dust, and diesel-emission particles. Chlorophyll was extremely effective at inhibiting the mutations of the various nitrogen compounds, aromatic amines, and hydrocarbons found in these substances. Chlorophyll also protected against harmful compounds in fried beef and pork, red grape juice, and red wine. Chlorophyll has also been used successfully to treat iron deficiency anemia and peptic ulcers.

Pure extracted liquid chlorophyll is available in health food stores. Always use chlorophyll that has been extracted from alfalfa or other plants; avoid the chemically manufactured variety. There is a benefit to consuming the plant itself as a source of chlorophyll, since grasses and algae offer their own additional properties. **I recommend taking 100 mg two or three times a day**.

Wheat and Barley Grass

Cereal grasses, such as wheat grass and barley grass, are high-chlorophyll foods. Commercially, they are available fresh and as supplements, in both powder and tablet form. It is also possible to grow wheat grass at home. Both have nearly identical therapeutic properties, although barley grass may be digested a little more easily by some. People with allergies to wheat and other cereals can usually tolerate these grasses since grain in its grass stage rarely triggers an allergic reaction.

These grasses contain about the same quotient of protein as meat, about 20 percent, as well as vitamin B_{12}, chlorophyll, vitamin A, and many other nutrients. Wheat grass is capable of incorporating more than 90 out of the estimated possible 102 minerals found in rich soil.

Wheat and barley grasses have been used to treat hepatitis and high cholesterol, as well as arthritis, peptic ulcers, and hypoglycemia. They are both effective in reducing inflammation and contain the antioxidant superoxide dismutase (SOD), which slows cellular deterioration, plus various digestive enzymes that aid in detoxification. **Combine one to two tablespoons of powdered wheat and/or barley grass (or one to two ounces of the fresh juice) in eight ounces of water per day.**

Microalgae

Spirulina, chlorella, and wild blue-green algae contain more chlorophyll than any other foods. These algae are aquatic plants, spiral-shaped and emerald to blue-green in color, and have been used medicinally for thousands of years in South America and Africa. Today they can be purchased, dried, in health food stores. They are also the highest sources of protein, beta-carotene, and nucleic acids of any animal or plant food, and contain the essential fatty acids omega-3 and gamma linolenic acid. The protein in spirulina and chlorella is so easily digested and absorbed that two or three teaspoons of these microalgae are equivalent to two to three ounces of meat. Further, unlike animal protein, the protein in algae generates a minimum of waste products when it is metabolized, thereby lessening the stress on your liver.

Spirulina detoxifies the kidneys and liver, inhibiting the growth of fungi, bacteria, and yeasts. Because spirulina is so easily digested, it yields quick energy. It is also strongly anti-inflammatory and therefore useful in the treatment of hepatitis, gastritis, and other inflammatory diseases. Spirulina strengthens body tissues and protects the vascular system by lowering blood fat. Athletes use spirulina for energy and for its cleansing action after strenuous physical exertion, which can stimulate the body to rid itself of poisons. **I suggest taking 1 to 2 tablespoons of spirulina, stirred into eight ounces of water per day.** Green foods are very concentrated, so start with a half dose and increase gradually to make sure it's well tolerated.

Chlorella is a well-known algae that is an especially effective detoxifier and anti-inflammatory agent, thanks to its high chlorophyll content, which stimulates these processes. Chlorella is notable for its tough outer cell walls, which bind with heavy metals, pesticides, and carcinogens such as PCBs (polychlorinated biphenyls) and then carry these toxins out of the body. Because of chlorella's growth factor, this algae also promotes growth and repair of all kinds of tissue. Animal studies show that it reduces cholesterol and atherosclerosis. **Take one tablespoon of chlorella in eight to 12 ounces of water.** Be sure to begin with a partial dose and increase gradually.

Wild blue-green algae grow in Klamath Lake in Oregon and are processed by freeze-drying. It is sold under various trade names, frequently as a mail-order product. Wild blue-green algae are very energizing and can improve an individual's mental concentration. However, a sign of overuse is weakness and a lack of mental focus, and certain forms are known to be highly toxic. **Try one tablespoon of blue-green algae in eight to 12 ounces of water per day.**

   Note: It is important to buy wild blue-green algae from a reputable company that processes the algae in an FDA-approved laboratory. To avoid certain wild blue-green algae that are highly toxic, never collect it yourself or consume any that you have gathered.

GLORIOUS GREEN FOODS

Spirulina and other green foods are nutrient-rich and promote alkalinity within the body. They are an excellent source of many easily absorbable, alkaline minerals as well as amino acids, vitamins, enzymes, and chlorophyll, and can be used to supplement your regular meals. The following is a list of green foods commonly found on the market:

- Spirulina and chlorella provide a concentrated source of protein containing all the amino acids and are a good source of minerals as well.
- Green magma, made from young barley leaves, supplies amino acids and minerals.
- Kyo-green (a combination of barley, wheatgrass, kelp, and chlorella) provides amino acids and many nutrients.
- Alfalfa is a source of abundant calcium, magnesium, phosphorus, and potassium in a balanced ratio that promotes absorption.
- Barley grass is an excellent source of all the amino acids, calcium, and iron.

Making the Transition

To help you make the transition from your current way of eating to one that supports your hormonal and overall health, I've put together this five-step plan.

Step 1—Identify Your Problem Foods

Look at the foods identified as either too acidic or too alkaline for your hormonal profile, then see if they match up with any in your diet. Use the pH chart on page 353 as your guide.

Step 2—Why Do You Eat Those Foods

Is it just a habit? Do you eat certain foods because they're part of your childhood and require little thought or effort, such as pizza and hamburgers? Do you eat the same foods day after day because it's simple and easy? I've often heard artificially-sweetened yogurt and pre-packaged slices of cheese described this way.

Or maybe you're addicted to it. Sugar and alcohol, for instance, can be quite addicting. Do you use the food or beverage to boost energy? Sugar, coffee, and products that contain caffeine often fall into this category.

Are you an emotional eater, using food to comfort or dull some emotion, such as eating chocolate or potato chips when you feel needy, fearful, upset, or angry?

Are you eating a food because you've been told it's good for you? As we've discussed, oranges may be healthy, but not for estrogen deficient-fast processors. Ditto for brown rice and estrogen dominant women and estrogen deficient-slow processors.

Make a brief note next to each food on your list from Step 1 about why you think you eat it.

Step 3—Prioritize Foods for Elimination

List the food(s) you're willing to give up first. Then, in decreasing order, the foods you'll eliminate over time until you have successfully transitioned to a new eating plan. This may take a month or even much longer. It's up to you. There's no right or wrong way to do this. It's better to be cautious than to make rapid changes that you'll discard some time later.

Step 4—Find Healthy Substitutions

Keep a copy of the list of food staples from page 404 in your purse, and shop your local health food store or even supermarket for these items.

When dining out, order mineral water instead of alcoholic beverages, bring an herbal tea bag for after dinner, or ask for some olive oil for your bread instead of butter. And don't feel shy about bringing a small bag of rice cakes to munch on while everyone else eats bread. After all, it's your body!

Step 5—Track Your Progress

Keep a food journal or diary. Track your symptoms and each change you make. Soon, you'll see real proof of progress. It will also help remind you how bad you felt if you're ever tempted to go back to your old ways.

Go at Your Own Pace

I've found that the speed with which many of my patients have felt comfortable making the lifestyle changes so necessary to regaining great health can vary greatly. Some women can change their lifestyle habits very quickly and easily and never look back.

One of my patients, "Ruth," suffered from painful headaches. I recommended that she eliminate foods from her diet that I was certain were triggering her symptoms. I also suggested that she take specific nutritional supplements that would give her some relief.

She told me that within one week, she was able to clear out her pantry and refrigerator of unhealthy foods and found it very easy to begin the program of nutritional supplements that I recommended to her. A week later, she told me she began to feel better and, within a month, she had noticed a dramatic reduction in her symptoms.

Some of my other women patients, however, have found it much more difficult and slow-going to change longstanding unhealthy lifestyle habits. But I have found that if they are determined to heal and persevere, they will eventually get there and enjoy every bit as dramatic and positive a recovery.

I still remember "Beth," a patient of mine who took nine months to finally give up the coffee habit that had been making her breast cysts so sore and tender that she disliked even touching them. When she reported to me that she was finally able to eliminate coffee permanently from her diet, she literally glowed with satisfaction and pride.

While you are making the lifestyle changes necessary to better support and heal your body, keep in mind that it's very common to oscillate between your old pattern of illness and your new pattern of health. In fact, when you're under stress, neglect to exercise, or go on a binge of eating foods that you know you should avoid, the healing process can be bumpy. You may go two steps forward and then take one step back into the discomfort, frustration, and limitations that illness can cause in your life. But don't give up, just keep persevering and you'll make it to the finish line of great health and well-being.

29 eating made easy

Throughout my medical career, I've dealt with every possible food issue women have, and I've had to make it work for all of them. Some of my patients ate at home, others ate out. Some cooked for themselves, others did so for large families. The busy career woman who eats in restaurants five days a week needs help on what to order, not how to shop. The at-home mother, in turn, needs to know how to get her children on board with her diet plan, but still be able to make quick and easy meals they will actually eat.

As a result, I've been customizing meal plans and dietary recommendations for more than 30 years. To meet the needs of each woman, I have to take into account her particular lifestyle.

For example, if she liked to cook but needed to adopt a more vegetarian diet, I suggested she make bean dishes like lentil or split pea soup, or beans and rice at home. If she worked outside the home and did not have the time to do much cooking, or simply didn't enjoy cooking, I recommended passing on high-fat lunches of hamburgers and lasagna and instead choosing salads with beans and hard-boiled eggs for protein.

Most important, I made sure that each woman agreed with and felt comfortable with the meal plan we put together before she left my office.

That is why I feel confident that this can work for you and your entire family, regardless of whether you live alone, have a spouse or significant other, or are feeding a troop of hungry kids. I've looked at all the issues and found answers for the dining out dilemma, the dual body chemistry types, the non-cooker, the culinary dabbler, and the gourmet chef. Whatever the problem, you now have a solution.

The Dining Out Dilemma

If you are like some of my patients who have tended to eat out frequently due to a busy work or social schedule (or simply because you don't like to cook), then this section should help to make your food selections much easier when you are dining out. While you are following a program to restore your body to a more alkaline pH, proper food selection is critical to avoid putting undue wear and tear on your already stressed buffer systems.

Whether you tend to be an overall acidic woman who is an estrogen deficient-fast processor or a more alkaline, estrogen dominant woman or estrogen deficient-slow processor, this can prove to be tricky when you are not the one preparing the food.

Traditionally, people have chosen mostly highly acidic dishes and entrées when eating in restaurants. Luckily, all-American, overly acidic fare such as the 16-ounce porterhouse steak, French fries, and rich, sugary deserts, and French cuisine with its heavy butter- and cream-based sauces have been replaced or supplemented in many restaurants by lighter, healthier, and less acidic, more alkaline dishes. This is true both in American restaurants and in those serving ethnic cuisines. The important thing is to know which dishes on the menu represent the less acidic, more alkaline options and to select a variety of these types of dishes when dining out.

International Cuisine

I have prepared the following list to assist you in making intelligent menu selections, particularly if you are working hard to restore your body to a state of healthy hormonal balance. In general, you will want to order salads, non-dairy soups, vegetable or bean appetizers and side dishes, and vegetarian or fish entrées. I've found that most restaurants are willing to make up vegetarian entrées and platters at your request, even if they are not on the menu. I frequently do this myself and have never had a problem.

- **American cuisine:** salad or salad bars, bean or vegetable soups, baked potatoes, rice, vegetable side dishes or platters, fish or shellfish entrées.
- **Italian cuisine:** escarole soup, bean or minestrone soup, white bean salad, Caesar salad, risotto, polenta (cornmeal) with a mushroom sauce, grilled eggplant entrée, fish or shellfish entrées.
- **French cuisine:** vegetable or seafood salads, nondairy soups, vegetable side dishes, stewed beans, fish or shellfish entrées.
- **Indian cuisine:** lentils, rice pilafs, cucumber salad, curried vegetable or shellfish dishes.
- **Chinese cuisine:** stir-fried vegetables, sizzling rice soup, tofu or bean curd dishes, steamed rice, shrimp and mixed vegetable entrées.
- **Japanese cuisine:** Japanese salads, miso soup, sticky rice, sushi, side dishes and soups made with vegetables and tofu.
- **Mexican cuisine:** mixed vegetable salads, tostada salad, bean and rice side dishes, bean or shrimp burritos, chicken or shrimp fajitas, bean or seafood tacos (skip the cheese and sour cream).

Dining With Your Opposite

Members of the same family can often have different hormonal make-ups and may require different food choices. One person may be estrogen dominant or an estrogen deficient-slow processor while the other is an estrogen deficient-fast processor.

This same issue can also arise when socializing with friends or business associates. Since the standard American diet is so prevalent, overly acidic people will often try to keep up with their more alkaline spouse or friend, much to their detriment. It is important to eat according to the needs of your basic constitution: You will feel better and maintain your health more readily if you stick to the diet best suited to your hormonal needs.

This is not as difficult as you might expect. When cooking at home, you can all share soups, salads, vegetable dishes, and starches. Your entrées, however, may differ. A more alkaline individual may choose to eat meat as an entrée much more frequently and often in larger portions. They may also want to add hotter, spicier seasonings such as ginger and peppers to their dishes. Remember, high-alkaline producers need to do this to maintain their level of energy.

Overly acidic people should avoid the acidic and spicy condiments and opt instead for more grain- and legume-based entrées instead with servings of omega-3–rich fish and free-range poultry eaten in smaller amounts. My overly acidic patients have reported that customizing entrées while keeping all of the side dishes the same is really not too difficult. Sometimes, they will even prepare food for the whole family—like spaghetti and meatballs, tacos, and casseroles—and simply not add the red meat to their portions.

In addition, overly acidic people may want to skip the vinegar marinades and dressings, wheat bread, wine, coffee, and dessert that their naturally alkaline dining partner(s) can enjoy in moderation. Luckily, these individuals can enjoy the many substitutions that are now available and not feel deprived. For example, when doing food preparation at home, slices of very tasty rice bread can be served alongside the wheat bread. You can even bring a few slices of your own wheat-free bread with you when you go out to eat at a restaurant or a friend's house. You can also cook up veggie burgers on the grill right next to the free-range, all-beef hamburgers.

Restaurant dining is somewhat easier when people with different acid/alkaline constitutions eat together, because a restaurant menu normally contains many more dishes than are prepared for one meal at home. On the negative side, diners have no control over the ingredients used to prepare a dish or the types of dishes offered.

While your naturally alkaline dining partner may choose to order a highly vinegary antipasti followed by steak with a glass of red wine and an apple tart for dessert, an overly acidic person can put together a tasty and varied meal by ordering a vegetable soup, salad, and several vegetable side dishes or rice- and legume-based dishes, or fish or poultry as an entrée. This allows for great flexibility in both ordering and eating.

And if you and your dining partner are willing to share your dishes, all the better. When you order a broccoli and beef dish in a Chinese restaurant, for example, the overly acidic, estrogen deficient-fast processor diner can eat most of the broccoli while the more estrogen dominant or estrogen deficient-slow processor type eats most of the beef.

TRAVEL WOES

When traveling, always keep your eye out for fresh, local fruits or vegetables. However, try to avoid highly acidic fruits like oranges and grapefruit if you are estrogen deficient-fast processor. Stop at a local market to stock up on high-enzyme foods like sprouts, carrots, celery, or papaya to snack on.

If you are eating in a restaurant and are estrogen deficient-fast processor, you should concentrate on including salads, steamed vegetables, whole grains, legumes, fish, and poultry. Be sure to order the less acidic, more alkaline fruits such as melons and papayas. Conversely, women who are estrogen dominant or estrogen deficient-slow processor can load up on spinach salads with vinegar- or lemon juice-based dressings, entrees with tomato sauce, spicy entrees, or healthy meat-based dishes.

I also recommend traveling with a brown-bag meal, particularly when you fly across time zones. For example, if you are flying from New York to Los Angeles and you arrive at your hotel at 9:00 P.M. (which for you is actually midnight), you will probably be too tired to go out for dinner—even if you have skipped the dinner served on the airplane and feel hungry.

Instead of raiding the room's refrigerator, which is often filled with nutrient-poor, enzyme-deficient, unhealthy options like potato chips, salted peanuts, and colas, reach into your own store of energy-rich foods that you brought from home. These can include raw, fresh vegetables with a flavorful dressing or dip, whole-grain crackers with almond butter, and a piece of fruit.

If you didn't have time to pack a snack before you left, look for salad and fresh fruit on the room service menu. This will make a great light supper that won't keep you up all night with indigestion. You'll wake up refreshed and ready to go in the morning.

Easy Meals for the Non-Cooker

I've had many female patients and friends who either don't have the time to cook, or simply don't like to cook. Fortunately, there are a myriad of options available that allow you to simply open a bag, toss something into the oven or microwave, or even pop open a can.

If you are **estrogen dominant or an estrogen deficient-slow processor**, then the following breakfasts would work great for you. In all cases, the most you'll have to do is boil water or open a bag or can.

- Plain soy or goat yogurt with fresh berries and two tablespoons of flaxseed
- A hard-boiled organic egg with a cup of pineapple
- A delicious, high-protein, high-fiber snack bar

If you are an **estrogen deficient-fast processor** and prefer to stay out of the kitchen, then these are the breakfasts for you. Again, the most you'll have to do is use the toaster or boil some water.

- Steel-cut oatmeal with mango and two tablespoons of flaxseed
- Half of a wheat-free bagel topped with almond butter
- Wheat-free cereal with soy milk and a banana

Snacks are also a breeze. A handful of almonds and a handful of berries, red peppers and hummus, or a cup of soy yogurt are all perfect for **estrogen dominant women or estrogen deficient-slow processors. Estrogen deficient-fast processors** can enjoy celery with almond butter or soy cream cheese, tuna on a rice cake, or sliced cucumbers with hummus, just to name a few.

SHOPPING MADE EASY

The best way to ensure you can adhere to your specific dietary needs is to make sure you always have a few staples on hand.

- A variety of dried herbs
- A salt-free herb blend such as Spike or Mrs. Dash
- Brown rice
- Raw almonds
- Raw walnuts
- Soy or almond milk
- Almond butter
- Herbal or green tea
- Mineral water
- Liquid stevia (flavored if you like)
- Pure maple syrup
- Honey
- Xylitol and/or erythritol
- Olive oil
- Bragg's Liquid Aminos
- Bagged organic lettuce
- Fresh fruits and vegetables (that fit your hormonal profile)
- Soy or goat yogurt
- Flaxseed

I've also found that the easiest way to make sure you have these staples on hand, as well as any other items you may need, is to organize your shopping trips. Before you head to the grocery store, plan out your meals for the next week, check your supply of the essentials I mentioned above, and make a list of the necessary ingredients to be sure you pick up everything you need.

For lunch or dinner, there are several options for women of all hormonal types. If you don't mind opening a few bags and cans, you can take some pre-washed organic lettuce and top with any of your favorite veggies and protein.

If you are **estrogen dominant or an estrogen deficient-slow processor**, you may want to sprinkle on some walnuts and broccoli, and top with some slices of poached salmon or peppered turkey and a little olive oil and balsamic vinegar. **Estrogen deficient-fast processors** can top with a can of wild-caught tuna in olive oil and some slices of avocado, or carrots, celery, kidney beans, and garbanzo beans. Sprinkle on a little pumpkinseed oil and you are all set.

Amazing Name Brand Products

For the ultimate in easy, Kimberly and I have compiled a list of our favorite brand-name items that fit the guidelines of my program. They are all wheat- and dairy-free. If you cannot find these items in your local grocery store, Whole Foods Market, or specialty store, we've included a Web site for you so you can buy them online. You can also visit Miss Roben's (*www.missroben.com*) for many sugar-free and wheat-free products all in one place.

Breakfast
- Lifestream Buckwheat or Flax Plus waffles
- Glutino plain or sesame bagels (*www.glutino.com*)
- Barbara's Puffin cereals
- Silk soy yogurt
- Redwood Hill Farms goat yogurt (*www.redwoodhill.com*)
- Milled Flaxseed (*www.drlark.com*)
- Galaxy Foods cream cheese (*www.galaxyfoods.com*)
- Justin's Nut Butter (*www.justinsnutbutter.com*)
- Pamela's pancake and baking mix (*www.pamelasproducts.com*)

Lunch/Dinner
- Imagine soups
- Health Valley Black Bean and Vegetable Soup
- Amy's Naturals Organic soups
- Walnut Acres Carrot-Ginger Soup and Sweet Potato Chowder
- SeaBear Wild Alaskan salmon (*www.drlark.com*)
- Carvalho wild-caught Albacore tuna (*www.drlark.com*)
- Lundberg brown rice pasta
- Bionaturae pasta
- Pastariso brown rice linguini

- Near East Lentil Pilaf mix
- Amy's frozen entrées
- Taj Ethnic Gourmet meals
- Food for Life brown rice bread and millet bread
- Cascadian Farms Vegetarian meals (frozen bags)
- Yves veggie chili

Snacks
- Ruth's MacaPower bars (*www.drlark.com*)
- Organic Food bars
- Arico snack bars (*www.aricofoods.com*)
- Kind fruit and nut bars (*www.peaceworks.com*)
- Native Kjalii chips and fresh salsas (*www.sfsalsa.com*)
- Paul Newman's wheat-free, dairy-free sandwich cookies
- Pamela's baking mixes (*www.pamelasproducts.com*)
- Cherrybrook Kitchen frosting mix
- Good Karma organic rice cream (dairy- and wheat-free) (*www.goodkarmafoods.com*)

Beverages
- Silk soy milk
- Pacific Breeze almond milk
- Rice Dream rice milk
- Luxe teas (*www.luxetea.com*)
- Zhena's Gypsy Tea (*www.gypsytea.com*)
- Teeccino herbal coffee (*www.teeccino.com*)
- Sweet Leaf flavored liquid stevia (*www.sweetleaf.com*)
- Ito En bottled, unsweetened green tea (*www.itoen.com*)

Condiments
- Nasoya Nayonaise
- XyloSweet xylitol (*www.xylosweet.com* or *www.drlark.com*)
- Z Sweet erythritol (*www.zsweet.com*)
- La Tourangelle nut oils (*www.latourangelle.com*)
- Mac Nut oil (*www.drlark.com*)
- Organicville dressings (*www.organicvillefoods.com*)
- Annie's Naturals Organic green garlic dressing (no vinegar)

The Culinary Dabbler

For those women who don't like to spend lots of time in the kitchen, but like to do a bit more than eat out for most meals or heat up something in the microwave, Kimberly and I have created several easy, two to three ingredient recipes that can help you bridge between the non-cooker and the gourmet chef. Enjoy!

Estrogen Dominant and Estrogen Deficient–Slow Processor "Recipes"

Scrambled Eggs with Salsa
Place 1 teaspoon olive oil in a small frying pan. Add two organic eggs and scramble. When cooked, top with your favorite salsa.

Power Shake
Place 1 cup almond milk, 2–3 tablespoons flaxseed, and ½ cup of your favorite berries into a blender. Mix well and drink.

Tomato and Basil Soup
Pour 1 cup of pre-packaged tomato soup in to a pot. Add 1 tablespoon fresh chopped basil or 1 teaspoon of dried basil. Cook on medium for 15 minutes. Enjoy warm.

Whipped Acorn Squash
Peel and cut one acorn squash into large pieces. Steam until tender. Place in blender with 2 ounces apple juice. Add ¼ teaspoon nutmeg and purée until smooth. Goes great with free-range chicken or beef.

Oven Fries
Cut a sweet potato into "disks." Spray a cookie sheet with canola oil and place potato disks in single layer on the cookie sheet. Spray the potatoes with the canola oil. Sprinkle potatoes with cinnamon and bake at 425°F for 20–25 minutes, turning halfway through the cooking time.

Easy Chicken
Grill or lightly sauté free-range chicken breast in 1 tablespoon olive oil. While it is cooking, cut a large tomato in half lengthwise. Top each half with pre-made pesto and broil until pesto browns. Dice pesto tomato and top chicken with the mixture.

Simply Spectacular Salmon

Grill or lightly sauté wild-caught salmon in 1 tablespoon olive oil. While it is cooking, mix ¼ cup diced pineapple with 1 tablespoon diced red onion and 1 teaspoon chopped fresh cilantro. Blend well and top salmon with the mixture.

Baked Apple

Core an apple, then cut in half from top to bottom. Place sliced almonds in the newly created trench. Sprinkle with cinnamon and bake at 375°F for 20 minutes or until the apple is soft.

Estrogen Deficient–Fast Processor "Recipes"

Scrambled Eggs with Dill

Place 1 teaspoon olive oil in a small frying pan. Add two organic eggs and ½ teaspoon of dill. Scramble and serve.

Power Shake

Place 1 cup soy milk, 2 tablespoons greens powder, and ½ a banana into a blender. Mix well and drink.

Miso Soup

Heat 1 cup of water in a pot. Add 1 tablespoon miso, 1 tablespoon sliced green onion, and ¼ cup diced tofu. Bring to a boil, then turn to low and simmer for 15 minutes. Eat warm.

Savory Bean Sprouts

Heat ½ cup vegetable stock over low for five minutes. Add ¾ cup bean sprouts and ½ cup sliced mushrooms. Simmer for 10 minutes. Makes a great side dish for halibut or mackerel.

Oven Fries

Cut a potato into "disks." Spray a cookie sheet with canola oil and place potato disks in single layer on the cookie sheet. Spray the potatoes with the canola oil. Sprinkle potatoes with Spike, Mrs. Dash, or your favorite no-salt dried herb blend. Bake at 425°F for 20–25 minutes, turning halfway through the cooking time.

Easy Tuna

Grill or bake wild-caught tuna. Mix 2 tablespoons cup dairy-free mayonnaise with 2 tablespoons diced celery and 1 teaspoon dried thyme. Top tuna with mixture and enjoy warm.

Broiled Trout with Dill
Slice 1 fresh, 8-ounce trout in half and bone. (This will make 2 fillets.) Sprinkle the fillets with 1 tablespoon lemon juice and ½ teaspoon dried dill. Broil for 5 to 6 minutes or until done.

Broiled Mango
Slice mango and lay on cookie sheet. Sprinkle with coconut flakes and broil until coconut turns brown. Enjoy warm.

The Healthy Gourmet

When it comes to great-tasting, healthy food, I trust Kimberly implicitly. She and I have collaborated on many food preparation projects, including recipes for my newsletter, special reports, and my recent book *Eat Papayas Naked*. In addition to acting as Executive Editor for *Papayas*, Kimberly also reviewed and tweaked all the recipes, even adding a few of her own.

Kimberly is unique because her desire to prepare healthy meals in no way lessens her demand that they be easy to make and extremely tasty too. In fact, Kimberly guarantees that all of her recipes have passed what she humorously calls the "Trip test."

Kimberly's husband Trip was raised by a mother who is, for all intents and purposes, a gourmet chef. As a result, he has come to expect great homemade food. Kimberly's challenge was to combine her love of health food with Trip's love of great taste. And she has definitely succeeded! In fact, I'm told that her sugar-free ice cream tastings caused near-riots when demand far exceeded supply.

Kimberly has been associated with nutritious food since her childhood, growing up with sprout sandwiches and carob rather than McDonald's and chocolate. While she did work in catering during high school and college, her most recent focus has been on food preparation from the point of view of the family food preparer rather than the restaurant or catering approach. This focus is responsible for her method of creating healthy meals that everyday people actually enjoy preparing and eating, and it's this focus that she brings to every issue of her online eLetter *Food for Thought: Quaffs and Cuisine for Decadent Health*.

So you can imagine my delight when Kimberly agreed to share several of her best recipes with you. In addition to one of the notorious sorbet recipes, you'll also find a wide variety of breakfast, soup, salad, dinner, and dessert options for your gastronomic pleasure.

Enjoy!

Recipes for Estrogen Dominance and Estrogen Deficiency-Slow Processor

BREAKFAST

Fabulous Fritatta   *Serves 2*

2 teaspoons extra virgin olive oil
½ onion, chopped
4 eggs, slightly beaten

1 can wild salmon
½ teaspoon dill
Black pepper to taste

1. Heat oil in 8-inch nonstick skillet over medium-high heat.
2. Add onion and cook until soft.
3. Add eggs, salmon, dill, and pepper. Stir often and cook until eggs are done.
4. Serve warm.

Nutritional Info (per serving): Calories 183, Total fat 13 g (Sat fat 3 g/Mono fat 7 g/Poly fat 2 g), Cholesterol 374 mg, Sodium 115 mg, Carbs 4 g, Fiber 1 g, Protein 11 g

Huevos Rancheros   *Serves 4*

(4) 6-inch corn tortillas
½ teaspoon cumin
16 ounces black beans, rinsed and drained
1 chipotle chile canned in adobo, diced

1 teaspoon olive oil
4 eggs
½ cup salsa
1 avocado, sliced

1. Preheat oven to 200°F (to warm).
2. Put tortillas on a baking sheet, cover with foil, and place in oven to warm.
3. In a small saucepan, mix cumin, beans, and chile for 5-7 minutes.
4. In a large skillet, heat the olive oil, then fry the eggs.
5. Place tortillas on individual plates. Top with equal amounts of bean mixture, one egg, ⅛ cup of salsa, and ¼ avocado slice.
6. Enjoy warm.

Nutritional Info (per serving): Calories 318, Total fat 15 g, Cholesterol 187 mg, Sodium 613 mg, Carbs 33 g, Fiber 9 g, Protein 15 g

Recipes for Estrogen Dominance and Estrogen Deficiency-Slow Processor

SOUPS AND SALADS

Spinach Salad   *Serves 4*

2 cups fresh spinach, torn
1 pint fresh raspberries
½ cup walnuts, chopped

2 tablespoons walnut oil
1 tablespoon balsamic vinegar
2 ounces dark chocolate, shaved

1. In a salad bowl, combine spinach, raspberries, and walnuts.
2. Add walnut oil and vinegar and toss
3. Top with dark chocolate and serve.
4. Serves four (serving size ½ cup spinach, ¼ pint raspberries, ⅛ cup walnuts, ½ tablespoon oil, and ½ ounce chocolate).

Nutritional Info (per serving): Calories 257, Total fat 20 g, Cholesterol 0 mg, Sodium 13 mg, Carbs 19 g, Fiber 6 g, Protein 5 g

Broccoli Salad   *Serves 4*

¾ cup nonfat mayonnaise
¼ cup erythritol
1 tablespoon white vinegar
1 large head of broccoli
1 onion, diced

4 pieces turkey bacon, cooked and
   crumbled
½ cup goat cheese, crumbled
¼ cup sunflower seeds

1. Combine mayonnaise, erythritol, and vinegar. Mix well, cover, and place in refrigerator for 1-2 hours.
2. Cut broccoli into small flowerettes. Add onion, bacon, goat cheese, and sunflower seeds.
3. Mix in dressing and serve.

Nutritional Info (per serving): Calories 159, Total fat 9 g, Cholesterol 18 mg, Sodium 564 mg, Carbs 23 g, Fiber 4 g, Protein 9 g

SOUPS AND SALADS

Momma Sue's Chicken Soup *Serves 6*

By adding more vegetables and taking out the rice, my mom's amazing chicken soup is now packed with all of the quercetin, beta-carotene, vitamin C, allicin, selenium, and protein you need to fight a cold at the first sign of a sniffle.

1 tablespoon olive oil	½ teaspoon dried thyme
1 medium onion, chopped	1 bay leaf
2 medium carrots, chopped	1 cup green beans, cut
2 medium celery stalks, chopped	½ cup baby spinach
1 teaspoon minced garlic	2 medium zucchini, sliced
8 cups free-range chicken broth	¾ pound free-range chicken, cooked
¼ cup fresh parsley	and cubed
½ teaspoon cayenne pepper	

1. Sauté onion, carrots, celery, and garlic in olive oil until soft.
2. Add chicken broth, parsley, pepper, thyme, and bay leaf. Bring to a boil.
3. Reduce heat, cover, and simmer 15-20 minutes.
4. Add green beans, spinach, zucchini, and chicken. Cover and simmer 15-20 minutes.
5. Remove bay leaf and serve.

Nutritional Info (per serving): Calories 213, Total fat 9 g, Cholesterol 37mg, Sodium 749 mg, Carbs 11 g, Fiber 3 g, Protein 24 g

Recipes for Estrogen Dominance and Estrogen Deficiency-Slow Processor

SOUPS AND SALADS

Turkey Chili   *Serves 4*

1 tablespoon olive oil
2 cups onion, chopped
1 cup red pepper, chopped
1 tablespoon garlic, minced
1 pound ground turkey
2 teaspoons cinnamon
2 teaspoons paprika
1 teaspoon chili powder
1 teaspoon cumin

½ teaspoon allspice
½ teaspoon marjoram
¼ teaspoon nutmeg
1 cinnamon stick
½ teaspoon sea salt
1 teaspoon pepper
2 cans low sodium tomatoes, chopped
   and undrained

1. Sauté onion, pepper, and garlic in olive oil.
2. Add ground turkey and cook until brown.
3. Add cinnamon, paprika, chili powder, cumin, allspice, marjoram, nutmeg, and cinnamon stick and cook 2-3 minutes.
4. Add salt, pepper, and tomatoes and simmer 45 minutes.
5. Serve warm.

Nutritional Info (per serving): Calories 275, Total fat 14 g, Cholesterol 90 mg, Sodium 360 mg, Carbs 18 g, Fiber 6 g, Protein 22 g

Strawberry Soup   *Serves 6*

2 pints strawberries, sliced
2 tablespoons orange juice
1 cup soy yogurt

½ teaspoon vanilla extract
1 cup soy milk
¼ cup xylitol

1. Place all ingredients into a blender and blend until smooth.
2. Serve chilled.

Nutritional Info (per serving): Calories 70, Total fat 1 g, Cholesterol 30 mg, Sodium 6 mg, Carbs 18 g, Fiber 3 g, Protein 2 g

SIDE DISHES

Green Beans with Roasted Onions *Serves 8*

2 pounds green beans, trimmed

1 red onion, peeled and halved

1½ tablespoons extra virgin olive oil, divided

½ teaspoon black pepper

½ teaspoon thyme

1 teaspoon dill

3 tablespoons white wine vinegar

1 tablespoon spicy mustard

1. Preheat oven to 400°F.
2. Steam green beans until tender but still a bit crunchy.
3. Drain and rinse green beans. Set aside and chill to room temperature.
4. Drizzle each side of onion with 1/4 teaspoon of olive oil. Sprinkle evenly with black pepper and thyme. Wrap in aluminum foil and bake for one hour.
5. Cool onion to room temperature, then chop and place in medium-sized bowl.
6. Add dill, vinegar, and mustard and mix well.
7. Add green beans to onion mixture and blend well.

Nutritional Info (per serving): Calories 64, Total fat 3 g, Cholesterol 0 mg, Sodium 33 mg, Carbs 10 g, Fiber 4 g, Protein 2 g

Roasted Vegetables *Serves 4*

1 red onion, cut in large chunks

1 red bell pepper, cut in large chunks

1 green bell pepper, cut in large chunks

5 cloves garlic

2 yellow squash, sliced

2 zucchini, sliced

2 tomatoes, cut in large chunks

1 tablespoon basil, sliced

1 teaspoon lemon pepper

2 teaspoons olive oil

1. Preheat oven to 425°F.
2. Add all vegetables to roasting pan.
3. Top with basil and lemon pepper.
4. Drizzle with olive oil and bake for 45 minutes.
5. Serve warm.

Nutritional Info (per serving): Calories 100, Total fat 3 g, Cholesterol 0 mg, Sodium 98 mg, Carbs 18 g, Fiber 5 g, Protein 4 g

Recipes for Estrogen Dominance and Estrogen Deficiency-Slow Processor

MAIN COURSES

Thai Turbot *Serves 4*

2 teaspoons sesame oil, divided
2 garlic cloves, minced
2 teaspoons fresh ginger, peeled and
    minced
1 cup red pepper, chopped
1 cup red onions, chopped
1 teaspoon curry powder
2 teaspoons curry paste
½ teaspoon ground cumin

4 teaspoons tamari sauce
1 tablespoon xylitol
22 ounces coconut milk, divided
2 tablespoons fresh cilantro, chopped
(4) 6-ounce wild turbot fillets
olive oil
3 teaspoons sesame seeds
2 cups quinoa, cooked in 2 cups water,
    2 cups coconut milk

1. Preheat broiler.
2. Heat 1 teaspoon of sesame oil over medium high heat.
3. Add garlic and ginger and cook for 1-2 minutes, until fragrant.
4. Add pepper and shallots and cook 2 minutes.
5. Stir in curry powder and cumin and cook 1 minute.
6. Add tamari, xylitol, and 14 ounces coconut milk and bring to a simmer.
7. Add cilantro and immediately remove from heat.
8. Brush fish with remaining teaspoon of sesame oil and sprinkle with sesame seeds.
9. Place on broiler pan brushed with olive oil and broil for 8 minutes (or until fish flakes easily).
10. Place fish on top of quinoa and top with sauce.
11. Serve hot.
12. Serves 4 (each serving ½ cup quinoa, one fillet, ½ cup sauce).

Nutritional Info (per serving): Calories 302, Total fat 24 g, Cholesterol 21 mg, Sodium 488 mg, Carbs 16 g, Fiber 4 g, Protein 11 g

MAIN COURSES

Bay Area Tuna Tacos *Serves 4*

¼ cup soy sour cream

¼ cup nonfat mayonnaise

2 tablespoons fresh cilantro, chopped

1 teaspoon chili powder

1 tablespoon lime juice

1 teaspoon extra virgin olive oil

2 cans canned tuna in water

4 large red leaf lettuce leaves

½ avocado

¼ cup onion

½ cup tomato

1. Mix sour cream, mayonnaise, cilantro, and ½ teaspoon chili powder in a medium bowl and set aside.
2. Preheat broiler and spray unslotted broiler pan with olive oil spray.
3. Mix ½ teaspoon chili powder, lime juice, olive oil, and tuna. Divide evenly into four "mounds" and place on broiler pan, about three or four inches from the heat. Cook for five minutes.
4. Place lettuce leaves on four plates (one leaf per plate).
5. Add one "mound" of tuna to each plate. Top with even amounts of avocado, onion, and tomato.
6. Add one tablespoon of sour cream mixture and serve warm.

Nutritional Info (per serving): Calories 183, Total fat 6 g, Cholesterol 25 mg, Sodium 477 mg, Carbs 11 g, Fiber 2 g, Protein 22 g

Recipes for Estrogen Dominance and Estrogen Deficiency-Slow Processor

MAIN COURSES

Shrimp and Scallop Kebabs   *Serves 4*

¼ cup tamari soy sauce

3 tablespoons xylitol

1½ tablespoons white wine vinegar

1 tablespoon fresh ginger, peeled and
   minced

¼ teaspoon cayenne pepper

½ teaspoon garlic, minced

1½ teaspoons cornstarch

1½ teaspoons water

16 large shrimp

16 sea scallops

16 broccoli flowerets

1 red onion, chopped

1. Combine tamari, xylitol, vinegar, ginger, cayenne pepper, and garlic in a small sauce pan and bring to a boil. Cook for 2-3 minutes.
2. In a small bowl, mix cornstarch and 1½ teaspoons water.
3. Add cornstarch mixture to tamari mixture and bring to a boil. Cook for 1-2 minutes, then remove from heat.
4. Thread 2 shrimp, 2 scallops, two broccoli flowerets, and 2 pieces red onion onto 8 skewers.
5. Brush each kebob with tamari mixture and grill for 3 minutes. Turn kebabs and brush with more tamari mixture. Grill for 2-3 minutes. Turn again, brush with tamari mixture and grill 1-2 minutes or until shrimp and scallops are thoroughly cooked.

Nutritional Info (per serving): Calories 133, Total fat 1 g, Cholesterol 21 mg, Sodium 50 mg, Carbs 21 g, Fiber 2 g, Protein 15 g

MAIN COURSES

Chicken Piccata   *Serves 4*

1 tablespoon olive oil

four 4-ounce chicken breasts

¼ cup shallots, chopped

1 cup low sodium chicken broth

1 tablespoon lemon juice

1 tablespoon parsley

1 tablespoon capers

1 teaspoon lemon zest

¼ teaspoon black pepper

1. Heat oil in large skillet over medium high heat.
2. Add chicken breasts and cook for 8 minutes on each side, until chicken is cooked thoroughly. Remove chicken from skillet and set aside.
3. Add shallots to skillet and cook for one minute.
4. Add broth and lemon juice and deglaze the skillet.
5. Stir in parsley, capers, lemon zest, and pepper. Simmer for 1-2 minutes.
6. Add chicken back to skillet and cook for 3-5 minutes, until chicken is reheat.
7. Serve warm.

Nutritional Info (per serving): Calories 152, Total fat 5 g, Cholesterol 53 mg, Sodium 210 mg, Carbs 3 g, Fiber trace, Protein 24 g

MAIN COURSES

Duck Stuffed Red Peppers   *Serves 4*

½ cup low-sodium tamari sauce	1 green pepper, diced
1 tablespoon lime juice	3 tablespoons garlic, minced
1 teaspoon garlic powder	2 cups tomatoes, diced
1 teaspoon cumin	½ cup low sodium chicken broth
1 teaspoon chili powder	1 tablespoon oregano
½ teaspoon salt	1 tablespoon cumin
½ teaspoon black pepper	1 teaspoon hot sauce
½ cup olive oil	2 tablespoons low-sodium tamari sauce
two 4-ounce duck breasts	½ teaspoon cayenne pepper
1 onion, diced	4 large red peppers

1. In bowl, add ½ cup tamari, lime juice, garlic powder, cumin, chili powder, salt, black pepper, and olive oil. Blend well.
2. Add duck breasts and coat thoroughly with marinade. Cover and place in refrigerator overnight.
3. In a large skillet, sear breasts in oil, about 5-6 minutes per side. Remove from heat and set aside.
4. Add onion, pepper, and garlic to the skillet and cook until tender.
5. Add tomatoes, broth, oregano, cumin, hot sauce, tamari, and cayenne pepper. Cover and simmer for one hour.
6. Preheat oven to 375°F.
7. Shred duck breasts with fork. Return meat to skillet and simmer (uncovered) for 15 minutes.
8. Cut off tops of red peppers and scoop out seeds and veins. Place peppers in shallow baking dish and bake in oven for 15-20 or until peppers are firm, but tender.
9. Fill red peppers with even amounts of duck mixture and serve warm.

Nutritional Info (per serving): Calories 446, Total fat 32 g, Cholesterol 44 mg, Sodium 795 mg, Carbs 28 g, Fiber 6 g, Protein 16 g

DESSERT

Blueberry Pomegranate Sorbet *Serves 6*

¾ cup xylitol

½ cup filtered water

2 cups pure pomegranate juice

1 cup fresh, puréed blueberries

Extra blueberries (optional)

1. Combine xylitol and water in saucepan and stir over medium heat until xylitol dissolves.
2. Bring to a boil, then remove from heat.
3. Cool completely.
4. Whisk in pomegranate juice and puréed blueberries.
5. Place in ice cream maker and freeze according to manufacturer's instructions. If you don't have an ice cream maker, place in freezer-safe container, and freeze.
6. Serve with extra blueberries.

Nutritional Info (per serving): Calories 196, Total fat 0 g, Cholesterol 0 mg, Sodium 18 mg, Carbs 67 g, Fiber 1 g, Protein 1 g

DESSERT

Gingerbread *Serves 9*

½ cup coconut oil, melted
½ cup erythritol
1 egg
½ cup light molasses
1½ cups Pamela's baking mix

¾ teaspoon salt
¾ teaspoon baking soda
½ teaspoon ginger
½ teaspoon cinnamon
½ cup boiling water

1. Preheat oven to 350°F.
2. Cream coconut oil and erythritol for 30-45 seconds.
3. Add egg and molasses and beat thoroughly.
4. In a separate bowl, sift together baking mix, salt, baking soda, ginger, and cinnamon.
5. Add dry ingredients to egg mixture, alternating with boiling water, until well blended.
6. Pour mixture into a lightly greased 8x8 pan and bake for 40 minutes, or until toothpick comes out clean.
7. Serve warm or at room temperature.

Nutritional Info (per serving): Calories 241, Total fat 14 g, Cholesterol 23 mg, Sodium 491 mg, Carbs 26 g, Fiber 1 g, Protein 3 g

Recipes for Estrogen Deficiency-Fast Processor

BREAKFAST

Grandma Ginny's Granola *Serves 20*

4 cups oats

2 cups soy flour

1 cup almonds, sliced

1 cup sunflower seeds, raw

1 cup coconut, unsweetened

1 cup flaxseed, ground

⅔ cup olive oil

⅔ cup honey

1 teaspoon vanilla

1. Preheat oven to 350°F.
2. Grease 13x9-inch baking dish.
3. Combine oats, flour, almonds, sunflower seed, coconut, and flaxseed in a large bowl. Set aside.
4. Combine oil, honey, and vanilla in a small bowl. Pour over oat mixture and blend well.
5. Pour mixture into baking dish and bake for 40-45 minutes or until browned. Stir mixture every 10-15 minutes.
6. Cool on baking rack. Can be stored in the refrigerator in an air-tight container.

Nutritional Info (per serving): Calories 339, Total fat 21 g, Cholesterol 0 mg, Sodium 7 mg, Carbs 29 g, Fiber 7 g, Protein 10 g

Mango Banana Smoothie *Serves 2*

1½ cups soy or rice milk

3 tablespoons ground flax seeds

¾ cup aloe vera juice

¾ cup frozen mangos

1 banana

1. Combine all ingredients in a blender and process until smooth.
2. Serve chilled.

Nutritional Info (per serving): Calories 264, Total fat 9 g, Cholesterol 0 mg, Sodium 56 mg, Carbs 41 g, Fiber 9 g, Protein 10 g

Recipes for Estrogen Deficiency-Fast Processor

SOUPS AND SALADS

Veggie Quinoa Salad *Serves 4*

½ cup quinoa

1 cup water

1 green pepper

1 cup carrots, sliced

1 cup cabbage, chopped

1 cup broccoli flowerets

1 cup cauliflower flowerets

1 tablespoon olive oil

2 teaspoons Braggs Liquid Aminos

1. Combine quinoa and water in small saucepan. Bring to a boil, reduce heat, and cook for 10-15 minutes, or until all liquid is absorbed.
2. Put quinoa in a large salad bowl. Add green pepper, carrots, cabbage, broccoli, and cauliflower.
3. Add olive oil and Braggs Liquid Aminos and mix well.

Nutritional Info (per serving): Calories 148, Total fat 5 g, Cholesterol 0 mg, Sodium 34 mg, Carbs 23 g, Fiber 4 g, Protein 5 g

Ensalada Mixta *Serves 4*

3 tablespoons olive oil

1 tablespoon Braggs Liquid Aminos

½ teaspoon sea salt

½ teaspoon dried mixed herb blend

1 head romaine lettuce

4 red potatoes, boiled, peeled, and diced

2 hard-boiled eggs, cut in half

8 ounces lima beans, cooked

8 ounces artichoke hearts, drained

8 asparagus spears, cooked and drained

1. Mix olive oil, Braggs Liquid Aminos, salt, and mixed herb blend in small bowl and set aside.
2. Divide lettuce evenly between four plates.
3. Top each plate with one potato, one half egg, 2 ounces lima beans, 2 ounces artichoke hearts, and 2 asparagus spears.
4. Drizzle about 1½ tablespoons of dressing over each salad and serve.

Nutritional Info (per serving): Calories 317, Total fat 14g, Cholesterol 106 mg, Sodium 342 mg, Carbs 38 g, Fiber 12 g, Protein 15 g

SOUPS AND SALADS

Butternut Soup   *Serves 6*

1 cup red onion, chopped

2 teaspoons olive oil

1 teaspoon ground sage

½ teaspoon sea salt

3 cups low sodium vegetable broth

1 large butternut squash, peeled and cubed

1. In a soup pot, sauté onion in olive oil over medium heat until soft.
2. Add sage, salt, broth, and squash. Bring to a boil.
3. Reduce heat and simmer for 25-30 minutes, or until squash is soft.
4. Ladle ¾ of the soup in to a blender or food processor and purée.
5. Pour back into pot and reheat for 5 minutes.
6. Serve warm.

Nutritional Info (per serving): Calories 184, Total fat 2 g, Cholesterol 1 mg, Sodium 459 mg, Carbs 37 g, Fiber 7 g, Protein 9 g

Mushroom and Wild Rice Soup   *Serves 6*

¼ cup olive oil

4 large shallots, chopped

1 cup wild rice, cooked

3 medium carrot, chopped

3 cups mushroom, sliced

6 cups low sodium chicken broth

2 bay leaves

1 teaspoon sea salt

1. Heat olive oil in a large stock pot.
2. Add shallots and sauté until tender.
3. Add rice and cook for three minutes.
4. Add carrots, mushroom, broth, bay leaves, and sea salt and bring to a boil.
5. Reduce heat, cover, and simmer for one hour.
6. Remove bay leaves and serve warm.

Nutritional Info (per serving): Calories 254, Total fat 9 g, Cholesterol 0 mg, Sodium 848 mg, Carbs 28 g, Fiber 3 g, Protein 16 g

Recipes for Estrogen Dominance and Estrogen Deficiency-Slow Processor

SOUPS AND SALADS

Miso Soup *Serves 4*

4 cups water, divided
2 carrots, sliced
1 onion, sliced
1 cup tofu, cubed

4 tablespoons miso
2 tablespoons scallions, chopped
½ tablespoon fresh parsley, chopped

1. In a large pot, heat ½ cup water.
2. Add carrots and onion and cook for 8-10 minutes.
3. Add another ½ cup water and tofu. Cook for 5-7 more minutes.
4. Add the rest of the water and bring to a boil.
5. Lower heat, cover, and simmer for 15 minutes.
6. In a small bowl, add 2 tablespoons of boiled water to miso and create a thin paste.
7. Add miso paste, scallions, and parsley to pot and stir.
8. Cook for 5 more minutes and serve warm.

Nutritional Info (per serving): Calories 110, Total fat 4 g, Cholesterol 0 mg, Sodium 652 mg, Carbs 12 g, Fiber 3 g, Protein 8 g

SIDE DISHES

Zucchini and Eggplant Sauté   *Serves 4*

1 tablespoon olive oil
2 zucchini, sliced
½ eggplant, cubed

1 leek, sliced
1 tablespoon fresh basil, chopped
1 teaspoon oregano

1. Heat olive oil in large frying pan over medium high heat.
2. Add zucchini, eggplant, and leek and sauté about 15 minutes.
3. Add basil and oregano and sauté until vegetables are tender.
4. Serve warm.

Nutritional Info (per serving): Calories 73, Total fat 4 g, Cholesterol 0 mg, Sodium 9 mg, Carbs 10 g, Fiber 3 g, Protein 2 g

Steamed Flowerets   *Serves 4*

2½ cups broccoli flowerets
2½ cups cauliflower flowerets

4 tablespoons flaxseed oil
1 teaspoon herbes de Provence

1. Place broccoli and cauliflower in a steamer and steam for 10 minutes. Vegetables should be tender but still a bit crisp.
2. Place vegetables into a large bowl. Add oil and spice and mix well.
3. Serve warm.

Nutritional Info (per serving): Calories 148, Total fat 14 g, Cholesterol 0 mg, Sodium 31 mg, Carbs 6 g, Fiber 3 g, Protein 3 g

Recipes for Estrogen Deficiency-Fast Processor

MAIN COURSES

Seafood Bonanza *Serves 6*

2 teaspoons olive oil
2 carrots, sliced
2 stalks celery, sliced
1 red onion, chopped
3 cloves garlic, minced
2 cups low sodium vegetable broth

1 pound halibut, cut in ½" cubes
½ pound shrimp, peeled and halved
2 zucchini, sliced
2 yellow squash, diced
2 teaspoons herbes de Provence

1. Heat olive oil in a large stock pot.
2. Add carrots, celery, onion, and garlic and cook until tender.
3. Add broth and bring to a boil.
4. Reduce heat, cover, and simmer for 30 minutes.
5. Add halibut, shrimp, zucchini, squash, and herbes de Provence.
6. Cover and simmer for 15 minutes or until fish flakes easily.
7. Serve warm.

Nutritional Info (per serving): Calories 195, Total fat 4 g, Cholesterol 82 mg, Sodium 293 mg, Carbs 10 g, Fiber 4 g, Protein 29 g

Recipes for Estrogen Deficiency-Fast Processor

MAIN COURSES

Scallop Kebabs With Minted Quinoa   *Serves 4*

2 cups water

1 cup quinoa

2 tablespoons fresh mint, chopped

2 tablespoons basil

1 teaspoon sea salt

1 tablespoon olive oil

24 large scallops

2 red peppers, cut into 1-inch chunks

2 zucchini, sliced

2 yellow squash, sliced

1 sweet potato, sliced

1. Add water and quinoa to a medium-sized saucepan and bring to a boil.
2. Cover and lower heat.
3. Cook until all water is absorbed (should have about 2 cups of quinoa).
4. Add mint. Mix well and set aside, covered.
5. In a small bowl, combine basil, sea salt, and olive oil. Set aside.
6. Thread 3 scallops and 2 pieces each of red pepper, zucchini, yellow squash, and sweet potato onto 8 metal skewers.
7. Brush each kebab with basil-olive oil mixture and grill for 5-8 minutes per side.
8. Serve two kebabs with ½ cup minted quinoa.

Nutritional Info (per serving): Calories 351, Total fat 7 g, Cholesterol 30 mg, Sodium 639 mg, Carbs 50 g, Fiber 8 g, Protein 24 g

Recipes for Estrogen Deficiency-Fast Processor

MAIN COURSES

Tabouli Temptation   *Serves 6*

2 cups brown rice, cooked	8 ounces cooked tofu, cubed
1 cup parsley, chopped	1 tablespoon Braggs Liquid Aminos
½ cup fresh mint, chopped	2 tablespoons olive oil
½ leek, diced	1 teaspoon oregano
1 cup carrot, chopped	½ teaspoon cilantro
1 tablespoon pine nuts	¼ teaspoon sea salt

1. In a large bowl, add rice, parsley, mint, leek, carrot, pine nuts, and tofu. Mix well.
2. In a small bowl, mix Braggs Liquid Aminos, olive oil, oregano, cilantro, and salt.
3. Pour olive oil mixture over rice blend and mix well.

Nutritional Info (per serving): Calories 327, Total fat 9 g, Cholesterol 0 mg, Sodium 101 mg, Carbs 54 g, Fiber 3 g, Protein 9 g

Vegetarian Burritos   *Serves 4*

1 red pepper, diced	14 ounces vegetarian refried beans
½ small red onion, diced	½ avocado, thinly sliced
2 tablespoons olive oil	1 tomato, sliced
4 corn tortillas	½ cup chopped lettuce

1. Preheat oven to 200° F.
2. Sauté pepper and onion in olive oil for 4-5 minutes.
3. While they are cooking, warm tortillas in oven.
4. In separate pan, heat beans.
5. Place tortillas on a plate. Evenly distribute the onion/pepper mixture, beans, avocado, tomato, and lettuce on each tortilla.
6. Serve warm.

Nutritional Info (per serving): Calories 261, Total fat 12 g, Cholesterol 0 mg, Sodium 459 mg, Carbs 32 g, Fiber 8 g, Protein 8 g

MAIN COURSES

Portobello Quiche *Serves 6*

2 tablespoons olive oil	2 cups plain rice or soy milk
¾ cup red onion, diced	4 eggs
3 portobello mushrooms, thickly diced	¼ cup soy parmesan cheese
2 cups broccoli, chopped	1½ teaspoon garlic powder
¼ cup ground corn meal	2 teaspoons mixed dried herb blend

1. Preheat oven to 350°F.
2. Heat olive oil in skillet on medium high for several minutes.
3. Add onion and portobellos and sauté for 4-5 minutes.
4. Add broccoli and cook 3-4 minutes.
5. Add corn meal and mix thoroughly.
6. Place in a quiche pan or similar deep-dish pan and set aside.
7. In a separate mixing bowl, whisk milk with the eggs and parmesan cheese.
8. Add garlic powder and mixed dried herb blend.
9. Pour over the portobello mixture and bake for 40–45 minutes, until the center is set and firm.
10. Let stand 5–10 minutes before serving.

Nutritional Info (per serving): Calories 180, Total fat 11 g, Cholesterol 127 mg, Sodium 119 mg, Carbs 13 g, Fiber 4 g, Protein 10 g

Recipes for Estrogen Deficiency-Fast Processor

DESSERTS

Papaya-Mango Custard *Serves 2*

4 ounces soft tofu	1 cup mango
1 cup papaya	1 teaspoon honey

1. Place all ingredients into a blender until thick and pudding-like.
2. Serve chilled.

Nutritional Info (per serving): Calories 135, Total fat 3 g, Cholesterol 10 mg, Sodium 8 mg, Carbs 25 g, Fiber 4 g, Protein 5 g

Oatmeal Cookies *Makes two dozen*

½ cup canola oil	½ teaspoon sea salt
¼ cup erythritol	1 cup brown rice flour
1 egg	¾ teaspoon baking soda
2 teaspoons vanilla	2 cups rolled oats

1. Preheat oven to 375°F.
2. Mix oil and erythritol together in a large bowl.
3. Add egg and vanilla. Blend well.
4. In a separate bowl, mix together salt, flour, baking soda, and oats. Mix well with a whisk.
5. Add to oil and egg mixture and mix well. (Add a few tablespoons of water if you want to thin out the dough.)
6. With a tablespoon, scoop out dough and place onto a greased cookie sheet.
7. Bake for 12-15 minutes, or until slightly brown.

Nutritional Info (per cookie): Calories 94, Total fat 5 g, Cholesterol 8 mg, Sodium 82 mg, Carbs 12 g, Fiber 1 g, Protein 2 g

30 reduce stress, maintain hormonal health

I have yet to meet a woman who does not struggle with stress. In fact, 10 percent of the American population—between 20 and 30 million people—exhibit clinical signs of stress and anxiety each year, and another 10 percent struggle with depression severe enough to warrant medication. Women of all ages, from preadolescence to post-menopause, are affected by stress, anxiety, and depression, with no one age group more affected by stress than another. And I can promise you that Kimberly and I have both had our share throughout the years. Unfortunately, there is no way to eliminate it completely.

But the hectic pace at which many of us live our lives exhausts our adrenal glands and nervous systems and lowers our resistance to disease. Given all that, it's no wonder that stress often impedes a woman's ability to function optimally with co-workers, friends, and family.

Throughout the chapter, I'll explain what is going on in your body when you become stressed and how it affects your hormone production and overall health. I'll then give you a great and very useful self-quiz so you can gauge how much stress you have in your life. Once you learn where you fall on the stress meter, I'll introduce you to some of the most extraordinary people in the realm of stress reduction and personal growth, whose resources you can call on for your own use. I'll also share my own calming, soothing program for stress reduction with you.

What is Stress?

Stress is defined as a demand on physical or mental energy, as well as the distress this demand causes. Stress can be emotional, psychological, social, chemical, and/or physical in origin. It can be acute and sudden, as when a car cuts in front of you on the freeway. There are also persistent, chronic forms of stress, such as loneliness or the demands of raising children or caring for an aging parent. Changing jobs, getting a parking ticket, meeting new people, going away on vacation, competing in a tennis match, or giving a speech can all cause stress.

What you perceive as stress is purely subjective. A situation that one person considers manageable, another person may see as dangerous or threatening. People's perception of stress depends on their attitude toward challenges and change, their emotional and psychological coping skills, and their physical capability to respond to stress and recover quickly.

Unfortunately, millions of people lack the ability to effectively handle stress. As a result, we often trigger an output of chemicals within our bodies meant to help cope with stress. These chemicals have a profound effect on our physiology, affecting how we breathe, how blood circulates throughout the body, and even our level of muscular tension. If these stress chemicals are triggered only occasionally, the body does not suffer physical damage from their release. However, when triggered repeatedly, these chemicals may exhaust the body, causing unpleasant symptoms and, eventually, physical breakdown and disease.

Specific physical symptoms of stress include fatigue, insomnia, shortness of breath, heart palpitations, sweating, light-headedness, a craving for sweets, alternating constipation and diarrhea, low blood pressure, and blood sugar disturbances. Emotional signs of stress include anxiety, nervousness, and mood swings.

Stress-related symptoms may occasionally be so intense that they can interfere with a person's ability to function. For example, anxiety disorders such as claustrophobia (fear of closed or narrow spaces) and agoraphobia (fear of open or public places) may actually cause affected individuals to avoid social and work situations that can trigger their fears. I have had patients who reported having panic episodes when driving their car on a freeway or when presenting a speech before a large audience. If this sounds like you, believe me, you are not alone. Nearly 10 percent of the U.S. population—that's 20 to 30 million people—experience phobias, panic attacks, and other anxiety disorders in any given year.

What is Your Body Trying to Tell You?

Whether your stress is triggered by a crazy commute, a busy household, an angry spouse or child, a demanding job, a difficult neighbor or family member, or even a poor self-image and too much self-criticism (which are very common issues for most of us), every woman has a point where the strain and anxiety start to take their toll. The problem is many women don't hear the warning messages their bodies send out—partly because they're too stressed out to listen, and partly because they don't know what the messages are.

Most women know that irritability, loss of sleep, appetite changes, tense muscles, and a tendency to catch whatever "bug" is going around can be signs of stress. But did you know that excessive stress can increase your risk of developing infectious diseases, including genital herpes and bladder infections? Researchers have even seen a relationship between stress and occurrences of psoriasis, a chronic skin disease.

In fact, many studies have shown that extreme stress can increase your susceptibility to virtually every major category of disease. For example, stress is one of the top risk factors for heart disease. A study from the *Journal of the American Medical Association* showed that negative emotions can even trigger a reduction in blood flow to the heart.

In my own medical practice, I've seen excessive stress worsen every possible hormone imbalance, whether the woman was estrogen dominant, estrogen deficient-fast processor, or estrogen deficient-slow processor. It aggravates the symptoms inherent in each of these hormonal imbalances.

Stress can exacerbate virtually every female problem, from PMS through post-menopause, by interfering with normal hormone production and function. I've seen this time and again in my practice. Women come in with severe PMS symptoms, fibroid tumors, and endometriosis, as well as hot flashes and insomnia. When I talk to them about what is going on in their personal life, more often than not, they tell me about an extremely stressful situation they are dealing with.

Unfortunately, even if you are eating the perfect diet, exercising every day, and taking the recommended nutritional supplements religiously, excessive stress can literally neutralize the benefits of everything positive that you are doing. But the good news is that the reverse is also true. You can create miracles by handling stress in a positive, self-nurturing, life-enhancing manner.

By discovering and taking the emotional and spiritual journey towards a stress-free life, you'll begin to notice several amazing changes. Your mood will lift and even out, you'll feel much more loving and joyful, you'll begin to sleep like a baby, you'll experience more positive dreams, and you'll have a new appreciation for your friends and family. What you may not also realize is that your health will greatly improve too, particularly your hormonal health.

So now that you know the emotional and physical ramifications of too much stress, let's determine your current level of risk.

WHERE DO YOU SQUIRREL AWAY YOUR STRESS?

Just like a squirrel has a favorite hiding place for its chestnuts, you most likely have a place on your body where you store stress. It may be tension or tightness in your shoulders, neck or throat, upper or lower back, arms, or stomach. Some women I know develop horrible headaches, complain of eyestrain, or grind their teeth when stress gets the better of them. Do any of these areas or pains ring a bell for you?

This accumulation of stress can lower your energy and increase fatigue. Next time you feel the tell-tale signs of increased pressure in your "storage area," stop what you are doing and begin to breathe deeply. This will often alleviate the pressure. If the stress is too great and this isn't effective, try one of the stress reduction exercises found later in this chapter.

How Stressed *Are* You?

To properly assess your level of stress, you have to look at the type of stress you are dealing with. Is it macro or major stress or is it micro or daily, everyday stress?

Major stress includes important, life-changing events such as marriage, birth of a child, divorce, death of a spouse or parent, or loss of a job. According to Dr. Thomas Holmes and his team at the University of Washington Medical School, major stress is not a one-at-a-time thing. He maintains that major stress can be cumulative. For this reason, he developed the Life Change Index. I have developed my own version of this type of index, based on my own study of the research on stress, coupled with decades of feedback from my patients. This evaluation tool assigns a number to certain stress events. You mark all of the changes you've had over the course of two years, and then add up the values. If you have a score of 300 or more, you have serious major life stress. If your score is between 200 and 299, you have medium risk. A score of 199 or lower indicates low risk.

Test Yourself

Here's a modified version of Dr. Holmes' Life Change Index. What's your tally? Remember to include all events that have taken place in the last 24 months.

Value	Score	Life Event
100	_____	Death of a spouse
73	_____	Divorce
65	_____	Separation from your spouse
63	_____	Death of a close family member
53	_____	Personal injury or illness (serious)
50	_____	Newly married
47	_____	Fired from your long-time job
45	_____	Marriage reconciliation
45	_____	Retirement (from work)
44	_____	Change in health of a family member
40	_____	Discover that you are pregnant
39	_____	Difficulty with sexual activity
39	_____	Gaining a new family member
39	_____	A major job readjustment
38	_____	A radical change in finances
37	_____	Death of a close relative
36	_____	Career change
35	_____	Increase in number of marital arguments

31	_____	Incur a loan/mortgage of more than $100,000
30	_____	Foreclosure of a mortgage or loan
29	_____	Change in responsibilities at work
29	_____	Son or daughter leaving home
29	_____	Irritating trouble with your in-laws
28	_____	Recognition for outstanding achievements
26	_____	Spouse starts or stops work
26	_____	Begin or end schooling
25	_____	Undergo a change in living conditions
24	_____	Revise your personal habits
23	_____	Experience trouble with your boss
20	_____	Work hours or conditions are different
20	_____	Change your residence
20	_____	Change your school or major subject
19	_____	Major changes to recreational activities
19	_____	Church or club activities change
18	_____	Social activities change
17	_____	Incur a loan/mortgage of less than $100,000
16	_____	Change your sleeping habits
15	_____	Change the frequency of family get-togethers
15	_____	Alter your eating habits
13	_____	Go on vacation
12	_____	Year-end holidays occur
11	_____	Commit a minor violation of the law

The Little Things

Next, take a look at those micro or minor areas of stress in your life. Evaluate for yourself the little tensions that creep up on a daily basis.

Work Stress

_____ **Pushing beyond your limit.** You press yourself too hard, trying to get it all done and done well.

_____ **Boredom.** Work is not stimulating you. You are bored and wish you were doing anything else.

_____ **Time crunch.** You are always against the clock and rushed.

_____ **Boss pressure.** Your manager or supervisor is too demanding or picky.

_____ **Unpleasant physical surroundings.** Lights are fluorescent, too bright, or too dim. The noise level is uncomfortable, there are noxious smells or chemicals, and/or there is an overwhelming amount of activity going on around you.

Spouse/Significant Other or Family/Home Life

_____ **Poor communication.** You don't discuss feelings, hopes, and desires. You hold in emotion and thrive on negative drama. Arguments are frequently loud and abrasive rather than calm and quiet. One person talks while the other clams up.

_____ **Affection.** One or both of you withhold affection (hugs, kisses, hand-holding, etc.) from the other, or are not comfortable with the level of affection your partner demands.

_____ **Sexuality.** You are not on the same page. You may want more or less than your partner.

_____ **Children.** They are too loud and boisterous. They demand too much of your time and attention.

_____ **Organization.** Your home is poorly organized, dirty, and/or messy. Chores are rarely finished, if even started.

_____ **Time.** You have too much to do and not enough time to do it.

_____ **Responsibility.** You need more assistance, some help with the many demands of your time and energy.

Negative Self-Talk

_____ **Too anxious.** You worry about every little thing and what may or may not go wrong.

_____ **Playing victim.** You think everyone is out to get you, hurt you, or take advantage of you.

_____ **Poor self-image.** You don't like yourself and continually find faults and flaws.

_____ **Too critical.** You continually judge and find fault with others.

_____ **Cannot relax.** You are tightly wound and have difficulty relaxing.

_____ **No down time.** You don't take time to unwind and relax.

_____ **Lack of sleep.** You don't sleep well or often enough and are frequently tired.

Like any major change, identifying the problem is the first step. Now that you've determined your current level of stress, let's see how that stress is affecting you physically.

The Physiology of Stress

In this section, I discuss the physiology of stress and the actual chemical changes that occur within the body in response to stress. If you would rather skip this material, as it is more technical in its description, you can go on to page 441, where I discuss how stress affects your hormones.

Stress has an incredibly profound effect on performance and health. When you sense serious danger, a sequence of biological events called the "fight-or-flight response" occurs. This response is a cascade of chemical and electrical processes meant to increase your ability to survive in the natural world. The fight-or-flight response occurs with any perceived threat, whether it is physically real, psychologically upsetting, or even imaginary; it can even occur simply when you are excited by a positive event if you have a sensitively wired nervous system.

The fight-or-flight response occurs first in the nervous system, beginning in your brain, moving down the spinal cord, and then to the peripheral nerves. The nervous system is divided into two parts—the voluntary nervous system and the involuntary, or autonomic, nervous system (ANS). The voluntary nervous system manages activity in the conscious domain, such as when you touch a hot stove and quickly pull your hand away. In contrast, the ANS regulates functions of which most people are unaware, such as pulse rate, circulation, and glandular function.

The ANS is also divided into two parts, which oppose and complement each other: the sympathetic and the parasympathetic nervous systems (SNS and PNS, respectively). The sympathetic nervous system tends to speed up the responses to your muscular and internal organs to help you deal with stressful situations. In contrast, the parasympathetic nervous system helps to slow your physiological responses down. For example, if excitement speeds up the heart rate too much, it is the parasympathetic nervous system's job to act as a control circuit and slow it down. But if the heart slows down too much, then it is the sympathetic nervous system's job to speed it back up.

In response to a stressful situation, the sympathetic nerves secrete a chemical called norepinephrine, which directly enters into the target tissues of organs such as the heart, the abdominal organs, the sweat glands, and the pupils of the eyes. Stimulation by norepinephrine causes an excitatory response within these tissues, which allows your body to react and protect itself from a stressful situation. For example, sympathetic stimulation increases blood flow to vital organs and the muscles. The end results are such stress-relieving and performance-enhancing qualities as increased muscular strength and enhanced mental alertness. However, the effect on the target tissues of norepinephrine from the sympathetic nerves is short-lived, lasting only a few seconds, because its reuptake and diffusion away from the tissues is rapid.

The Stress–Adrenal Connection

Your adrenal glands work in tandem with the SNS as part of your stress response system. The adrenals are triangular-shaped organs resting on top of each kidney. Each gland consists of two parts, the medulla (the central section) and the cortex (the outer section). The SNS sends nerve impulses into the adrenal medulla causing it to secrete the same type of chemicals as the sympathetic nerves themselves—the hormones epinephrine (commonly referred to as adrenaline) and norepinephrine (or noradrenaline). However, while the SNS secretes these chemicals directly into your tissues, the adrenal medulla secretes them into the bloodstream, which transports them to various target tissues, also in response to stressful situations. Thus, your body has two overlapping systems to manage stress—the production of epinephrine and norepinephrine by both the SNS and the adrenal medulla.

However, while only a small percentage of cells in the body are stimulated by the epinephrine and norepinephrine produced by the sympathetic nerves, these same chemicals, when secreted by the adrenal medulla (especially epinephrine) are carried in the bloodstream to tissues and organs throughout your body. Even the time that these chemicals remain active in the tissues differs, depending on their source. The norepinephrine secreted by the sympathetic nerves is active for only a few seconds, while the same chemical, when secreted by the adrenal medulla, remains active in the tissues for one to several minutes.

When the alarm response is triggered, epinephrine increases arterial pressure, as well as blood flow to specific muscles needed for vigorous activity. It also increases the rate of metabolism, the concentration of glucose in the blood, the conversion of sugar to energy in muscles, muscle strength, and mental activity. All of these physiological responses are necessary for you to perform effectively in a challenging situation.

The adrenal cortex, or outer portion of the adrenal gland, also produces hormones that help you to manage stress, called glucocorticoids and mineralocorticoids. (The adrenal cortex also produces a third class of hormones, the sex steroids, particularly dehydroepiandrosterone, or DHEA, which is discussed in Chapter 20.) Adrenal hormones are primarily produced from acetyl Coenzyme A (acetyl CoA) and cholesterol. Acetyl CoA is a chemical produced in the liver, made from fatty acids and amino acids. It provides an important source of energy for the body as well as being a building block from which hormones are made. Cholesterol is a waxy, white, fatty material, widely distributed in all body cells. The cholesterol in the body is supplied by animal foods in the diet, such as eggs and organ meats, and the liver also produces a certain amount of cholesterol.

Glucocorticoids are especially important in allowing an individual to withstand various kinds of stress. The secretion of cortisol accounts for at least 95 percent of adrenal-glucocorticoid activity. Cortisol is the primary stress hormone. In an attempt to buffer the effects of stress, cortisol is released when the body is threatened by extreme conditions such as infection, intense heat or cold, surgery, and any kind of trauma. Cortisol acts as a natural anti-inflammatory when the body is assaulted by an injury, arthritis, or allergy. Cortisol also affects carbohydrate and fat metabolism, promoting the conversion of stored sugars and fat into energy, as well as hormone production.

The Stress–Neurotransmitter Connection

Besides those chemicals produced by the adrenal glands and sympathetic nerves that create the stress response described above, there are a myriad of other substances produced by the body that affect your susceptibility to stress, including serotonin, dopamine, estrogen, and progesterone.

As we've discussed throughout this book, serotonin and dopamine are neurotransmitters, naturally occurring chemicals that relay electrical messages between nerve cells throughout your body. Serotonin is part of the inhibitory pathway, while dopamine is part of excitatory pathway. Because these two pathways oppose and complement one another, imbalances in either serotonin or dopamine can make a person more sensitive to everyday stress than someone who is able to produce these neurochemicals in more balanced and appropriate amounts.

Serotonin is one of your brain's principal neurotransmitters. Its action on the nerves is inhibitory, relieving stress and calming the mind. Serotonin also regulates appetite, influences mood, and promotes healthy hormone production.

Dopamine is a neurotransmitter that stimulates and energizes the body. In fact, dopamine is actually a precursor to substances made by the adrenal medulla and sympathetic nervous system that regulate the stress response within the body. High levels of dopamine have been linked to such traits as mental alertness, physical energy, and vitality, as well as aggressive drive and libido. Dopamine is synthesized by the adrenal glands and is converted by the body into the stress hormones epinephrine and norepinephrine, which also stimulate hormone production. Before ages 40–45, dopamine levels remain fairly stable, but they then decrease by about 13 percent per decade.

As levels of these neurotransmitters begin to decline with age, your body's ability to handle stressful events can change. Depressed serotonin levels can trigger mood imbalances, sleeplessness, and food cravings. For example, women who suffer from PMS may have a tendency towards low serotonin levels. That's one reason why women with PMS often respond to stressful events in an exaggerated manner. Irritability, anger, tension, and upset are common responses in the second half of the menstrual cycle to such usually small stresses as a nagging child, a minor disagreement with a spouse, or a work deadline. Women who suffer from a serotonin imbalance often feel like a firecracker about to explode for one to two weeks out of each month.

In contrast, when levels of the stimulatory neurotransmitter dopamine are depressed, epinephrine and norepinephrine production is also diminished. This is more common in women who are frequently fatigued, lethargic, and lack vital force and joy of life.

Stress and Your Hormones

Women produce two major sex hormones, estrogen and progesterone. These hormones regulate the menstrual cycle, with estrogen reaching a peak during the first half of the cycle, while progesterone output occurs after midcycle, when ovulation has already occurred. Estrogen causes the growth of the sexual organs at puberty and thickening of the lining of the uterus before it receives a fertilized egg. Estrogen also causes fluid and salt retention in the tissues, which helps to plump up the skin. In contrast, progesterone has a maturing and growth-limiting effect on the tissues of the body, including the uterus, and functions as a diuretic, preventing retention of excess fluid in body tissue.

These two hormones also help to keep in balance the various functions of the nervous systems, and they can have a strong impact on how a woman responds to stress. For example, estrogen tends to affect the levels of serotonin and acts as a natural mood elevator, whereas progesterone affects the levels of dopamine and has a sedative or calming effect. When these hormones (and subsequently, neurotransmitters) are out of balance in relation to one another, stress symptoms can be aggravated.

Stress and Estrogen Dominance

Additionally, stress itself can cause or aggravate hormone imbalances. In fact, it can interfere with your ability to ovulate, thereby blocking progesterone production and pushing further into estrogen dominance. This can lead to severe PMS, menstrual cramps, anxiety, fibroids, endometriosis, and infertility. I've even seen fibroid tumors themselves get larger in patients with chronic stress.

Studies from journals as varied as *Human Stress, Psychosomatics,* and *Acta Psychiatry Scandinavia* have all shown that women with stressful lives are much more likely to experience PMS symptoms. In fact, a study from the *Archives of Family Medicine* found that women who suffered from PMS scored four times higher on a stress scale than other women.

Another Scandinavian study looked at baboons living in captivity. Researchers found that those who developed endometriosis had higher stress levels and were less able to react positively to stress as compared to baboons in the wild.

Finally, according to a study from the *British Medical Journal,* excessive stress can increase your risk of breast cancer. Researchers tested 119 women aged 20 to 70 who had been biopsied for breast cancer. They found that severe and stressful life events significantly increased the likelihood of a cancer diagnosis. Non-stressful and non-serious life events were not associated with a cancer diagnosis.

CARRIE'S STORY

"Carrie," a 44-year-old founder of a small business, came to me for help managing terrible PMS and cramps. She also suffered from the aches and pains she was experiencing from stiffness associated with rheumatoid arthritis, as well as digestive complaints due to irritable bowel syndrome.

After talking for a short time, I discovered that she had no time for herself. By simply setting aside a few hours each week to relax and renew herself, and beginning a daily walking program, Carrie was able to considerably reduce all of her health complaints.

Stress and Estrogen Deficiency

Like their estrogen dominant sisters, estrogen deficient-fast processors must also manage stress carefully. Not only can stress reduce estrogen levels, but it can reduce production of all sex hormones. This can lead to a worsening of menopausal symptoms, including hot flashes, insomnia, depression, and vaginal and tissue dryness, as well as other related issues, such as heart health.

A study from the journal *Menopause* looked at more than 400 women between the ages of 37 and 47 who were still menstruating. Researchers gave the participants an anxiety test at the start of the study and again six years later. By this time, many of the women were experiencing irregular periods and hot flashes.

The researchers found that those women with the highest anxiety levels had almost five times as many hot flashes as the less anxious women. Women with moderate anxiety had three times as many hot flashes. A second study from the *Maternal and Child Health Journal* found that vaginal dryness (also a common symptom of estrogen deficiency) was significantly associated with high emotional or psychological stress.

Lastly, a study from the *Annals of Internal Medicine* found that excessive stress was associated with increased risk of high blood pressure. Researchers found that stress reduction techniques such as deep breathing, biofeedback, meditation, yoga, and hypnosis all helped to reduce blood pressure.

LUCY'S STORY

"Lucy," in her mid-50's, came to me for a consultation. As she began to share her health history with me, she turned pink and started to perspire. While I've often seen menopause-related hot flashes occur during an office visit, they are usually triggered by the stress of seeing a doctor. However, in Lucy's case, it was obvious that several other issues were causing her distress. Her elderly father had recently moved into her home, and she was very concerned about his declining health. Plus, her husband was having a difficult time adapting to the loss of his privacy.

While Lucy had gone into menopause earlier that year, she had only suffered from the occasional hot flash. However, since her father's arrival, she had begun to experience frequent hot flashes during the day and night sweats while sleeping. She also began to feel tired and short-tempered as she struggled to help take care of her father, pacify her husband, and maintain her busy job. For Lucy, the final blow came when she had a complete health evaluation done shortly before she consulted with me. At that time, she was diagnosed with low bone density and low thyroid function. Clearly she needed to get her stress under control.

TANYA'S STORY

When I first met "Tanya," a 48-year-old mother of two, she was going through an extremely difficult time in her life. She was in the process of an ugly divorce and was deeply concerned about her finances and her future. The stress was affecting every aspect of her life, especially her sleep. She had not had a decent night's sleep in several weeks.

She was mentally and physically exhausted, and I could tell just by looking at her that the stress and sleeplessness were taking a huge toll on her health. I quickly determined that Tanya's situation was a classic example of insomnia caused by an imbalance in her autonomic nervous system.

JENNIE'S STORY

"Jennie" is a 64-year-old retired nurse. She came to me complaining of terrible hot flashes, chronic fatigue, depression, and difficulty sleeping at night. I quickly learned that her husband had passed away, and she was concerned about going back to work.

I encouraged Jennie to practice deep breathing and appreciation for the time she had with her husband. In a few short weeks, Jennie found a job she loved. Her mood has improved and her hot flashes have abated.

31 my program for stress reduction

When we began to work on this chapter, Kimberly and I wanted to create the most loving, nurturing, supportive intentions we could create within ourselves to give to you. I chose to put myself in a loving, meditative state, while Kimberly chose to go for a run, one of her preferred stress-relieving activities. This allowed both of our bodies to become free of stress and tension, and open to the creative and loving spirit.

One of the best things you can do for yourself is to discover that stress-reduction technique or techniques that are most beneficial to you. Regardless of your hormonal type, I've found that the foundation of any stress reduction program is to master the arts of deep breathing and meditation. Next, I advocate using positive, life-affirming emotions to bring about renewed hormonal health. Specifically, we'll look at how prayer, love, gratitude, appreciation, laughter, happiness, optimism, positive self-image, forgiveness, and generosity can support and harmonize your health and hormones, relationships, job, and overall life and well-being.

Practicing Deep Breathing and Meditation

I have taught deep breathing and meditation to patients for several decades now. Without fail, they tell me that they become much calmer, more patient, and happier after practicing these exercises. Best of all, a calm mind creates a calm body, and a calm body allows your autonomic nervous system to balance and slow down, your body chemistry to normalize, and your hormones to regain a much healthier state of balance.

To get ready for any stress reduction exercise, it's important that you take the following steps to prepare yourself:

1. Separate yourself physically and mentally from your normal, daily environment. Maybe designate a space in your home specifically for relaxation. It can include soothing pictures, a comfortable chair or couch, and possibly a sound machine.

2. Make sure you are wearing loose, comfortable clothing. Sit or lie down in a comfortable position. Try to make your spine as straight as possible and be sure to keep your arms and legs uncrossed.
3. Focus all of your attention on the stress reduction exercise you choose. Don't allow anything to distract you. Close your eyes and take a few deep, abdominal breaths. Focus on how the air goes in and out of your body.

These steps will help you separate your problems and concerns of the day from your relaxation practice so you can quiet your mind and begin to ease your mind, body, and soul.

General Relaxation Exercises

Regardless of their hormone status, the following exercises can benefit all women of any age. They include deep breathing, reducing muscle tension, and meditation.

Deep Breathing

Deep breathing is the foundation for any kind of stress relief. I have found that you must be able to control and be aware of your breathing if you want to relax your mind, body, or spirit. When you're physically or emotionally stressed, your breathing becomes more rapid and shallow. You may stop breathing altogether for brief periods without even realizing it. These changes in breathing patterns bring less life-sustaining oxygen into your lungs. At the same time, stress makes your muscles tense up, constricts your blood vessels to restrict blood flow, makes your heart beat faster, and stimulates the output of stressful chemicals from your adrenal glands.

All of these reactions decrease the amount of oxygen available to your cells, tissues, and organs. Poor oxygenation compromises a multitude of chemical reactions that are necessary for cell growth, maintenance and repair. Energy production, waste removal, digestion, and other essential body processes are impaired. You feel fatigued, your body becomes less able to fight illness, and degenerative processes accelerate.

By breathing deeply, you are able to take in large amounts of oxygen. From your lungs, oxygen moves into your bloodstream where it binds to red blood cells and is transported to all the cells and tissues in your body. Oxygen helps your cells produce and utilize energy. When you exhale, waste products (carbon dioxide) are removed from your body through your lungs. This helps to optimize the oxygen levels throughout your body. Your muscles relax, your blood vessels dilate to increase blood flow, and your equilibrium returns, making you feel more energetic and balanced.

Similarly, your brain uses 20 percent of the oxygen in your body. If you don't get enough oxygen, mental clarity fades and you'll have barely enough energy to get by, and you'll lack your natural zest for life.

Next time you're stressed out—or feel stress coming on—try this deep abdominal breathing exercise:

1. Lie flat on your back with your knees pulled up. Keep your feet slightly apart. Try to breathe in and out through your nose.
2. Inhale deeply. As you breathe in, allow your stomach to relax so that the air flows into your abdomen. Your stomach should balloon out as you breathe in. Visualize your lungs filling with air as your chest swells out.
3. Imagine that the air you inhale is filling your body with energy.
4. Exhale deeply. As you breathe out, let your stomach and chest collapse. Imagine the air being pushed out, first from your abdomen and then from your lungs.
5. Imagine that the air you exhale is carrying away fatigue, concerns, and upset.
6. Repeat the process for three to five minutes, keeping your attention on your breath.

Reducing Muscle Tension

When stressed, most women store the tension in a certain group of muscles. Use this exercise to discover where the tension is, then to release it from your body. This sequence is particularly important for women with emotional distress, such as anxiety and nervousness.

1. Lie on your back with your arms at your side, palms down.
2. Raise your right arm and keep it elevated for 15 seconds. Notice if your forearm feels tight and tense, or if the muscles are soft and pliable.
3. Let your arm drop back down to your side and relax. Your arm muscles should relax too.
4. As you lie still, pay attention to other parts of your body that are tense, tight, or sore. Do any of your muscles have a dull ache?
5. Next, inhale deeply. As you breathe in, allow your stomach to relax so that the air flows into your abdomen. Let your stomach balloon out as you breathe in.
6. Imagine the breath is filled with love and relaxation. Let this positive energy travel and fill your muscles.
7. On your next exhalation, take the tension from your muscles and push them out of your body.
8. Continue this pattern of breathing in relaxation and breathing out tension until all of the tension in your muscles has melted away.

Meditation

Meditation allows you to create a state of deep relaxation, which is very healing to the entire body. Metabolism slows, as do physiological functions such as heart rate and blood pressure. Muscle tension decreases. Brain wave patterns shift from the fast beta waves that occur during a normal active day to the slower alpha waves that occur just before falling asleep, or in times of deep relaxation.

Try any or all of the following meditations:

Peace and Calm

1. Sit or lie in a comfortable position.
2. Close your eyes and breathe in and out deeply. Let your breathing be slow and relaxed.
3. Focus all of your attention on your breathing. Notice the movement of your chest and abdomen in and out.
4. Take yourself to a calm and peaceful place deep inside of you, and as you inhale, say the word "peace" to yourself. As you exhale, say the word "calm." Draw out the pronunciation of these words, so that they last for the entire breath.
5. Repeat this exercise for three to five minutes.

Golden Temple

1. Lie on your back in a comfortable position. Inhale through your nose and exhale slowly and deeply through your mouth.
2. Visualize a beautiful green meadow full of lovely fragrant flowers. In the middle of this meadow is a golden temple. See the temple emanating peace and healing.
3. Visualize yourself entering this temple. You are the only person inside. It is still and peaceful.
4. As you stand inside, you feel a healing energy fill every pore of your body with a warm, golden light. Every cell in your body that is in need of repair and healing is nourished by this light. This energy feels like a healing balm that relaxes you totally. All stress dissolves and fades from your mind. You feel totally at ease. Remain in this temple for as long as you wish.
5. When you are ready to leave, open your eyes and continue your slow, deep breathing for a few more cycles.

Oak Tree

1. Sit in a comfortable position, your arms resting at your sides.
2. Close your eyes and breathe deeply. Let your breathing be slow and relaxed.

3. See your body as a strong oak tree. Your body is solid like the wide, brown trunk of the tree. Imagine sturdy roots growing from your legs and going down deeply into the earth, anchoring your body. You feel solid, strong, and able to handle any stress.

4. When upsetting thoughts or situations occur, visualize your body remaining grounded, like an oak tree. Feel the strength and stability in your arms and legs.

5. You feel confident and relaxed, able to handle any situation.

ANGELA'S STORY

"Angela" came to see me several years ago for relief from stress and anxiety. The last two years of her life had been marred by emotional and physical turbulence. She seemed very shaky and frightened, and her gestures were nervous and jumpy. As we sat together and talked, she shared with me that she felt as if her life was falling apart, as her moods degenerated from tenseness into frequent bouts of anxiety.

One major trigger for Angela's anxiety appeared to be quitting a job that she had previously enjoyed for seven years. At that time, Angela's old boss left the company and was replaced by a new manager who constantly found fault with Angela.

She found a different job and, astonishingly enough, discovered that she had an equally negative situation with her boss at the new company. She also had problems with her roommate and was forced to move to a new apartment—which threw her equilibrium further off balance.

The final straw for Angela occurred when she began to date a man who, on the surface, seemed perfect. He fit all her fantasies of a tall, dark, and handsome "dream partner." He appeared to have a wonderful, calm demeanor, in contrast to her own tenseness and edginess. However, her whole perfect picture collapsed when he confessed on their third date that he too was suffering from acute anxiety and panic attacks—and could only stay calm by using anti-anxiety medication and even street drugs.

All of a sudden, Angela felt like she was looking in a mirror at her own reflection. She realized at that point that she needed to own up to her problems with anxiety. Her instincts were telling her that she really needed to strengthen her body, mind, and spirit to better handle and become more resistant to the many stresses in her life.

She decided that she would commit to using only natural, complementary health care methods. Angela and I worked together over many months to help her get a handle on her anxiety. As she learned to nurture herself and take care of her own inner needs, I was pleased to see her self-confidence and ability to handle stress improve significantly over time.

Stress Reduction for Different Hormonal Types

In addition to practicing the general relaxation exercises I described above, there are specific exercises you can do if you are estrogen dominant, estrogen deficient-fast processor, or estrogen deficient-slow processor. With estrogen dominance or an estrogen deficient-slow processor, you need to speed up your metabolism without becoming overly revved up. You can do this by varying the breathing exercise to include color. In your case, you'll want to breathe in heating, warming colors such as red and orange.

For estrogen deficient-fast processors, you need slower, more meditative options. When you vary the breathing exercise described above, you should use more cooling hues like violet, blue, or green.

You can also use a combination of affirmations and visualizations to reduce your stress load. Affirmations are positive statements describing how you want your mind, body, and soul to be. By describing how you want your body to be, affirmations constructively align your mind with your body. Your state of health is determined in part by the interaction between your mind and body, via the thousands of messages you send yourself every day. Therefore, it is essential that you cultivate a positive belief system and a positive body image as a critical part of your stress management program.

Visualization transports your mind to a calm and peaceful place, free from stress and anxiety. When you practice visualization, close your eyes and create a picture in your mind that you find soothing and relaxing. Try to make the image as detailed as possible. If you're on a beach, feel the sand between your toes, smell the seawater, luxuriate in the caress of the breeze on your sun-kissed skin.

By using the following affirmations and visualizations, your estrogen dominant, estrogen deficient-slow processor, or estrogen deficient-fast processor symptoms can begin to abate and even dissolve away.

Affirmations for Estrogen Dominance

Sit in a comfortable position and repeat the following affirmations. If any are particularly relevant for you, you may want to repeat those three times each.

- My body is strong and healthy.
- My hormones are balanced and normal.
- My body chemistry is balanced and normal.
- I go through my menstrual cycle with ease and comfort.
- My body is able to regulate my menstrual flow.
- I never spot between menstrual cycles.
- My ovaries and uterus are healthy.

- My vaginal muscles are relaxed and comfortable.
- My cervix and uterus are relaxed and pain-free.
- My adrenal glands are healthy and help promote healthy hormone balance.
- My thyroid is healthy and helps regulate my menstrual flow.
- My lower back muscles feel supple and pliable with each menstrual cycle.
- I am relaxed and at ease as my period approaches.
- My mood is calm and even throughout the month.
- I handle stress completely and competently.
- I eat a well-balanced and healthy diet.
- I eat only those foods that are good for my body type.
- I perform the perfect type and amount of exercise for my body type.
- I love my body and feel at ease in my body.
- My body is pain-free and relaxed.

Visualization for Estrogen Dominance

This visualization exercise is particularly helpful for reducing stress and easing the pain and discomfort of menstrual cramps, fibroids, and endometriosis. The entire exercise should take two to three minutes.

1. Sit in a comfortable chair or lie down on your bed or favorite couch.
2. Close your eyes and begin to breathe deeply. Inhale and exhale slowly. Notice as your body begins to relax.
3. Imagine that you can look through a magic mirror deep into your body. Focus on those areas that are tight, contracted, or cause you pain. See any knotted muscles, lesions, cysts, tumors, or scarring.
4. Next, picture a large eraser coming into your body. See the eraser rubbing away the knots, lesions, cysts, tumors, or scars. See as they begin to loosen, shrink, and disappear.
5. Now, look at your ovaries and uterus. Notice their healthy, pinkish color. They are relaxed and supple. Your uterus has perfect blood circulation and your ovaries are healthy and balanced with the perfect levels of hormones.
6. Look at your abdominal and lower back muscles. Your back is pliable, flexible, and has great muscle tone. Your abdomen is flat and free from bloat.
7. Look at your entire body and enjoy the sense of peace and calm running through your body. You feel wonderful.
8. Begin to withdraw from the visualization and return your focus to your breathing, inhaling and exhaling slowly.
9. Now open your eyes and luxuriate in the peace and relaxation.

Affirmations for Estrogen Deficient-Fast Processors

Sit in a comfortable position and repeat the following affirmations. If any are particularly relevant for you, you may want to repeat those three times each.

- I go through menopause easily and effortlessly.
- My body is strong and healthy during the life change.
- My body is healthier and healthier every day.
- My hormones are perfectly balanced and regulated.
- My body chemistry is balanced and regulated.
- My skin temperature feels comfortable all day and night.
- I sleep well every night.
- My mood is calm and relaxed.
- My thyroid is healthy and full of vitality.
- My bones and joints are strong and healthy.
- My heart is strong and healthy.
- I feel wonderful as I go through menopause.
- Menopause is a beautiful time to grow and change as a woman.
- I am respectful and careful with myself during this transition.
- I love to nurture myself.
- I practice the relaxation methods I enjoy.
- I eat a well-balanced and healthy diet.
- I eat only those foods that are good for my body type.
- I perform the perfect type and amount of exercise for my body type.
- I love my body and feel at ease in my body.
- My life is fun and exciting.

Visualization for Estrogen Deficient-Fast Processors

This visualization exercise helps you create a mental picture of how you would like your body to look and function after menopause. As you see your body radiate health and vitality, you stimulate chemical changes within your body to help make this condition a reality. The entire exercise should take two to three minutes.

1. Sit in a comfortable chair or lie down on your bed or favorite couch.
2. Close your eyes and begin to breathe deeply. Inhale and exhale slowly. Notice as your body begins to relax.
3. Imagine that you can look through a magic mirror deep into your body. Look at your female organs. They are healthy and vital. Your ovaries and uterus are healthy. Nutrients and oxygen flow freely to them and toxins are swept away. Your vagina is moist and healthy. You are able to enjoy a healthy and active sex life.

4. Look at your thyroid, just below your Adam's apple in your neck. It is the perfect size and texture. It regulates your metabolism perfectly.
5. Look at your bones. They are strong and sturdy. They are full of calcium and other critical nutrients.
6. Look at your heart. It is strong and powerful and pumps your blood with ease.
7. Now, see your face. You are smiling. Your mood is wonderful as you realize you can handle any difficulties with grace and ease.
8. Next, notice your skin. It is soft and moist. You lovingly bathe it with moisturizer and sunscreen. It is lovely.
9. Look at your entire body and enjoy the sense of peace and calm running through your body. You feel wonderful.
10. Begin to withdraw from the visualization and return your focus to your breathing, inhaling and exhaling slowly.
11. Now open your eyes and luxuriate in the peace and relaxation.

Affirmations for Estrogen Deficient-Slow Processors

Sit in a comfortable position and repeat the following affirmations. If any are particularly relevant for you, you may want to repeat those three times each.

- I go through menopause easily and effortlessly.
- My body is strong and healthy during the life change.
- My body is healthier and healthier every day.
- My hormones are perfectly balanced and regulated.
- I don't retain fluids or experience bloating.
- I lose weight easily and effortlessly.
- I have lots of vital energy and stamina.
- My mental function is sharp and I have great mental acuity.
- My vagina is moist and elastic with good circulation.
- I have sexual relations as often as I desire.
- I love to nurture myself.
- I practice the relaxation methods I enjoy.
- I eat a well-balanced and healthy diet.
- I eat only those foods that are good for my body type.
- I perform the perfect type and amount of exercise for my body type.
- I love my body and feel at ease in my body.
- My life is fun and exciting.

Visualization for Estrogen Deficient-Slow Processors

This visualization exercise helps you create a mental picture of how you would like your body to look and function after menopause. As you see your body radiate health and vitality, you stimulate chemical changes within your body to help increase your yang reserves and decrease your yin excess. The entire exercise should take two to three minutes.

1. Sit in a comfortable chair or lie down on your bed or favorite couch.
2. Close your eyes and begin to breathe deeply. Inhale and exhale slowly. Notice as your body begins to relax.
3. Imagine that you can look through a magic mirror deep into your body. Look at your female organs. They are healthy and vital. Your ovaries and uterus are healthy. Nutrients and oxygen flow freely to them and toxins are swept away.
4. Look at your thyroid, just below your Adam's apple in your neck. It is the perfect size and texture. It regulates your metabolism perfectly. You lose and maintain your weight easily and effortlessly.
5. Look at your bones. They are strong and sturdy. They are full of calcium and other critical nutrients.
6. Look at your heart. It is strong and powerful and pumps your blood with ease.
7. Now, see your face. You are smiling. Your mood is wonderful as you realize you can handle any difficulties with grace and ease.
8. Look at your abdominal and lower back muscles. Your back is pliable, flexible, and has great muscle tone. Your abdomen is flat and free from bloat.
9. Look at your entire body and enjoy the sense of peace and calm running through your body. You feel wonderful.
10. Begin to withdraw from the visualization and return your focus to your breathing, inhaling and exhaling slowly.
11. Now open your eyes and luxuriate in the peace and relaxation.

Create Female Health With Positive Emotions

The philosopher Plato spent much time teaching his students that there was no healing of the body without simultaneous healing of the mind. Today we have psychoneuroimmunology, a fancy word for a field of study created in the 1970's to address the growing awareness in medicine that your physical, mental, emotional, and spiritual health are inextricably intertwined.

In modern times, thousands of studies have been done that give scientific validity to the age-old wisdom that what you do with your mind and emotions has a powerful effect on your health. This is why I advocate focusing your time, attention, and energy on those positive emotions that build you up and enhance the quality of your life and your life force instead of breaking you down and spiraling you down into ill health. These include prayer, love, gratitude, appreciation, laughter and happiness, optimism, a positive self-image, and generosity.

The Power of Prayer

Several years ago, my dear friend Lew discovered that he needed to have cataract surgery on both of his eyes. He met with several doctors in the San Francisco Bay area, but didn't feel comfortable with any of them. He shared his concerns with his mother, who had had cataract surgery in Florida. Not only was she thrilled with her results, but she felt that the doctor had a particularly comforting bedside manner.

Lew flew down to consult with surgeon Dr. James Gills. Dr. Gills explained that Lew would not need sutures, and that the cost of the surgery was less than half what the Bay area doctors wanted to charge. Lew scheduled himself for surgery immediately, but nothing had prepared him for the unique and tremendously comforting bedside manner that his mother had referred to.

When Lew arrived at Dr. Gills' clinic the morning of the surgery, they were met by a nurse who asked them if it was alright if she prayed with them before the surgery. Lew immediately agreed, and the two of them prayed for Lew to have a safe, uneventful surgery. Lew then went into the surgical suite, where Dr. Gills greeted him. From the moment he entered the suite—and throughout the entirety of his procedure—he was pleased to find that there was a tape recording of passages being read from the Bible.

Lew's surgery went extremely well. His post-surgical healing took place so quickly that he was literally astonished. He is convinced that the prayer and spirituality aspects of his doctor's care played a role in the great success of the procedure.

The role of prayer in the field of medicine has been hotly debated for centuries. Not only are there some who believe that medicine and spirituality should be separate, but many question the real, measurable effectiveness of prayer in healing. I firmly believe that spirituality absolutely has a role in medicine, and the evidence surrounding the power of prayer in healing is as clear as Lew's vision.

JANE'S STORY

Some years ago, my friend "Jane" came to me for help for severe fibroids. She had not been able to effectively shrink her tumors, and needed to have a hysterectomy. She asked me, as well as her friends and family, to pray for her before and during her surgery.

Jane later told me that when she was being taken to the operating room, she could feel the energy of the prayers and that she was strengthened and fortified by them. As a result, her surgery was uneventful and she healed wonderfully.

Research Confirms the Power of Prayer

Studies from around the world are proving the healing power of prayer. One study in particular looked at the cardiac care unit in San Francisco General Hospital. Researchers divided the unit of nearly 400 patients into two groups. The patients in the first group were prayed for and those in the second group were not. Researchers found that those people who had prayers said for them had less risk of congestive heart failure and cardiac arrest, and fewer of them needed diuretics and antibiotics, as compared to the group that was not prayed for.

Similarly, a group of 40 AIDS patients were divided into two groups—one that was prayed for 6 days a week for 10 weeks and one that was not prayed for at all. Again, researchers found that the prayed-for group did considerably better than the others. They had significantly fewer new AIDS-related illnesses, saw their physicians less often, and spent less time in the hospital.

In a study from of the *Journal of Reproductive Medicine*, researchers tested nearly 200 women who were undergoing in vitro fertilization at a clinic in Seoul, Korea. All were of similar age and had similar fertility concerns. They were divided into two groups. Several prayer groups from the U.S., Canada, and Australia were given photographs of the women in the first group and prayed for the women for four months. Neither the women nor the researchers knew who was being prayed for and who wasn't. At the end of the four months, twice as many women who were prayed for became pregnant as compared to the women in the control group.

In a similar double-blind, placebo-controlled study published in the *American Heart Journal,* researchers divided 150 heart patients (all of whom were scheduled for angioplasty) into five groups. One group received guided imagery therapy, the second had stress relaxation, the third had healing touch, the fourth were prayed for, and the last received no complementary therapy. Neither the patients, physicians, staff, nor family members knew which patients were being prayed for. After the procedures, those patients who were prayed for had fewer complications than patients in any of the other groups. Researchers were so amazed at the outcome that they have since enrolled over 300 more people for additional studies.

Today, more than half of the medical schools in the United States now offer courses in prayer and medicine. And according to a 1999 *USA Weekend* poll, more than 75 percent of adults believe that spirituality and prayer can help you recover from an illness or injury, with 56 percent of these same adults saying that they personally have been helped by faith and prayer. And when asked how they felt about having their doctor discuss spirituality, nearly two-thirds felt that it would be a good idea.

But given all this, the reality is that only 10 percent of physicians address spiritual beliefs and needs with their patients. I am proud to say that I am—and have always been—in the 10 percent of doctors that address the spiritual needs and concerns of their patients. As a physician, I have found that asking patients about their faith helps me understand any emotional and spiritual blocks that need to be cleared. I am also able to learn more about the patients' support network, which helps me to ensure that they have the type of care that will enable them to heal and resume living a full and vital life.

Blessings to You

I wrote these blessings for my newsletter subscribers and want to share a few with you.

- May love, kindness, and compassion fill your heart each day. May you recognize the light of God in everyone close to you and in everyone you encounter in life's journey. May love, kindness, and compassion soften and illuminate your heart, casting a warm glow on the world around you.
- During difficult times, you need to be able to draw upon your inner strength to help you successfully meet the challenges in your life. You need to rely on your inner reserves of courage and self-confidence to help you make the right choices and decisions. At the same time, you need to be flexible in your approach, willing to change course, and allow yourself to find new and even better solutions when confronted with road blocks or seemingly insurmountable obstacles.
- Remember that each day is a fresh beginning. Your life, your health, and your sense of well-being benefits immeasurably when you live each day joyfully, filled with the positive expectation of the many good things that flow to you. It is with this positive attitude that you align yourself with Divine light and love.

Love Lessons

At the deepest spiritual and emotional level, our purpose in life is to express our love and appreciation for ourselves, our family, friends, co-workers, and the entire world and all of God's creatures that we share this world with. Love has tremendous healing power. It is an emotion you should strive to feel within yourself and express to those around you as often as possible. There is no other emotion that is more immensely self-nurturing and self-healing.

As a physician, I have seen the healing power of love many times. I have always been touched by the great care and acts of helpfulness that many of my women patients show to their children, spouses, other family members, and friends when they're ill. It has always heartened me to see families gather together and support a loved one who is ailing.

I've also found that people tend to heal much faster and more completely when they're supported by love and caring. This is not just my own belief; many studies attest to the importance of love and positive relationships in creating health and wellness.

Conversely, feelings of fear, anxiety, loneliness, resentment, or other such emotions can have a tremendously negative impact upon one's health. I've seen intense negative emotions literally wreak havoc on patients' physical and chemical well being. Many patients I work with have themselves linked their poor immunity, menstrual disorders, digestive upset, high blood pressure, aching joints, and a host of other ailments to the negative and upsetting emotions they were feeling at the time. Many research studies also confirm the negative health effects that emotions like anger, depression, and loneliness cause. These studies find social isolation and lack of close relationships—the inability to connect with others in a loving way—also increases the likelihood of illness.

Follow Your Heart

Follow your heart in everything you do. It is important to make all of your choices out of love, kindness, and joy. These heartfelt emotions are just as important in making decisions about your life as the logical arguments and rationalizations generated by your mind. It is the love that is centered in your heart that responds to the deepest yearnings of your soul—enabling you to create a happy and meaningful life.

The crucial role your heart plays in creating your consciousness differs from the principles of conventional Western medicine, which greatly favors your brain. However, the ancient wisdom found in Eastern medicine deems the heart as the seat of the consciousness and the mind. Much fascinating medical and scientific research is now confirming this connection.

Love Meditations

These heart-felt, warm, loving meditations came to me from an angel whose love touched me deeply, and I want to share them with you. She is a nurturing mother who loves and cares for you and all her children. When you do these or any meditations, find a safe, quiet place where you can sit comfortably. Close your eyes, and let your arms rest easily at your side. As you take a deep breath, focus on the area of your heart (located just to the left of the center of your chest).

At One With Life

No matter where love comes from or how it manifests, dear one, it is important for you to remember who you are. You are the sweet aspect of God, in human form, in a human life. You are interconnected with all life. The trees send you their love by cleaning your air, you send them your love by breathing in their air. There is sweetness for you and the trees in every breath. You send the flowers your love by noticing them through sight, through smell, through touch, and even incorporating them into your physical being. Your love comes from life, life comes from your love. Send your love to every blade of grass, every bird, every tree, and every raindrop, and you will truly know God.

True Meaning of Love

You know when you have loved and when it has always been "I totally love you." You have loved your dearest friend this way, a beautiful garden, or your favorite pair of shoes. You have also loved other people this way as well. But true "love" is not about thinking; love is a sense of being. Love is who you are.

When you are being love, all your organs sing to you, all your organs love being part of you. This is the place where healing takes place. There is always in every molecule of love a piece of God, and there is no thinking or conditions or demands from and with God. There is only love.

Accepting Love

For most of your lifetime, dear one, the giving of love has been easier than the accepting of love. In human thought, love can be tied to vulnerability. And, in this sense, oh what a scary place it can be. Love itself cannot harm you. If it comes attached with conditions, requirements or demands, then it is not true love. Those are the human wanderings. Love is intention, it is opening up. It is relaxing into your own life, your relationships, and your world.

A Loving Visualization

I also want to share a visualization on love with you. It's perfect for those times when you feel too rushed, too busy, and too overwhelmed with your day-to-day tasks and responsibilities. It is meant to enhance and support your health and well being by giving you a few minutes to turn inward and get back in touch with yourself through self nurturance, healing any upsets you may have accumulated throughout the day. It will also help you reconnect with the healing power of love.

To do this visualization, find a quiet spot where you can sit or lie comfortably. As you take a deep breath, focus on the area of your heart (located just to the left of the center of your chest).

1. As you inhale and exhale slowly and deeply, close your eyes and envision your heart as a luminous, emerald-green jewel glowing with love and sending out brilliant light from behind your breastbone, where your heart resides.
2. Imagine you're filling your heart with love. Feel the area surrounding your heart soften and expand as you fill it with loving and peaceful energy.
3. As you continue to breathe in and out slowly and deeply, send love and appreciation to all of your family, friends, city, country, and entire Planet Earth.
4. Now gently open your eyes and slowly begin to move around again. Enjoy the feelings of love, peace, and gratitude you have created.

Embrace Gratitude and Appreciation

As a healer, I have been so impressed by how much feelings of gratitude and appreciation can greatly improve the health, well-being, and life quality of many of my patients over the years. These are positive qualities that I always strive to find in myself and express to everyone around me on a daily basis. However, I did not discover any real research that had been done in this area until the mid-1990's. At that time, I was serendipitously introduced to the innovative and groundbreaking work taking place at the Institute of HeartMath (IHM) in Boulder Creek, California.

Early one morning I received a call from DiagnosTech International, a laboratory in Seattle, that wanted to introduce me to their facilities and services. In the course of the conversation, they told me about very exciting research they were doing with the Institute. Specifically, laboratory testing was confirming that individuals who used techniques developed by the Institute to help them alleviate their feelings of anger and upset, and convert these emotions to feelings of gratitude and appreciation, were having dramatic improvements in several important chemical indicators of good health. From a medical perspective, these findings had amazing implications.

I was so intrigued by the work being done at the Institute that I called and requested their literature and research studies. After carefully reading their findings and conclusions, I was even more convinced of what I had been observing for years with myself and my patients—that there is a very strong, medically sound connection between positive emotions, such as gratitude, and good health.

The researchers at the IHM found that the heart plays a far more central role in stress, mental and emotional balance, and perception than previously thought. They found that the heart initiates most of the repetitious patterns within the body, and has a much more intricate communication pattern with the brain than does any other major organ. Plus, the heart not only responds to any stimulus the brain processes—from thoughts and emotions to light and sound—it also generates many times more electrical power than the brain. The signal is so strong that the current sent out by the heart radiates throughout the body. For all these reasons, the heart is in a unique position to connect the mind, body, and spirit.

To test this theory, researchers fed two groups of rabbits a diet that was high in fat. However, rabbits from the first group were held, petted, and talked to, while those in the other group were treated normally and were not shown any affection. They found that the rabbits that had been treated lovingly developed significantly less atherosclerosis than those rabbits that had not.

Based on this and other research, the IHM developed specific techniques to stop negative thoughts and convert them to positive feelings or emotions. By learning to generate feelings of sincere love, gratitude, and appreciation, a person's pulse, respiration, and brain wave frequencies are better able to synchronize.

In order to examine the health benefits of these techniques, the researchers then did a series of fascinating studies in which they taught these techniques to volunteers, then measured changes in various physical and chemical parameters. The results were very promising, as volunteers had more harmonious and efficient functioning of their cardiovascular, immune, and hormonal systems.

Most telling is that the people who have become adept at using these techniques have reported dramatic increases in the ability to solve problems and handle stresses such as conflicts on the job, rush hour traffic, and rebellious children.

The IHM found that appreciation can significantly increase your body's production of the steroid hormone DHEA. This is particularly exciting for women wanting to improve their hormonal health and balance. Researchers took DHEA samples from 28 volunteers, then asked them to listen to music specifically designed to promote a sense of peacefulness and emotional balance every day for one month. At the end of the month, researchers took a second DHEA sample from the volunteers. The results were impressive. Among all volunteers, DHEA levels increased, on average, 100 percent; for some, the levels tripled and even quadrupled. This is extremely important for female hormonal balance, since DHEA is converted by your body into estrogen and testosterone.

In addition, the researchers found that feelings of care and appreciation can boost levels of an immune antibody called IgA, which is an important part of your body's defense against bacteria and viruses. And while anger is known to suppress your immune system, they discovered that even remembering a previous angry experience had a negative, long-term impact on immune function.

Conventional Medicine Weighs In

Interestingly, the *American Journal of Cardiology* also featured a study that found that gratitude and appreciation might be positively associated with a reduction in blood pressure. However, it was several years before another mainstream medical journal would present additional support for the Institute of HeartMath's findings. In a study from the *Journal of Social and Clinical Psychology*, researchers divided volunteers into three groups. The first group kept a daily log of five complaints, the second group wrote down a daily list of five things they were better at/did better than their peers, and the third group kept a daily log of five things they were grateful for. After three weeks, those who kept the gratitude journal reported increased energy, less health complaints, and greater feelings of overall well-being as compared to the participants in the other two groups.

This finding was corroborated in the *Journal of Personality and Social Psychology* when researchers found that many of their subjects used gratitude as a positive way to cope with acute and chronic life stressors.

Express Your Gratitude

Journaling is a fantastic way to express your feelings of gratitude and appreciation. In her book *Simple Abundance*, author Sarah Ban Breathnach talks about a "gratitude journal." She recommends that you write down at least five things each day that you are thankful for, thereby forcing you to focus on what is going right in your life rather than what is going wrong. I couldn't agree with her more. Regardless of the type of journal you choose to keep, there are a few things to keep in mind:

- Select any kind of journal you want. Some women have used spiral notebooks, others a loose-leaf notebook, still others a gold-trimmed, bound book. What you choose is up to you.
- Make an appointment with yourself for fifteen minutes to half an hour each day to write.
- Choose a safe, calming location where you can write freely, without being disturbed.
- Do not censor yourself as you write – write down your emotions, good and bad. Once the thoughts and feelings are on paper, you can always throw them out if you choose to. The important thing is to get them out.
- Do not worry about punctuation or grammar.
- Finally, be free, be honest, be candid—be yourself!

Similarly, one of my favorite books is *The Art of Thank You: Crafting Notes of Gratitude* (Beyond Words Publishing, Inc.). This beautiful book suggests sending thank you notes as a way to show generosity, gratitude, and kindness to others. Why not show the same consideration to yourself? Why not start each day thanking and appreciating your body? Your soul? Your family and friends?

Write these positive thank yous and appreciative thoughts as affirmations in your journal, say them out loud in the privacy of your bedroom or office, or even visualize sending loving messages to your body each day. Over time, releasing more and more of your own toxic emotions and replacing them with kind and loving thoughts to yourself will help to diminish the load on your body, mind, and spirit. Then your body will begin to be filled with the most wonderful light, radiance, and health.

Love and Gratitude Meditation

This is a great meditation to do when you feel too rushed, too busy, and too overwhelmed with your day-to-day tasks and responsibilities. It will enhance and support your health and well being by giving you a few minutes to turn inward and get back in touch with yourself through self nurturance, healing any upsets you may have accumulated throughout the day. It will also help you reconnect with the healing power of love, forgiveness, and gratitude.

1. Find a quiet spot where you can sit or lie comfortably.
2. Close your eyes, and let your arms rest easily at your side. As you take a deep breath, focus on the area of your heart (located just to the left of the center of your chest).
3. As you slowly inhale and exhale, imagine you're filling your heart with love. Feel the area surrounding your heart soften and expand as you fill it with loving and peaceful energy.
4. Now, direct your breath into all of the parts of your body, starting with your feet and moving up through your body, finally into your head and neck. Notice any areas where you have stored any negative or upsetting emotions such as frustration, anger, or other feelings that make certain parts of your body feel tense, tight, heavy, or devitalized. Keep breathing love into those parts of your body until they, too, relax and soften. By the time you're done, you should feel much more quiet and peaceful.
5. Now visualize your love radiating out from you and touching everyone you love and care about. If you choose to, you can send your love and the spirit of healing to your community, to our country, and even the entire earth.
6. Now gently open your eyes and slowly begin to move around again. Enjoy the feelings of love, peace, and gratitude you have created.

Practice Forgiveness

In my practice, I've seen conditions as diverse as heart disease, high blood pressure, arthritis, inflammation, allergies, and immune disorders aggravated by frequent and constant feelings of anger. I've also seen unresolved and unexpressed anger contribute to menstrual problems and excessive weight gain.

In fact, several studies have also linked anger to neck and back aches, muscle tension, elevated homocysteine levels, and increased progression of coronary atherosclerosis. If you too suffer from unresolved anger and illnesses that can result from keeping it bottled up inside, then take heart. It is possible for you to release the offensive feelings and move forward with your life.

> ## CAROL'S STORY
>
> I was recently chatting with my friend "Carol," and she told me how amazed she was at how easily younger women, specifically her daughter and daughter-in-law, expressed their concerns, fears, annoyances, and anger. "It's not that they're confrontational," Carol clarified, "Just honest about how they feel." She also admitted that anger was the one emotion she was always afraid to express.
>
> Several decades ago, Carol's mother and aunt had a major disagreement. They didn't speak to one another for years, and never had the opportunity to reconcile before the aunt's death. Over time, Carol began to equate expressing anger or upset with a loss of love or friendship. As a result, she has held in any resentment or frustration she has felt toward those close to her rather than express her feelings to her family or friends.
>
> The irony is that the only one affected is Carol. While the people she is angry with go about their daily lives completely unaffected by Carol's hurt feelings, she suffers from worsening hot flashes, chronic headaches, digestive upset, and emotional paralysis. By learning to express her emotions, she was able to ease her physical symptoms.

Strange as it may sound, many women are hesitant to let go of their anger and resentment. Not only is it hard for many of us to forgive others, but it is difficult to forgive ourselves for our own personal faults and weaknesses. Frequently, anger becomes a comfortable, familiar barrier between you and disappointment or upset. But trust me when I tell you that the only way for good, positive changes to come into your life is for you to take action now to forgive the person who wronged you, forgive yourself, and move on.

Once you empower yourself to take charge of and responsibility for your emotional responses, the rewards will come pouring in. You may reconcile and heal relationships that have been tainted by resentment, anger, and pain. Marriages, families, and friendships that have been strained for years may improve. You could lose unwanted weight or lessen the frequency of debilitating headaches. But most importantly, your quality of life will drastically improve, providing you with greater peace, contentment, and optimism in your life and in your relationships.

If you have a problem dealing with or letting go of resentment, anger, and pain—and forgiving yourself and those you perceive as having hurt you—here are a few suggestions to help you start turning that pattern around quickly and effectively:

1. When you feel upset, learn to express your feelings quickly, in a way that allows you to find positive solutions to your grievances. This will help you to resolve situations that you may have felt stuck in for years, and regain more hope and joy in your life with all of your relationships. Then learn to focus on your appreciation of others, rather than on what angers or upsets you.

2. The most powerful antidotes to anger are the words "I forgive you," "I appreciate you," and "thank you." Learn to say and feel these words often to the people and situations in your life.

3. Look at the positive aspects of your life rather than feeling angry and resentful for what you feel you don't have or what you lack. This will also help you to heal long-standing hurts.

4. If your relationships with certain people or situations turn out to be unworkable and only trigger anger and upset rather than happiness or pleasure, consider gently and lovingly letting them go from your life rather than staying stuck in constant anger or upset.

Change the Anger to Appreciation

The following affirmations take about one minute to do, but can have lifelong benefits. Keep them nearby and repeat them any time you feel anger and resentment building up inside of you.

1. I enjoy focusing on and giving thanks for all of the many positive people and situations in my life.

2. When people or situations cause me to feel upset, I look for positive ways to deal with my grievances so that I feel pleased with the outcome.

3. I seek to deal with the upsets and challenges in my life with a sense of calm and peacefulness.

4. I communicate my feelings of anger and upset when necessary in a kind and thoughtful way that will do no harm to myself or others.

5. I let go of resentment and don't allow it to accumulate inside of me.

6. I enjoy finding new ways to make my life even more positive and joyful.

7. I forgive all of those people who have caused me to feel upset and angry in the past.

8. I forgive myself.

A Blessing for Appreciation

Each day, you should give appreciation to those you love and cherish. I recommend sharing the following words of gratitude:

- Thank you for being there for me.
- Thank you for caring.
- Thank you for listening to me during my times of need.
- Thank you for your kind touch.
- Thank you for your love.

Live for Laughter

I absolutely love to laugh. I think it's one of the most powerful and effective healing tools there are. There is no doubt that positive emotions like laughter and joy have tremendous health benefits—plus, they make your life more wondrous and enjoyable.

I've found that boosting your daily laughter is a great way to relax the tensions we are holding. That's why I developed the stress-to-laughter index. It comes from observing the stories my patients have shared with me over the years, as well as examining my own life and those of my friends and family. And what I've seen is that this index can really help you judge how effectively you are providing stress relief for yourself.

If you have too much heaviness, seriousness, responsibilities, worries, or concerns and not enough fun and laughter in your life, it's time to flip the scales in the other direction. I've seen thousands of cases of people getting flare-ups of illnesses, such as colds, flu, immune breakdowns, worsening of menopause symptoms, menstrual cramps, PMS, and painful arthritic episodes immediately following periods of too much stress and heaviness in their lives.

Often, just by flipping into a state of laughter and fun, you can help to bring yourself back into a state of optimal health. That's because your immune system functions better, your hormones are more likely to be in balance, and pain is reduced when you laugh and have fun, thanks to a whole cascade of positive chemicals within your body that are released during times of joy and fun.

To this point, I can distinctly remember a time I was working too much. I noticed that it began to have negative effects on my body. I was waking up in the morning feeling stiff, my neck was tense, and my muscles were tight. I also noticed that I wasn't digesting my food quite as well. In short, I was pushing myself to a place of too much stress. I quickly realized that it was time for me to give myself a big dose of laughter, fun, and pleasure to bring myself into healthy balance.

It just so happened that my daughter Rebecca was home from college, so we decided to go to our local toy store and have some fun. I felt this would be as wonderful an opportunity for her as it was for me. It was fun to propose that she and I do something together to play with our inner child. So, like two conspirators, we went to the toy store, pretending that the marbles, tops, and other toys we were buying were for children, when they really were for us!

We came home and laid our treasures out on the dining room table, then spent the entire evening playing with our toys and games. It was definitely the right antidote for me and helped me get back into balance and support my perspective about giving myself equal doses of seriousness and fun. I started to regain the balance, and noticed that when I laughed, my muscles immediately started to loosen up and feel better. The next morning, I woke up and felt much more refreshed, light, and energetic. I even found that I was digesting my food normally again. In short, laughter truly is the best medicine.

Mainstream Medicine Has a Sense of Humor

The healing power of laughter has been the subject of many, many studies. According to an article published in *Family Practice News*, children laugh, on average, about 400 times a day, while adults only laugh about 15 times a day. This is a sad state of affairs, because when laughter is your automatic response to stress, trying times are less likely to threaten your health and well-being.

Dr. Norman Cousins introduced this concept to medicine after he was diagnosed with a severe health condition called ankylosing spondylitis. He was determined to find a treatment for his disabling condition, and essentially cured himself by listening to recordings of laughter, watching lots of funny movies, and taking large doses of vitamin C.

More recently, research studies have provided scientific confirmation of this phenomenon. Laughter has been shown to lower the stress hormone cortisol, as well as blood pressure and heart rate, and to increase mood-elevating beta-endorphins—natural, feel-good chemicals produced by your body that are 200 times more potent than morphine.

And when it comes to smiles, it turns out they really are contagious. Researchers at the University of California at San Francisco determined that there are 19 different kinds of smiles, all of which are extremely contagious! In addition, Russian research has found that frequent smiling helps people heal from a host of degenerative diseases.

JEFFREY'S STORY

"Jeffrey" was a joyful, fun, amusing person. He was a successful businessman who was devoted to taking care of his health. However, the pressures of owning his own business had begun to take their toll. He developed insomnia, pain in his lower back, and high blood pressure.

He quickly went from being a happy-go-lucky, joyful person to being serious, grim, and overly-stressed. It was a surprise to see how much he changed with all that stress and lack of laughter, joy, and fun in his life. The last time I saw him at a social function, I had an ominous feeling in the pit of my stomach. The next day, I heard he suddenly passed away from a stroke. Again, this was a very disciplined man who followed a good supplement program, exercised, and ate well, but the stress and lack of fun and laughter cost him his life.

Jeffrey taught me an important lesson—if your stress-to-laughter quotient is tipped too far to the stress side, your health can seriously suffer. That's why I'm a huge proponent of getting as much laughter and fun into your life as you can, however you choose to do it.

Whatever your sense of humor calls for, indulge it. Go on a laughter odyssey and discover what tickles your funny bone. Whether you like to watch silly movies, read funny books, tell or listen to jokes, visit a comedy club, play games, or go to the toy store, I strongly recommend that you enjoy a little levity as often as possible. And always try to see the humor in the little frustrations and minor disasters that occur every day. It can greatly improve the quality of your life, and just might even save it!

Hold On to Happiness

Your state of health is very closely tied to how truly happy you are. A study on this important subject, published in the *Proceedings of the National Academy of Sciences*, found that people who consider themselves happy are more likely to be healthy and resistant to disease. They also have lower levels of the stress hormone cortisol and a reduced risk of heart disease. This study joins an ever-growing body of research that proves the importance of creating a life in which positive feelings of love, happiness, joy, and optimism predominate over negativity.

There is one particular study I love. Researchers studied the longevity of a group of 178 Catholic nuns from a convent in Milwaukee. The nuns lived together and taught in the same school. They had the same daily routine, ate the same food, didn't smoke or drink alcohol, had the same financial situation, and had identical medical care.

The researchers then looked at the writings each nun did prior to taking her vows. A separate team of psychologists then assessed the positive and negative comments made in the writings, and divided the sisters into different classifications based on the degree of joy and satisfaction in their letters.

The researchers then took these classifications and matched them against the life spans of each of the nuns. They found that 90 percent of those nuns who fell into the "most happy" category were still alive at 85 years old. Conversely, only 34 percent of those who were categorized as "least happy" lived to be 85.

Other studies have shown comparable results. A two-year study of 2,000 Mexican-Americans over the age of 65 found that the mortality rate of those people who expressed the most negative emotions was twice as high as those who expressed positive emotions. Similarly, a study from Finland discovered that of the 96,000 widowed people surveyed, the surviving spouse's risk of dying doubled in the week following their spouse's death.

What Happy People Do

In her book *The 15-Minute Miracle*, Jacquelyn Aldana (see page 475) has a wonderful list of attributes for truly happy people. She has generously allowed me to share the list with you. If you don't recognize yourself in at least three or four, aim to practice these principles so you can become "One of the Happiest People You Know."

1. They look for the good in life, *regardless* of prevailing circumstances.
2. They appreciate what they *already* have before asking for anything else.
3. They have a genuine sense of self-worth and look for the good in others.
4. They allow themselves to feel all of their feelings so they can choose which ones to keep and which ones to release.
5. They view life through the eyes of awe and wonder like a small child who knows beyond a shadow of a doubt that all things are truly possible.
6. They find something to love and admire about everything—and everyone—in every moment. They find creative ways to fall in love with Life, and everything in it—including themselves.
7. They embrace ALL aspects of life because they understand that contrast is an extremely valuable tool. By briefly acknowledging what they don't want, they can more easily identify what they prefer instead. Contrast creates clarity.
8. They totally release and let go things that no longer serve them, things like resistance, resentment, anger, rage, negative judgment, criticism, guilt, blame, shame, fear, depression, attachment to outcomes, etc. When you release and let go of these emotional burdens, they quickly release and let go of YOU!
9. They hold the space for themselves and others to regain their balance in just the perfect time in ways that bless and benefit everyone. This is one of the most loving and supportive things you can do for yourself or anyone else.
10. They love others, even when others are less than loving toward them. When other people do something that could be considered offensive, they just say to themselves, "That's just him (or her) not knowing a better way at this time. If he (or she) *could* do better, he (or she) certainly *would* do better." This concept is what we call "unconditional love at its very best."

Accentuate the Positive

I'm sure you've heard the expression "do unto others as you would have them do unto you." I think this is a wonderful credo to live by. Unfortunately, in my experience, many women seem to have an easier time with "unto others" than with "unto yourself."

So often I hear women say things about themselves, their bodies, and even their talents, which seem to be self-denigrating. We are constantly criticizing ourselves for not being good enough, smart enough, beautiful enough, or thin enough. My women friends are always jokingly offering to give each other transplants of their most disliked body parts—usually the breasts, behinds, and stomachs—which they often feel are too large.

I've had to work on myself for a very long time to make sure I don't do this. I try to stop any self-denigrating thoughts when they start to come up. But it makes me wonder why this trait is so common among women, and what, if anything, we can do to treat ourselves in a more accepting, caring, and nurturing way.

Much of this stems from childhood, when women are often programmed for self-criticism by hearing their own mothers' subtle (or not so subtle) messages of feeling somehow unworthy in their own lives—no matter how accomplished we or our mothers actually are. This is how deeply negative programming can reach!

Add to this society's impossible standards regarding how a woman should look—rail-thin, with flawless skin and perfectly coiffed hair—and it should come as no surprise that most women are in a constant self-dialogue of criticism and scorn.

Stop the Madness

When this type of negative self-talk becomes the norm rather than the exception, it can become downright abusive. I'm not referring to physical abuse, but a tendency for a woman to turn emotional violence on herself. Before you wave this off as something that doesn't apply to you, ask yourself these questions:

1. Do you set impossibly high standards for yourself?
2. Do you have higher expectations of yourself than of others?
3. Do you see a friend as "pleasantly plump," but yourself as obese?
4. Do you fixate on a particular aspect of your appearance that most people probably don't even notice?
5. Do you find that if a friend or loved one makes a mistake, or does something hurtful or unwise, you have compassion for her, but if you do some thing similar, you think of yourself as "stupid," "a loser," or a "failure"?

If you can take an objective look in the mirror and admit that you are harder on yourself than you are on anybody else in your life, then you are at an emotional fork in the road. And there's more at stake than your self-esteem. In fact, the path you choose may determine your *physical* health.

Research has repeatedly linked self esteem to physical and emotional well being. According to a study published in the *Journal of Aging and Health*, positive psychological states and self image were actually protective against health problems in older adults. Similarly, research from the *Journal of the American Medical Association* found that negative emotions, such as self-criticism, can cause a reduction in blood flow to the heart. And, a study in the *British Journal of Psychiatry* found a higher risk of depression in women with a negative self image.

Start Loving Yourself

For optimal mind and hormone health, it's important that you send positive messages to your body that reinforce your sense of self worth and self love. Try to put to rest any emotional issues you have that are chronic and self-destructive in nature, such as self-criticism and setting yourself up for a lifetime of failures by setting standards that no woman could possibly achieve.

The trouble is most women have tried to live up to unrealistic expectations for so long that the concept of self-deprecation has become deeply ingrained in their minds. As a result, even when you intellectually understand that you need to stop being so hard on yourself, in many cases you find that you simply *can't* stop. The habit of putting yourself down is so embedded in your mind that the self-destructive thought processes and behaviors have become an involuntary reflex.

My colleague "Stacey" is a good example. Stacey is a highly accomplished and success-ful woman. She has an Ivy League doctoral degree, seven published books, hundreds of magazine and scholarly journal articles to her credit, and has been happily married for more than 30 years. She also has a negative and sad secret: *She believes she's unworthy and not good enough.* She thinks she's the only one who knows, and she works hard to keep it that way. If someone asks her a question, she diligently researches the answer rather than admitting she doesn't know. If she makes a mistake, everything she's ever done right pales in comparison. If someone criticizes her, she can't get it out of her mind.

Contrast Stacey with "Rachel," the mother of one of my college friends. When you were around Rachel, she made you think she was absolutely the most beautiful woman in the world. However, she wasn't particularly attractive in a conventional sense. In fact, some people might have considered her dowdy and plain.

A wise and perceptive woman who was a close friend of the family told me a bit about Rachel's background. She grew up poor, with parents who had very little education. Yet she was an extremely accomplished woman in both her professional and personal life. She had several advanced academic degrees, a high-powered career, and a husband, family, and friends who adored her. Most fascinating to me, however, was the sheer joy she took in her-self and everyone around her. It was infectious, and she made us all feel good when we were in her presence. Her secret? According to the family friend, Rachel's parents had told her from day one how beautiful, capable, and intelligent she was, and how she could achieve anything she wanted. It was a wonderful, positive programming that imprinted Rachel in the deepest way.

As these two stories show, the key to loving yourself is to reprogram your mind with a new reflex. To do this, you need to redefine your circle of loved ones to include one very spe-cial, important, and hard working person—YOU!

Self-Loving Affirmations

Here are a few of the affirmations I use for loving and honoring myself. I like to say them at least once a day. I encourage you to use them to enhance your feelings of self-love and value.

To begin, place your hands in prayer position over your heart. Close your eyes and fill you mind with the most beautiful, peaceful image you can.

Repeat the affirmations five times each. When you feel emotion welling up in your eyes, you'll know that the message got in.

1. I honor and love myself.
2. I am enough.
3. I treat myself with kindness, gentleness, and nurturing.
4. I am worthy.
5. The Divine light of God protects and nurtures me in every way.
6. Every day, I fill myself with feelings of love for God, my friends and family, and all people and creatures on Earth.
7. Kindness and compassion for myself softens and illuminates my heart, casting a warm glow on the world around me.
8. I recognize the light of God in myself, those close to me, and in everyone I encounter on my life journey.
9. I rely on my inner reserves of courage and self-confidence to help make the right choices and decisions.
10. My heart is filled with appreciation and gratitude for all of the blessings that have been bestowed upon me.

Self-Love Visualization

This wonderful visualization allows you to get in touch with the fact that you are loved, nurtured and intertwined with Mother Earth. You are part of the planet and are loved by the trees, oceans, and air around you. Feel the love from the earth nurturing you and use that love to help love and nurture yourself as Mother Earth loves you.

1. Picture yourself at the beach, barefoot in the warm sand. Just before you get into the warm Caribbean water, you hear and see the waves, you hear and feel the rhythm of Mother Earth. You are content and at peace with yourself, your life, your universe.
2. Feel the warm loving embrace of Mother Earth. Smell the ocean breeze, breathe it into your lungs. You're fully immersed in the love of Mother Earth.
3. Now picture yourself floating there by moonlight. You feel the sweet embrace of the moon, as well as Mother Earth and the beautiful Caribbean sea. The water surrounding you flows gently and warmly, just like the water within you flows gently and warmly. There's no part of you that is not loved every single day. Your heart beats lovingly for you every single day. The beating of your heart creates the rhythms inside of your body lovingly. Just like the moon creates the rhythms of all the flows of all the waters in dear Mother Earth, in her

oceans, her rivers, inside the blood of the animals, the people. You are enveloped in your heart floating there by the moon in the warm Caribbean Sea.

4. Whenever your life feels unkind or doesn't flow smoothly, remember floating in the warm Caribbean Sea, soothed during the day by the sweet sun, soothed at night by the sweet moon. Nurture yourself as the sea nurtures you, fully supportive without conditions, just enveloping and supporting you in all aspects of you. If you need to call on this beautiful Caribbean Sea, in all its turquoise splendor, to support you in any and all aspects of you and the life you have chosen, and even the parts of life you have not chosen, the warmth and buoyancy and the sweetness of this sea supports you fully.

The Gift of Giving

Generosity is a quality that comes naturally when you feel that your own needs are met and you can pass the overflow onto others. An act of generosity implies trust that there is enough to go around, as well as confidence in your own inner emotional abundance. But if demands become overwhelming—which they are bound to do from time to time—your "helper's high" can turn into "just plain tired out," complete with all of the harmful stress hormones that accompany it.

When you hold on tightly to what you have, there's no room left for more to come in. On the other hand, if you give away everything, you can't take care of yourself, let alone take care of others. That's when it's time to be generous with yourself, even if it's just to pause and take a few deep breaths.

You'll find that this give-and-take applies to every aspect of sharing and caring. The most valuable coin in the realm of generosity is the one that's spent wisely. And at any point in time, you choose how you will spend yours.

My friend "Lisa" is a great example of knowing how and when to spend your generosity coins. As you'll see, just withholding a negative comment can be one of the greatest acts of generosity. Lisa stopped at the local restaurant on her way home from work to pick up dinner for her family. She was feeling guilty about feeding them fast food for the third time that week, she was running late, her husband was due at a meeting in an hour, and she'd had a particularly hard day. When she arrived at the counter, the young girl who was supposed to be taking her order was chatting on her cell phone. Lisa could tell that the girl had seen her out of the corner of her eye, but she just kept on talking. Finally, after what seemed like an eternity later, she hung up, turned to Lisa and said, "What can I get you?"

At this point, Lisa was so angry that she wanted to verbally assault the girl, but she realized that she had a window of opportunity to make a choice: She could fire off a sarcastic comment, or she could shift into neutral. She also knew that if she verbalized her self-righteous anger, it would take everything up a click, physically and emotionally, and unleash a flood of stress hormones into her system. She realized that her blood pressure was already too high, her stomach was in a knot, and she didn't need her headache to get worse. She also knew that she'd feel bad about losing her temper later on. As soon as she acknowledged that there was nothing in it for her or the young girl, she took a deep breath and placed her order. By the time she left with her food, she was feeling much better about herself and the world in general.

Lisa's response was generous to both herself and the girl taking the order. It was generous to be understanding and not to strike out verbally. It was generous to spare herself the consequences of a flood of stress hormones and remorse. And it was generous to her family not to bring home dinner with a side order of anger and resentment energetically contaminating the food. Instead, she made a positive offering of love and gratitude to the food for her family and herself.

The Research Tells the Story

Harvard researchers have studied the effects of altruism by taking before-and-after measurements of immune system markers in the saliva of volunteers who watched three films: the first on gardening, the second about the Nazis, and the third about Mother Teresa. There was no change in immune markers before or after the first two films, but after the third one, a marker for improved immune function rose dramatically. In other words, just watching someone else be generous is good for your health.

In another landmark study, a researcher from the University of Michigan followed 2,700 people for more than a decade to determine how their social relationships affected their health. He found that more than any other activity, doing volunteer work improved health and increased life expectancy.

Psychologists Allan Luks and Howard Andrews collected surveys from more than 3,000 student volunteers and found that their "helper's high" was followed by a second stage they called the "healthy-helper syndrome." They defined this stage as "a longer-lasting sense of calm and heightened emotional well-being…that is a powerful antidote to stress, a key to happiness and optimism, and a way to combat feelings of helplessness and depression."

You Get What You Give

Generosity has a ripple effect—it's contagious. When you give to someone else, they're more likely to give to others. Small acts of generosity, those practiced during your mundane, day-to-day life, have a more far-reaching impact than you could ever imagine. When you wave someone in ahead of you during rush hour traffic, the feel-good endorphins you just created for yourself and someone else will be passed on, possibly to hundreds or even thousands of others. If you could actually follow the ripple effects of your acts of generosity, you would see that they go on forever. In essence, you've just thrown your coin into the cosmic river of life!

Five Exceptional Healers

When it comes to relaxation, stress reduction, and meditation, there are five women that stand out above the rest—Linda Eastburn, Jacquelyn Aldana, Brooke Baggett, Evelyn Oliver, and Artemas Yaffe.

Linda Eastburn

My friend and colleague Linda Eastburn is a renowned medical intuitive. Her book, *Riding the Intuitive Wave: Learn to Listen to What Your Body Already Knows* (Endue Publishing, Springfield, MO) is one of my personal favorites. In it, she explains that it takes time, patience, and practice to develop your intuition. But once you do, you will discover hidden talents, your true self, and experience the healing miracles that you've been waiting for your entire life.

Linda often lectures at universities and conferences, and has even founded the International Academy of Intuitive Arts, a distant learning school, as well as IntuitiveCare, a line of holistic professional courses, many of which are accredited for continuing education. Additionally, she is frequently featured guest on radio and television programs all over the world. Plus, her own radio and television program, *Anomalies*, was also broadcast worldwide.

Recently, Linda and I were talking about the rise in the incidence of breast cancer. In her opinion, breasts related to the nurturing aspects of life. When a woman is not feeling nurtured, either by herself or those around her, the breasts tend to become more susceptible to disease. She then proceeded to tell me about two female clients of hers that exemplified this theory. I'd like to share their stories with you.

Mindy's Story

"Mindy" was 11 when her parents split up. While she was close to her father, a kind and loving man, Mindy lived with her mother, who clearly resented raising two children on her own. Throughout her childhood and even into adulthood, Mindy's mother was not able to show her love. Not surprisingly, Mindy went on to marry an unaffectionate man.

When Mindy learned she had breast cancer, she was left to deal with the disease as she had dealt with everything in her life—alone. As a result, she sought a more spiritual understanding of her disease. Linda worked with Mindy to intuitively and energetically understand what it was Mindy needed. Mindy soon reached within herself and out to her friends and found the emotional and nurturing support that had been missing throughout her life.

Carrie's Story

"Carrie" lost both of her parents at a very early age, and was raised by an aunt that didn't seem to want a child. As a result, Carrie frequently felt lost, unloved, and unwanted. Determined to overcome this, she married and had two children of her own. She nurtured them and allowed them to nurture her in return.

However, she became quite dependent on the love and interaction she had with her children. When they left home, Carrie resorted back to her old feelings of fear and loneliness. Shortly thereafter, she too developed breast cancer.

I was quite taken with these stories. I've always believed and seen in my patients how the heart chakra is so deeply tied to love, nurturing, and breast health. It was such a pleasure to be able to talk about these experiences with a colleague, and share thoughts on how to educate women about these types of connections. After several of these types of conversations, Linda and I decided to produce a series of CDs together to help women heal hormones and other health issues.

For information about these CDs, you can visit *www.DrLarksHormoneRevolution.com*. To learn more about Linda and her classes, log on to *www.intuitiveacademy.com*. For a private consultation with Linda, you can call 417-863-1377.

Jacquelyn Aldana

My dear friend Jacquelyn Aldana is the author of *The 15-Minute Miracle*™. Several years ago, she experienced what she calls "the lowest ebb of her entire life." Her husband was dying of Stage IV non-Hodgkins lymphoma, her marriage was on the rocks, and her business was nearly bankrupt.

She cried out to the heavens for help and demanded to either "be shown a way to experience joy" or to be put out of her misery. She then wrote down everything she desired for herself and her life. Shortly thereafter, a series of positive shifts occurred that completely transformed her life. Her husband beat his cancer, their marriage was the best it had ever been, and her business began to generate more revenue than she'd seen in 20 years.

She attributes this amazing turnaround to a simple technique she calls *The 15-Minute Miracle*™. This easy, fill-in-the-blanks journaling process allows you to accomplish your goals and realize your dreams by raising your vibrational frequency, making you an irresistible magnet for miracles! It takes only 15 minutes, and works wonders for most anyone who merely experiments with it. Results are typically so dramatic and life-changing that many people refer to their experiences as "miracles." In fact, thousands of people all over the world have used the technique to dramatically improve their health, relationships, and overall quality of life.

There are two stories in particular of women who have used Jacquelyn's program very effectively that I'd like to share with you. The first is about Cheri. Cheri was an estrogen dominant type. She had been a self-proclaimed "self-help junkie," flitting from counseling to seminars to books and workshops for more than 30 years. However, nothing brought her the promise or purpose she was looking for. After attending one of Jacquelyn's weekend workshops, Cheri's entire life turned around "at the speed of thought." Her 15-year struggle with acne rosacea completely disappeared, as did her negative self-image. She set all-time high records in her business, and experienced incredibly high levels of energy and enthusiasm. She even met the man with all of the positive qualities that she had been dreaming about.

The other story is about Janette, an estrogen deficient-fast processor type who was in significant physical and financial pain. She had terrible arthritis in her knees and had a job she didn't like. After learning about *The 15-Minute Miracle*™ and practicing it in her life, Janette began to experience greater energy, more motivation, and even improved flexibility. It was the change in her health that particularly astounded her. Today, Janette runs her own very successful business and enjoys a virtually pain-free life.

Jacquelyn's approach works on the level of the Law of Attraction, which maintains that "What you think about is what you bring about," and "What you fill your mind with your life is full of." Therefore, say it or believe it, and it will be so. If you say, "I can do this," you will be right. Conversely, if you say, "I cannot accomplish this," you will also be right. By staying focused on what you desire to experience, and by communicating with positive words and actions, you can unlock the secret to your life's limitless potential.

I love Jacquelyn's story and technique for so many reasons, but mostly because it demonstrates how, at the highest spiritual level, ill health and disease tend to occur, in part, when you lose your inner light and become energetically filled with the darkness of stress, unhappiness, and upset.

To release this darkness and rediscover your Divine Light, try this wonderful meditation excerpted from Jacquelyn's book:

"Imagine yourself as a beautiful, long-stemmed glass filled with sparkling *crystal clear water* from the *purest source* in the Universe… The pristine water in the glass represents *YOU* when you are in the *flow* of Life, appreciating even the smallest of things—*YOU* when you are *happy* and *grateful* for what you *already* have, while looking forward to even *more* wonderful things.

"If you are like most people, however, you probably experience times that are less than ideal. Allowing yourself to become negatively focused for very long is equivalent to putting a drop of *black ink* into your glass. If you keep looking at what's *not working*, what you *don't like*, and what you want to *get rid of*, your pure glass of water will soon become quite *murky*. You are likely to become *discouraged* and *overwhelmed* trying to find ways to extract all those yucky black molecules out of the water… Where do you start?

"The answer is so simple… Instead of struggling to remove the darkness, simply *reconnect* with your Divine Source. Just place your glass under the faucet of *love* and *light* and allow the pure magnificence of *life* to fill your glass to overflowing, thereby completely *displacing* the darkness of negativity and *replacing* it with the light of life… Choosing to focus upon feelings of *love, joy*, and *appreciation* is like inviting the Red Sea to part, thereby making it *possible* for you to reach that long-awaited 'shore of fulfillment.' "

You can learn more about Jacquelyn and *The 15-Minute Miracle*™ by visiting her Web site at *www.15MinuteMiracle.com* or calling 408-353-2050.

Brooke Baggett

Another amazing healer that I am fortunate to call a very good and close friend is Brooke Baggett. Not only is she an accomplished Reiki Master healer and acupuncturist, but she is also a BodyTalk practitioner.

The main premise of BodyTalk is that the body can heal itself. It is a way of tapping into the body's communication system to assess whether any of the lines are down—which can hinder healing from an illness or an injury. It is based on the fact that every living thing is made of energy. When that energy is properly tuned and there are no blockages to its flow, then direct and efficient communication runs freely within your body—between one organ system and another, and between your body, mind, and spirit. It's only when all the lines of communication are fully open that everything can function together for optimal health.

BodyTalk practitioners communicate with the body by using neuromuscular biofeedback, or muscle testing, which allows the practitioner to have a dialogue with the innate wisdom of each individual's body. Communication is reestablished between the various parts of the body by tapping specific points over the head and heart to recreate the healthy energetic linkages.

The key to the BodyTalk system is *order*. Every cell within your body, every spark of emotion, every belief system, every one of your thought processes—all these things must be able to communicate together in an orderly fashion, so your body can coordinate the billions of bioelectrical, chemical, and energetic events that support life.

When something goes wrong, this rapid-fire internal dialogue allows the body's own wisdom to determine the order in which repairs should be made, and then directs the body's energy to heal the trouble spots in the most efficient manner. For example, your body may not want to detoxify its overly burdened liver *until* the digestive problem in the small intestine is healed—otherwise, toxins liberated from the liver can flood into the small intestine and be rapidly absorbed by the body through its raw, unhealed lining. This cart-before-the-horse type of treatment is typical of many medical approaches, and it can create what is often referred to as a "healing crisis." Conversely, the BodyTalk system taps into your inner wisdom to find out where the problem is and which lines need to be re-linked—helping your body heal itself quickly, efficiently, and completely.

Brooke has since integrated BodyTalk into her practice with great success. She has found BodyTalk to be very helpful for a variety of health issues—including hormonal and reproductive disorders, asthma, allergies, chronic fatigue, infections, digestive disorders, Parkinson's disease, anxiety, depression, learning disorders, back pain, and arthritis.

Mary's Story

Brooke told me about one case in particular that was simply incredible. "Mary" was a 42-year-old woman who exercised daily, ate healthfully, and seemed quite emotionally balanced. However, she had daily migraines that were so severe she needed to take prescription medication.

Brooke started Mary on a regimen of weekly acupuncture treatments, which temporarily alleviated the migraine pain. However, she reached a point where there was no more relief, and she was still suffering and taking her medication a few times a week.

That's when Brooke suggested BodyTalk. Mary agreed, and what transpired was nothing short of miraculous. Brooke discovered that Mary had imbalances relating to Mary as a 12-year-old girl, grief, home and family, and maple and pine trees. After a bout of tears, Mary told Brooke that she had lost her mother when she was 12. Her mother had died from brain cancer, which at the time the doctors were treating as migraines. During her grieving process, she spent much time among the maples and pines near her home.

Several days later, Brooke checked in with Mary and was thrilled to hear that she hadn't experienced any more migraine pain. The same was true a few weeks later.

Bonnie's Story

Another amazing story involves "Bonnie," a career woman with two children. Bonnie held a prominent position in her company, which required travel as well as public presentations in front of large groups of people. Her main reason for coming to Brooke's office was to reduce her anxiety issues, which she had experienced for most of her life. Compounding her anxiety was her fatigue, which was due, in large part, to her youngest child "Katie," who would wake in the middle of the night screaming in terror.

After just a few sessions, Bonnie had a major lecture out of the country, and it was preceded with unmatched ease. She was so pleased with the veritable disappearance of her anxiety that she decided Brooke should also begin to work with Katie.

Katie was a delightful baby with a gentle disposition. However, in the middle of the night, after several hours of sweet dreams, Katie would wake up screaming. Bonnie could not find any rhyme or reason for Katie's sudden shrieks.

What came up through Katie was incredible. The first thing Brooke looked at was Katie's prenatal life, the three months between fall and winter. It seemed that there was a lot of anxiety in Bonnie's life during her pregnancy with Katie that caused Bonnie to wake every night in terror during those three months.

We are all aware of the gift of connectedness between a mother and child, however, that connection begins long before birth, as this session demonstrated. Bonnie's anxiety transferred onto the baby and revealed itself in the baby's first life experience in the interim between fall and winter.

Just as her mother had done, Katie would wake up in terror every night screaming for her mother's comfort. Bonnie was amazed to learn that the source of Katie's distress was found with such ease and effectiveness in just one session. Bonnie now reports that Katie sleeps soundly and happily.

Using BodyTalk

I find the BodyTalk System to be exciting because not only is it completely safe, but some people see dramatic results in as little as one session. It can be used as a stand-alone treatment, or to enhance the effectiveness of other therapies. In addition to its ability to affect physical, emotional, and spiritual healing, I particularly like the fact that this healing modality is respectful of the body's wisdom.

If you're interested in trying BodyTalk and would like to find a qualified practitioner near you, visit *www.bodytalksystem.com*. If you want to contact Brooke Baggett directly, log on to *www.mosaichealingarts.com* or call 408-202-3444. You can opt to work with Brooke either in person or remotely via telephone.

Evelyn Oliver, PhD

I've known and loved Eve since she was the Director of Counseling Services at my clinic nearly 30 years ago. To call Eve a medical intuitive is only half the story. She does a transformative type of therapy that is unbelievably effective and powerful. Her work allows you to create the life of your dreams and get beyond whatever blocks (physical, emotional, and spiritual) you may still be struggling with despite years of conventional counseling.

Eve is widely recognized as one of the premier Medical Intuitives in the U.S. As such, she is frequently interviewed on radio and television. She does telephone consultations from as far away as Australia, Columbia, England, and Russia. Famous names in Hollywood, as well as infamous criminals, have been among her clientele.

Along with her husband Prof. James Lewis, Eve has co-authored two books: *The Dream Encyclopedia*, and *Angels A to Z*, She is also the author of *Dream Yourself Awake*. In recent years Eve has been lecturing on "Energy Medicine in Healing," "How the Brain Works in Conversation," and "Human Energy Field & Auric Cleansing" at the University of Wisconsin. While residing in California, she lectured at the Stanford University Medical School, Division of Family Practice on how to utilize intuition in the emergency room and other crisis situations.

Amazing Cases

More amazing than the details of Eve's career are the stories from the people she has helped. There are more testimonials than I could possibly include, so I chose only two that I found particularly profound to share with you:

Kit's Story

"Kit" grew up in a chaotic and emotionally stressful home with two alcoholic parents. She had vivid memories of experiencing gross sexual imposition during her adolescent years. At different crisis points, she had participated in individual and group therapy, and had directed some healing on her own when therapy reached a plateau. Even with the remarkable progress she had made from a panicky, reactive, insecure girl who could not adequately manage even low levels of stress to a highly functioning, independent woman, there remained a core of pain and anger that was outside her consciousness, but continued to create difficulties in her personal and working relationships.

When Eve worked with Kit, she was able to non-intrusively pinpoint the damaging link between the emotions and cognitions underlying Kit's pain and anger in a loving, safe, and creative manner, and to introduce an alternative healthy link garnered from Kit's own goals and dreams for her life. Literally, in a matter of minutes, Kit felt instant relief, emotionally and physically. Her physical symptoms, which had been worsening and had been unsuccessfully treated by medical doctors, were unexpectedly alleviated as well.

Months later, the emotional and physical relief allowed her to approach the many challenging circumstances in her life in a more appropriate, focused, and optimistic frame of mind. This, in turn, generated further change in her ability to think clearly, trust her own intuition, and act with purpose.

Julie's Story

"Julie's" life was falling apart around her. She had difficulty communicating. As a result, her marriage, finances, and career were suffering. She also battled depression and substance abuse for years, including the prescriptions her medical doctor gave her to muffle her emotional pain. At the time, that sounded like the perfect fix. Julie had been to psychiatrists and marriage counselors, but talking didn't seem to help. She walked into their offices expecting them to read her mind and tell her how to fix her problems.

The reality was Julie was desperately missing happiness and joy in her life. Her self-esteem was low, and she sensed a complete lack of spirituality. Her first conversation with Eve was the beginning of the most amazing transformation in her life. When she spoke with Eve for the first time, she felt like she was talking with her best friend who knew everything about her. One of the things that went right to her heart was when Eve told her that Julie didn't want to be a mother right now, and that it was okay. It wasn't that Julie didn't love her children; in fact, she loved them very much. She was simply afraid she was going to ruin their lives and have them grow up to be like her—miserable, lonely, and depressed. Julie quickly realized she needed to start taking better care of herself.

With Eve's guidance, Julie was able to find the right direction. Her internal map now leads anywhere her heart desires. Today, Julie can honestly say she loves herself. For the first time in her life, she is secure with who she is. Julie says she has reclaimed her power and is more meaningfully in touch with her life since her four sessions with Eve.

In addition to dozens of wonderful testimonials like the two you just read, many psychologists and therapists have also written glowing letters about new and insightful directions Eve has offered in support of their work with patients. Over the past thirty-five years I have seen Eve assist people from all walks of life, with their business concerns as well as their personal issues.

Eve has an uncanny ability to accurately intuit the underlying cause of an individual's issue. She is a real detective in this way.

She described to me how reverently she honors the issues people want to be rid of because holding on to such issues is a strategy for protecting themselves from experiencing more of the same kind of pain. Eve says, "A client is ready for my work when the pain to remain the same has become greater than the pain to change."

Eve's work is deep and swift. She says, "I like to work as fast as my client will allow to accomplish what 'they' want, the way 'they' want it—not the way I or anyone else thinks it should be."

Contact Eve

Dr. Oliver's clients have created a description of her life-changing work: "Hit the Nail on the Head; Strategies to Fix & Repair Your Life." Eve's telephone number is 715-343-6171 or you can e-mail her at *docoliver@charter.net*.

Artemas Yaffe

Artemas is a dear friend and one of the most empathetic medical intuitives I have ever met. A gifted healer, Artemas has an extremely well-developed Third Eye, and has an unusual ability to "see" her clients' problems, even when the issue is unclear to them.

After earning a Medical Science degree in respiratory therapy, as well as many years of experience as a certified therapist in the intensive care unit, critical care unit, emergency room, and neo-natal unit, led Artemas to realize that she was meant to work personally with individuals, healing their negative beliefs, emotions, body chemistry, relationships, and family patterns, as well as clearing present and past life traumas.

Artemas trained under teachers globally in bodywork, pranic and psychic healing, meditation, bio-energy balancing, acupressure, cranial sacral therapy, counseling in death and dying, medical intuitive scanning, Zero Balancing, color therapy, gem healing, and many other modalities.

By combining all of these healing modalities into her own unique form of therapy, Artemas is able to gently, lovingly, and tenderly help her clients transform disease into health through spiritual and emotional growth. When this occurs, physical and spiritual flowering emerges, and clients' lives turn around, opening the door for health and joy.

Artemas also works with patterned energies within the body. Checking these energies allows her to find and heal hormones, organs, and systems that are unhealthy, blocked, or devoid of normal patterns. By clearing these types of latent distortions within physical, emotional, mental, or spiritual bodies, she allows internal and external harmony to manifest.

Artemas uses her inner knowing to locate and heal these types of core issues. One great example of this gift is "Cathy," a young mother with a three-month-old daughter who screamed whenever she saw a doctor. Through muscle testing, Artemas found that the infant's reaction was due to an event that had occurred when Cathy was four months pregnant. Cathy had forgotten to tell Artemas that she had an emergency appendectomy at that time. Since the womb is thin, her then pre-natal infant witnessed the doctors cutting through Cathy and thought they both were being attacked! By offering healing energies to both the infant and womb space, Artemas was able to clear the problem. Today, Cathy's daughter no longer screams when she sees a physician.

If you would like to set up an appointment with Artemas, give her a call at 650-365-3248.

FREE TELECONFERENCES
I am pleased to tell you that I will be offering free, periodic teleconferencing with colleagues such as Brooke, Jacquelyn, Linda, Eve, and Artemas. These meditation support groups are designed to lead women in many of these exercises to support hormone and overall health. Visit *www.DrLarksHormoneRevolution.com* for days and times, and additional information.

---

* * *

As you can see, stress really throws your hormones out of balance. But, with the right mindset, a willingness to slow down, and a loving, appreciative attitude towards yourself, others, and life in general, you can diffuse stress, redirect your energy, change your reactions to the upsets and frustrations of daily life, and restore your healthy balance to create a life that is extremely and consistently happy and fulfilling.

Throughout this chapter, you've discovered many different ways to reset your mind and body to help your hormones and health stay balanced and healthy. I suggest trying all of the ones that appeal to you at least once. When you find the one, two, or more that work best for you, be sure to practice them every day.

I've found that the more time you spend practicing stress reduction and the more frequently you do it, the more you'll convert your negative emotional vibrations and frequencies into positive ones that support your health. Your mood, your hormones, and your body will thank you immensely.

32

exercise your right to great hormonal health

It is often said that the simplest things in life bring the most benefit. In the case of exercise, this is certainly true. Regular physical activity allows a discharge of physical, mental, and emotional tension, helping to prevent the accumulation of stress that can lead to a state of chronic stress and anxiety and other health problems, including hormone imbalances.

Exercise also improves circulation and oxygenation throughout the body, improves the functional capability of your major organs, loosens and limbers up your joints and muscles, promotes emotional grounding and stability, improves stamina and endurance, and boosts your vigor and energy level. Most importantly, exercise plays a huge role in maintaining your hormonal health, supporting healthy production and balance of hormones, as well as easing the side effects associated with hormone imbalances.

To ensure you are getting the full benefits exercise provides, you should aim for 30 to 60 minutes a day five to seven times a week during every phase of your hormonal life. Whatever your hormonal type—whether you are estrogen dominant, estrogen deficient-slow processor, or estrogen deficient-fast processor—regular exercise is essential to help you move towards improved hormonal balance.

The best way to stick to this type of program is to vary your routine by incorporating equal amounts of aerobic activity, weight bearing exercises, and stretching and flexibility, especially in the form of yoga, Pilates, Feldenkrais, or T'ai Chi.

Let's look at each of these groups in more detail. We'll discover why they are so fantastic for your hormonal and overall health, as well as which forms of exercise are best for you.

Walk (or Run) Your Way to Health

The statistics regarding aerobic exercise and health are really impressive. According to a recent article in *Newsweek*, physically inactive people are 40 percent more likely to be diagnosed with colon cancer, 45 percent more likely to have coronary artery disease, and nearly 60 percent more likely to develop osteoporosis. And yet, less than one-third of all adults over the age of 18 participate in any form of regular exercise. No wonder America is in such a health crisis!

Fortunately, just a few minutes a day several times a week can turn your health, especially your hormonal health around. To this point, a study in *Age and Ageing* showed that regular moderate aerobic exercise and a physically active life enhanced higher production of DHEA in older people. Remember that DHEA is one of the "mother" hormones from which other hormones like estrogen and testosterone are produced.

You'll not only be increasing your DHEA levels, but helping to promote better oxygenation and blood flow to all the tissues of your body. The oxygen you breathe in during aerobic exercise is an alkaline gas, and the carbon dioxide we breathe out is an acidic waste product of our body. This helps regulate pH by allowing the acidic carbon dioxide circulating in your blood to be expelled and enabling alkaline oxygen to be better absorbed by the body. Aerobic exercise is especially beneficial as you age, since your lungs become less efficient at extracting oxygen from the air and delivering it to your cells.

In addition to boosting oxygen levels and DHEA, aerobic exercise supports the health and balance of all hormones. Let's take a look at how you can personally benefit.

Lift Your Spirits With Exercise

Regardless of where you fall on the hormonal scale, exercise can be a potent defense against depression. When you move, you greatly improve blood flow and oxygenation to the brain, which in turn increases the production of beta-endorphins, the body's natural painkillers that give you a sense of euphoria and well-being. While you may be familiar with this concept of exercise alleviating depression, you may not know that research has shown that it's as effective as commonly prescribed antidepressants.

According to a study from the *Archives of Medicine*, exercise was found to be as effective as medication in reducing depression among patients with major depression. Researchers randomly separated more than 150 men and women over the age of 50 with major depressive disorder into three groups. One group was given the antidepressant sertraline (Zoloft), the second group either rode a stationary bicycle, walked, or jogged for 30 minutes three times a week, and the third group received the antidepressant as well as the exercise regimen. All subjects underwent extensive evaluations for depression. After 16 weeks, researchers found that there was equal improvement in depressive levels between the groups.

A study from the *American Journal of Epidemiology* took these findings one step further and set out to determine if exercise could actually prevent depression. Researchers studied nearly 2,000 adults aged 50 to 94 for more than 5 years, and rated their physical activity on an eight-point scale, with eight indicating the highest level of physical activity (activities included walking, swimming, etc). They found that every one-point increase in activity lowered a person's risk of being depressed by 10 percent, and cut their risk of becoming depressed by 17 percent. Researchers concluded that physical activity did indeed have a protective effect on depression for older adults.

Similarly, a study from the University of Virginia observed depressed college students. Those who jogged regularly during the study period showed a significant reduction in symptoms of depression, while those who did not exercise showed virtually no change in their symptoms.

In the *President's Council on Physical Fitness and Sports Research Digest*, researcher Daniel Lánders examined several studies that have been conducted on the relationship between exercise and anxiety. His findings are impressive. One study looked at 27 narrative reviews that had taken place between 1960 and 1991. On average, 81 percent of the authors concluded that exercise was significantly related to decreased anxiety.

Landers also evaluated six additional meta-analyses that looked at the effect exercise had on anxiety levels. These meta-analyses ranged from 159 studies to just five studies. All six of these meta-analyses found that across all of the studies they looked at, physical activity was significantly related to a reduction in anxiety.

While it is clear that all women can benefit emotionally from exercise, there are also tremendous specific physical benefits for women with estrogen dominance and estrogen deficient-slow processors, as well as estrogen deficient-fast processors. However, the *types* of exercise in which each group of women should be engaging are dramatically different. Let's take a closer look.

Estrogen Dominant and Estrogen Deficient-Slow Processors

Kimberly is your typical estrogen dominant type, and follows my guidelines for this type of hormonal profile when it comes to exercise. She keeps her hormones properly balanced with high-intensity activities such as running, triathlons, and tennis. She has even been known to power walk and try her hand at ballroom dancing, especially the tango and swing. In other words, she's more the "hare" than the "tortoise."

This is exactly the right type of exercise for Kimberly and other women who lean towards estrogen dominance or are in menopause and have abundant yin. These types of women tend to be instinctively drawn to strenuous types of exercise that are more contractive, more acidifying, and more yangizing to counter their natural tendency towards alkalinity and expansiveness. These types of exercises are more likely to deplete both the oxygen content and the natural buffering agents contained within the muscles, as well as to generate lactic acid. That's why physical activities such as jogging, weight lifting, competing in triathlons, competitive cycling, and mountain climbing are best for them. The key for these women is to generate more yang energy by heating up their bodies, sweating, and ridding themselves of excess yin (as edema, bloating, or excess weight).

Many estrogen dominant women and estrogen deficient-slow processors can maintain this level of intense physical activity well into their later years, provided that their other chemical functions remain reasonably intact. It is not unusual to see these women participating in triathlons and doing bodybuilding and long-distance swimming well into their 70's, 80's, and 90's.

My friend Cecile, who is in her mid-70's, is typical of this type of woman. She has plenty of yin reserves, and works out daily in the gym lifting weights and riding a stationary bike at a very fast and furious pace to generate the vital energy, heat, and yang that she is missing. She tells me that she feels less tired and sluggish after her great workouts.

The Experts Weigh In

The research on the benefits of exercise for estrogen dominant women is overwhelming. Intense, aerobic activity has been found to ease menstrual cramps, decrease the risk for endometriosis, shed excess weight, and even reduce the risk of breast cancer.

Researchers have learned that women who exercise regularly, starting at an early age, have a decreased risk for endometriosis. They've also discovered that women who are a little older and began an exercise program later in their reproductive life also report having less painful menstrual periods.

A study from the *Journal of Psychosomatic Research* showed that women who exercised regularly had fewer PMS-related mood and pain symptoms than those women who were more sedentary. In terms of menstrual cramps, a study from the *American Journal of Obstetrics and Gynecology* found that women who exercise enjoyed a nearly 90 percent reduction in menstrual pain. A similar study from the same journal found that girls between the ages of 14 and 18 who exercised saw between a 76 and 92 percent reduction in menstrual pain.

A third study, this time from the *Journal of the American College of Health*, supported these finding. Researchers found that women who either ran or jogged over the course of 12 weeks reported significantly less severe menstrual symptoms.

Aerobic exercise is also one of the most powerful tools to help correct the metabolic imbalance of "middle fat," insulin resistance, and diabetes. According to a study from the *Archives of Internal Medicine*, women who had successfully completed a three-month weight loss program were more likely to keep the weight off and maintain a trimmer waistline when they added a walking regimen to their routine.

Similarly, in a study published in the *American Journal of Clinical Nutrition*, researchers observed that postmenopausal women who walked three times a week for 24 weeks enjoyed an 8 percent decrease in their body weight and an 8 percent increase in their aerobic capacity. They also noted a decrease in mid-thigh fat and an increase in mid-thigh muscle, as well as a 6–24 percent decrease in total glucose and insulin, an 8 percent increase in HDL ("good") cholesterol, and a 19 percent decrease in triglycerides.

Lastly, researchers have found a direct correlation between frequent moderate to vigorous exercise and a reduced risk of breast cancer. A study conducted at the Harvard Medical School and the Harvard School of Public Health looked at data provided by 166,388 women.

Researchers were looking at self reports of physical activity (most often walking), the frequency and vigor of exercise, and the incidence of breast cancer.

They found that women who engaged in moderate or vigorous activity for seven or more hours per week had a nearly 20 percent lower risk of breast cancer, compared to women who exercised at the same level of activity but for less than one hour per week. Additionally, they also found that it's not the vigor, but the frequency that yields the protective benefits.

THE PCOS PRESCRIPTION

When it comes to polycystic ovarian syndrome (PCOS), a condition affecting many estrogen dominant women, the best prescription I could give is a pair of running shoes.

Studies have shown that exercise not only helps women with PCOS gain better control over insulin and glucose, but also promotes hormonal balance. Plus, exercise helps reduce stress, which is an aggravating factor of PCOS.

Estrogen Deficient-Fast Processors and Exercise

To keep myself in healthy hormonal balance, I follow the exercise plan for estrogen deficient-fast processor women, even though I still have menstrual periods. I follow this program because it enhances yin, peace, and calm, which really helps to keep me in balance, given my fast-paced, high-intensity life. This is necessary because I am a petite woman who has maintained the same weight since I was in college. I never really have to diet, so too much expansion isn't an issue for me. I also work very hard and intensively on a lot of projects like this book, so I have a naturally very fast-paced, yangizing, and contractive career. To keep my hormones in healthy balance, and to counter the great contractive intensity of my life, I need to slow down every day with my meditation and exercise program. I need the balance that this program provides to my mind and body. Being more peaceful, calming, and yinizing allows me to remain in the great health I enjoy.

I am an avid walker, and have been since medical school—nearly 30 years ago! I walk at a moderate pace, breathing slowly and deeply to maximize the alkalinizing benefits. Walking also allows me to reflect on the day while enjoying the fabulous health benefits of regular exercise, which is why I do it nearly every day. The days I'm not able to get out, I can literally feel a subtle drop in my energy level, and my mood isn't as cheery and bright. Walking also helps to keep me limber and has kept my weight virtually the same as when I was in medical school.

Unlike our estrogen dominant sisters, estrogen deficient-fast processors don't want to heat up their bodies and sweat. It is more important to maintain your yin reserves of fluid with slower, more expansive and relaxing aerobic activities that are moderately strenuous and can be done in a relaxed and leisurely way. Activities in this category include golf, swimming, walking, and bicycling at a leisurely pace. You can also try gardening and ballroom dancing, particularly the waltz. In other words, be more the "tortoise" than the "hare."

With these types of exercise, you will tend to breathe more deeply and slowly. Over time, this helps to improve the elasticity of your lungs and relaxes the diaphragm and chest muscles, thereby allowing you to inhale more oxygen. Moderate aerobic exercise also relaxes, dilates, and expands the network of blood vessels in the body, and enables the heart to work more efficiently. Better circulation and oxygenation improve the health of all your organs, including your ovaries and uterus.

Researchers Support Exercise's Medicinal Benefits

For estrogen deficient-fast processors, exercise has been shown to benefit a whole host of health conditions, including menopausal symptoms, bone and heart health, libido, memory and cognitive function, postmenopausal weight gain, and fibromyalgia.

A study from the *Journal of Obstetrics and Gynecology* in Scandinavia found that just 21.5 percent of postmenopausal women who exercised regularly experienced hot flashes, as compared to 43.8 percent of women who lead a more sedentary life. Moreover, researchers discovered that those women who had no hot flashes at all exercised, on average, more than three hours a week. Those who exercised between two and three hours a week had moderate to severe hot flashes.

Another benefit of physical activity is the dilation (expansion) of the network of blood vessels so blood reaches the muscles and vital organs as well as the small capillaries. This can help reduce your risk for heart disease, as seen in a study from the *New England Journal of Medicine*. Researchers found that middle-aged and older women who walked just three hours per week cut their risk of heart disease by 30 to 40 percent.

I have also found that aerobic exercise, as well as a healthy diet, can enhance sexual desire and performance. Specifically, poor circulation can have a negative effect on libido and sexual performance. By increasing your level of aerobic activity, you are not only keeping your heart strong and healthy (a key concern for postmenopausal, estrogen deficient-fast processors), but you are ensuring a steady supply of blood flow to your entire pelvic region, including your vagina, which enhances sexual desire and vaginal lubrication.

Physical activity can improve mental alertness and cognitive function as well. It does this by opening up and dilating blood vessels of the head and brain, and by improving oxygenation and circulation to the brain and nerves. Thus, more nutrients can flow into this vital system, and more waste products can be removed.

An abundance of research shows that adults engaged in an active exercise program have better concentration, clearer thinking, and quicker problem-solving abilities. And a recent study in the *Journal of Internal Medicine* found that regular walking improved memory and reduced signs of dementia. The threshold for this positive effect was about 1,000 steps, or a little over a mile a day.

The Journal of the American Medical Association has also found that exercise helps women lose weight after menopause, thereby neutralizing the increase in breast cancer risk that accompanies even a small postmenopausal weight gain. This is supported by a study published in the *Journal of Gerontology*, which found that people between the ages of 60 and 70 who walked or jogged for 45 minutes several times a week for 9 to 12 months lost an average of 7 pounds, with the majority of the weight lost in the midsection. A positive association between reduction of abdominal fat and a decreased risk of heart disease and diabetes was also noted.

Several studies have shown that exercise is extremely helpful in easing osteoarthritis symptoms. According to research published in *The Gerontologist*, older patients with osteoarthritis in their lower extremities who engaged in an exercise program (flexibility, walking, and resistance training) for two to 12 months enjoyed statistically significant improvement in lower extremity stiffness and pain.

A similar study from the journal *Physical Therapy* divided 134 patients with osteoarthritis of the knee into two groups. Over the course of four weeks, the first group received supervised exercise, individualized manual therapy, and a home exercise program. The second group received the same home exercise program, as well as an office visit after two weeks. Researchers found that both groups had clinically and statistically significant improvement, with 52 percent improvement in the first group and 26 percent improvement in the second group.

Finally, exercise is extremely useful in relieving the symptoms of fibromyalgia. In fact, a study published in *Arthritis and Rheumatism* found that women with fibromyalgia who participated in a strength training and walking program for 20 weeks improved their muscle strength, endurance, and overall ability to function without aggravating their symptoms.

My Advice

Regardless of where you fall on the hormonal index, set aside 30 to 60 minutes each day to engage in regular aerobic exercise. If you've been sedentary, start with 10 minutes a day and work your way up to 30 minutes to an hour a day.

If you are estrogen dominant woman or estrogen deficient-slow processor, choose high-intensity exercises like running, power walking, or faster-paced dancing. If you are an estrogen deficient-fast processor, aim for slower, more meditative exercise such as walking, moderately-paced bike rides, or gardening.

Whichever activity you select, you will be vastly improving your hormonal health and overall well-being.

EXCEPTIONAL HEALER DAVID DWORKIN

An amazing book by physicist Steven Rochlitz entitled *Why Do Music Conductors Live Into their 90s?* showed that regular upper body movement, such as that of conductors, greatly benefits your cardiovascular system by opening up the chest and allowing for fuller, deeper breathing.

Based on this and similar research, Maestro David Dworkin, a longtime music conductor and musician, developed a fantastic exercise program called Conductorcise®. David studied as a clarinetist at The Juilliard School in New York, then attended Columbia University to do graduate work in conducting.

After realizing how elated he felt after each conducting experience, he discovered that his elation was not just based on the fact that he was doing something he loved, he was also benefiting from the endorphins he generated by getting a great workout. Based on this uplifting and positive feeling, he started Conductorcise, so he could share the benefits and enjoyment he experienced each time he conducted an orchestra with other people.

One of the best things about Conductorcise is that no one is too young or too old to practice it. Participants have included chair-bound people who have Alzheimer's disease or have suffered from strokes, as well as children at schools and hospitals. In fact, David himself is 73-years-old and he spends his days dancing around to the beat of Mozart or Brahms.

David starts each Conductorcise performance or class, with light stretching and Qigong. He then passes out batons to each participant and teaches them a basic conducting pattern. He then starts the music, which ranges from marches by John Phillip Sousa to ballets or operas by Mozart and Tchaikovsky, and he lets the class loose. As the music plays and his audience moves to the beats, David points out particularly beautiful sections of the music and encourages everyone to really listen to and move with the music.

For David, the best part is people's reaction to the class. He finds, "It makes people happy. These people come up to me and give me a huge hug and a kiss, and they say, 'God bless.'" After every class, someone approaches him and tells them how they smiled for the first time in months, or moved and swayed for the first time in a year. And, the participants don't just receive a great workout, they enjoy tremendous stress relief as well. It allows them to combine music therapy with aerobic exercise. What could be better!

If you want to learn more about David and Conductorcise, or would like to try a class, visit *www.conductorcise.com* or call 914-244-3803. If you want to try Conductorcise at home, click on the marketplace section of his Web site for information on his Conductorcise instructional DVDs.

Before You Start, Be Prepared

As you can see, the power of exercise is far reaching—from helping to alleviate PMS and prevent breast cancer to easing hot flashes and decreasing your risk for heart attack—there isn't a system in your body that doesn't rejuvenate itself with regular exercise.

However, launching headfirst into a vigorous exercise regimen without giving your body an opportunity to adapt to this new routine is a setup for failure.

Exercise should be a lifestyle change, not a weekend romp. If you start slowly, include proper hydration, and treat injuries quickly and correctly, you'll be more likely to not just adopt a new exercise routine, but also stick with it.

Warm Up and Cool Down

The two most critical aspects of any exercise routine are what you do immediately before and after your actual workout. The "warm up" involves coaxing your body from a state of inactivity to one of motion. Warming up gets your body in gear, helping all your systems get ready for exercise.

To warm up, walk around gently swinging your arms and raising your knees. Gently stretch the muscles of your calves, the backs of your legs, your waist and back. Hold each stretching position for 30 to 45 seconds. Go to the point of tension but not pain; breathe deeply; and pay special attention to those parts of your body you will be exercising.

When you have finished your exercise, simply repeat this process to cool down.

Hydrate, Hydrate, Hydrate

The need to keep your body well hydrated before, during, and after exercise is critical. Especially when you consider that we all consist mainly of water—water makes up 82 percent of blood, 75 percent of muscle, 25 percent of bone, 76 percent of brain tissue, and 90 percent of lung tissue!

Everything in your body depends on water, and when you exercise, you lose it through your sweat, breath, and urine. Moderate exercise in a temperate climate results in the loss of half a gallon of water per day, while heavy training can leave you two gallons drier each day.

When you are exercising, be sure to drink water throughout your workout. And remember, this is *in addition* to the eight glasses you need each day for normal, healthy functioning.

Easing the Pain

While no one plans to hurt themselves, injuries can occur when you exercise regularly. If you do get a bruise, wrench a knee, or turn an ankle, there are some simple and easy things you can try in order to recover from minor injuries quickly.

Several supplements are very beneficial to the healing process. Studies done back in the 1960's found that citrus bioflavonoids greatly hastened the time of recovery from sports injuries. A placebo-controlled study reported in the *Medical Times* compared the effects of citrus bioflavonoids, ascorbic acid, citrus bioflavonoids and ascorbic acid together, and a placebo, on recovery from athletic injuries. The injury recovery rate in the bioflavonoid-treated groups was twice as rapid as the ascorbic acid and placebo controls.

Similarly, professional athletes routinely use pancreatic digestive enzymes to limit the extent of traumatic injury and promote healing. In two studies conducted in Germany and presented at the International Federation of Sports Medicine's World Congress, pancreatic enzymes were given to patients undergoing surgery for sports injuries. In the first study, half of the patients were treated with enzymes postoperatively. These patients had a more rapid reduction in edema and a more rapid return to complete mobility. In the second study, one group of patients received enzyme treatment beginning five days before surgery. They had significantly less edema both before and after the operation and notably less pain.

To keep yourself safe from pre- and post-injury, or to repair pre-existing trauma or injury, **I recommend taking 2,500–4,000 mg of citrus bioflavonoids daily. For digestive enzymes, I recommend papain (200 mg four times a day), pancreatin (300–500 mg four times per day), and/or bromelain (500–1,000 mg three times a day). All enzymes used for repair should be taken apart from meals.**

You can also try methylsulfonylmethane (MSM), one of the most powerful anti-inflammatories derived from natural foods, to counteract inflammation. According to several studies, MSM helps to prevent joint pain, muscle soreness, and fatigue. **I recommend taking ½–1 teaspoon of MSM granules a day, with meals, before any particularly strenuous activity.**

Finally, if you are an estrogen deficient-fast processor, you may find it useful to take moderate amounts of sodium bicarbonate (baking soda) before, during, and after exercising to reduce and even prevent stiffness and sore muscles. Just drinking one-half to one teaspoon of baking soda dissolved in an 8-ounce glass of distilled water will do the trick.

IS IT A STRAIN OR SPRAIN?

Although most people use the terms interchangeably, strains and sprains affect different parts of your body, but in much the same way.

Strains are damage of some part of the muscle, fascia, or tendon brought on by overuse (chronic strain) or overstress (acute strain). An acute strain results from violent stretching or rapid contraction. A *grade-1* strain is characterized by low-grade inflammation, swelling and mild discomfort. To treat this level of strain, simply apply ice.

With a *grade-2* strain, the site is inflamed, swollen, and may discolor from hemorrhaging. It will definitely hurt and there will be a loss of motion. In this case, apply ice and rest.

Grade-3 strains are all of the above, only worse. Consult your doctor immediately if you believe your strain is this severe.

A sprain affects your ligaments rather than your muscles or tendons. They happen when you stretch a joint beyond its normal range of motion. Again, there are gradations of injury from a grade-1 to a grade-3 sprain, with one being painful but benign, and three involving a complete rupture and loss of function that may require surgery. (See a doctor immediately if you suspect a grade-3 sprain, as you may have fractured a bone.)

Treat a sprain with **RICE** (rest, ice, compression and elevation) to deal with swelling and inflammation. Muscles surrounding the sprain often become tense from the trauma, pain, or from modifying movement patterns. A trained massage therapist can help to prevent adhesions and restore function.

To summarize, I want to ensure that you are most successful in starting and maintaining a regular aerobic exercise program. Be sure to start slowly, include proper hydration, and treat injuries quickly and correctly. That way, you'll be more likely to not just adopt a new exercise routine, but also stick with it.

The following tips will prime your body for peak performance, and help to keep you injury-free.

1. Invest in a good pair of comfortable shoes, such as Rykä—a wonderful brand of shoes made just for women. I like their shoes because they are designed to take into account a woman's narrower heels and wider forefoot. Rykä can be found in most Lady Foot Lockers or ordered online at www.ryka.com. Whichever brand you choose, make sure your sneakers offer plenty of support and cushioning. And to prevent ankle or foot injury, replace your shoes when you notice the heels wearing down—at least every four to six months.

2. Exercise outside if weather allows. Take time to rejoice in nature and the change of the seasons. If the weather doesn't allow for outside activity, move your routine to a nearby mall or try the treadmill at a nearby gym.

3. Continue to challenge yourself and add variety to your routine. If you start off walking for 10 to 15 minutes a day three days a week, try building to 20 to 30 minutes a day, then try to walk four or five days a week. Ideally, you should work towards a goal of walking for one hour a day, six to seven days a week. You can also include more hills in your walk, or gradually increase your rate of speed.

4. Finally, build a community around exercise. Find a walking partner or join a walking club. It is easy to find excuses for not taking your morning walk, but those excuses won't hold up if someone is waiting for you on the corner or at the gym.

WHAT'S STANDING IN YOUR WAY?

As wonderful as aerobic activity is, I know how difficult it can be to move even one step when faced with pain and discomfort. While it seems like rest would be your best bet, the truth is exercise almost always *accelerates* healing. So, whether you have a short-term or lifelong condition, I encourage you to find creative ways to *adapt* your exercise program so you can still get the health benefits, without stressing the parts of your body that need special consideration.

Here are some of the most common roadblocks that can stand in the way of lacing up those shoes, and helpful strategies on how to get around them.

Excess Weight

Obesity is an epidemic in this country, and exercise is the absolute best way to cure it. However, walking can be a challenge for women who are extremely overweight. A study published in the *Journal of Applied Physiology* found that one in four obese patients who started taking brisk daily walks suffered knee injuries, and one in four of those injured patients never returned to exercise, suggesting that walking is bad for your knees if you're overweight.

However, the walkers in this study covered more ground—2½ feet or more per stride—which significantly increases knee strain, especially if body weight is excessive. The same study concluded that when taking shorter strides, which allow for carrying on a normal conversation without getting winded, even obese walkers had no significant increase in risk of knee injury.

continued on next page

WHAT'S STANDING IN YOUR WAY? *continued*

If you're overweight, take shorter strides and walk at a slow, steady pace. Just don't give up—as the pounds melt off and your overall condition improves, your joints will become healthier and have less weight to carry. Then you can pick up the pace, if desired.

Knee Problems

The knees are the most commonly injured joints in the body, partly because the bones are secured by ligaments designed to hold them in position only when the knee is *not* under load. The bulky muscles around the knees—particularly the quadriceps (front of the thighs) and the hamstrings (back of the thighs)—are supposed to do the heavy work. But many women use those muscles only to propel themselves forward—and otherwise allow their quads and hamstrings to be passive, relying heavily on the ligaments.

Building up your quads and hamstring muscles and keeping them active are the best ways to protect your knees. If you have knee problems, I recommend consulting with a physician before starting any fitness routine. At the same time, consider using the supplement recommendations listed in the sidebar to keep you moving forward with exercise. And, to avoid damaging the cushion under the knee cap, be sure to step lightly when walking—don't pound your feet into the ground, especially when walking downhill.

Osteoarthritis of the Hip

For most women with this incredibly common condition, walking is the last thing on their agenda. But if you have some cartilage left in your hips, arthritis is usually a good reason to tie those shoes on. That's because joint cartilage—the hardest-working part of your joints—has no direct blood supply of its own. Instead, like a sponge, it soaks in nutrient-rich joint fluid and cleans itself by discharging wastes into that same fluid, which is constantly replacing itself.

Weight-bearing exercise compresses your cartilage, causing the joint fluid to squeeze out. And when you release the weight, the cartilage expands and soaks up fresh fluid. In other words, your footsteps are the "heartbeat" that drives your joints' circulatory system. Without exercise, the cartilage gets very little nutrition and becomes increasingly gritty with accumulated wastes.

So, with your physician's guidance, using a cane or walker if needed, start a walking routine at whatever level is appropriate for your condition. Even if you can only make one loop around a room, you'll be helping your hips immeasurably. Then gradually increase your frequency and duration at a pace that's comfortable.

continued on next page

Plantar Fasciitis

Plantar fasciitis, inflammation in the tissue connecting the heel bone to the toes, is the result of carrying your weight without proper foot support. It is often caused by chronic small tears that keep reoccurring due to overuse. It usually manifests as pain in the heel, especially after extended periods of rest, such as what you are experiencing first thing in the morning. Common culprits include spending all day on your feet and wearing high heels, which can triple the strain on those tissues.

If you continue to overstress this area, the repeated inflammation can result in new bone growth on the heel, often referred to as a heel spur. If you strongly suspect that this may be your problem, I recommend that you consult with a podiatrist who can examine your feet properly.

In the meantime, to get relief from plantar fasciitis, I recommend relaxing your feet with a 15-minute alkaline soak each evening. Make the soak by dissolving two or three teaspoons of baking soda in about 5 inches of warm water, in a dishpan-sized container. After soaking your feet, massage them for at least five minutes each by rolling them over a tennis ball.

And, as hard as it may be for some high-heel addicts, I recommend limiting the heel height of your shoes to two inches or less. Better yet, wear flat shoes. In addition, buy shoes in the evening, when feet are naturally a bit larger, and don't wear the same shoes all the time—this relentlessly stresses the same areas of the plantar fascia.

Bone-A-Fide Reasons for Strength Training

The next type of exercise that all women should engage in is strength or weight training. Regardless of whether you are estrogen dominant, estrogen deficient-fast processor, or estrogen deficient-slow processor, regular strength training will help to improve your posture and balance, and help to build and strengthen bone density.

Researchers have found that weight-bearing exercise generates a small electrical current in bone, which stimulates growth. Additionally, studies have shown that exercising for 30 minutes three times a week can help you slow bone loss. More amazingly, researchers have found that exercising for two hours every day can even build bone mass!

And these benefits have been proven, regardless of age or hormonal status. Studies from the *Journal of the American Medical Association*, as well as the *American Journal of Clinical Nutrition* have shown that exercise is essential to the development of healthy bones in adolescent and college-aged women.

Similarly, studies from the *British Medical Journal, the American Journal of Clinical Nutrition*, and the *American Journal of Physical and Medical Rehabilitation* have found that postmenopausal women in their 50's through their 80's and 90's all increased bone density by engaging in physical activity, especially weight-bearing exercise.

Getting Started

Strength training exercises help to build bone over time; they also improve your posture and balance. However, many women are intimidated by the idea of lifting weights, while others would like to but are limited by joint problems, arthritis, or osteoporosis. Fortunately, weight bearing exercises such as modified push-ups, wall push-ups, and leg lifts confer the same benefits as lifting weights.

If you want to use weights but don't want to invest a lot of money, you can use household items such as soup cans or laundry detergent bottles. Be sure to check the weight before attempting any exercise.

You can even combine strength training with your cardiovascular workout by using a weighted walking vest or ankle weights when you go out for your daily stroll, or doing arm and leg lifts in a pool, using the water's natural resistance in place of weights. I am particularly fond of the Gaiam Walkvest (*www.gaiam.com* or 877-989-6321). They also sell amazing anatomical leg weights (4 pounds each), that you slip over your calf. This puts less pressure on your ankle and distributes the weight evenly, meaning less chance for injury.

Be sure to check with your doctor before starting any strength training program.

Stretch Your Body and Your Mind

Whether you have problems with your feet, hips, back, knees, or no significant issues at all, it is crucial to stretch your joints and muscles every day. Stretching helps keep you flexible, limber, and pain-free, and it helps your muscles, ligaments, and tendons stay youthful in their function well into your older years.

When it comes to stretching, there are four types that I favor: Pilates, Feldenkrais, T'ai Chi, and yoga. As a rule, Pilates is best for estrogen dominant women and estrogen deficient-slow processors, as it tends to include more intense and faster-paced movements. For estrogen deficient-fast processors, the more meditative movements of Feldenkrais and T'ai Chi are ideal. In terms of yoga, different styles are more beneficial than others, given your particular hormone type.

That being said, let's take a look at yoga in more detail.

The Wonderful World of Yoga

Yoga is a wonderful practice for women. Not only does it calm and balance your mood, it also gently stretches all your muscles, builds strong bones and balance, and encourages you to breathe deeply. However, you do need to be aware of the type of yoga you are choosing. Estrogen dominant women and estrogen deficient-slow processors do best with Bikram, or hot yoga, as well as power yoga. Estrogen deficient-fast processors should choose the slower, more quieting hatha or anusara forms of yoga.

UNDERSTANDING YOGA

With all the different types of yoga offered, it can be difficult to distinguish one from the other. Therefore, to help you choose the right one for your hormonal profile, I created a little "cheat sheet for you."

- **Hatha**—the basis for most other forms of yoga. It is usually slower and geared toward those new to the practice.
- **Iyengar**—uses props, such as straps, blocks, blankets, etc.
- **Ashtanga**—involves synchronizing breath with movement. It is usually a pretty quick-paced practice.
- **Anusara**—built on impeccable alignment, which in turn helps develop the flexibility and muscle tone to support flawless body mechanics.
- **Bikram, or hot, yoga**—the teacher turns up the heat up in the room during the practice.
- **Power yoga**—more of a gym workout than a discipline. It's usually a combination of Ashtanga and Bikram yogas.

Grounded in Science

Yoga is commonly accepted for relieving stress and anxiety, but it has also been shown to help with a wide variety of physical health conditions, including menopausal symptoms, cardiovascular disease, arthritis, asthma, and lower back pain.

Researchers at Richard Stockton College of New Jersey in Pomona studied six perimenopausal and postmenopausal women between the ages of 44 and 62 who participated in a one-hour-long Iyengar yoga class twice a week for two months. The women were also given a home yoga program, and instructed to practice on the days they were not in class. At the end of the study, five of the six women had fewer and less severe menopausal symptoms, including hot flashes and night sweats.

According to a study performed at Hanover Medical University in Germany, participants who practiced yoga, meditation, and ate a vegetarian diet had significantly lower blood pressure and cholesterol levels. Similarly, a randomized, controlled clinical trial published in *Stroke* found that African Americans with high blood pressure who performed transcendental meditation (often used in conjunction with yoga) for 20 minutes twice a day for just over five months actually reduced the thickness of their artery walls by nearly one millimeter. This translated to an 11 percent decreased risk for heart attack.

A study from the *Journal of Rheumatology* found that patients with osteoarthritis of the hands who practiced yoga enjoyed a significant reduction in pain and tenderness and greater range of motion in their fingers than those people who didn't do yoga.

Another study from the Northern Colorado Allergy Asthma Clinic in Colorado found participants who did 45 minutes of yoga three times a week for 16 weeks reported significantly better relaxation and attitude, and less dependence on their inhalers than the control group.

Finally, a small study conducted by Vijay Vad, M.D., a specialist in sports medicine at the Hospital for Special Surgery in New York, tested the benefits of yoga on 25 participants with lower back injuries. They gave the patients a series of poses and exercises, mostly supine, to practice three times a week at home. The participants then took a more challenging back-focused class three times a week at a yoga studio. A second group of lower back patients were given two different pain medications, but no yoga program.

After six months, 80 percent of those people who practiced yoga had significantly decreased pain, as compared with just 44 percent of the people taking the medications. Better yet, only 12 percent of the yoga practitioners had another acute episode of their injury, as compared to 56 percent in the medication group.

Yoga Resources

There are a wide variety of yoga books and CDs that you can purchase to do yoga at home. For estrogen dominant women and estrogen deficient-slow processors, I suggest the following:

- Ashtanga Yoga: The Definitive Step-By-Step Guide to Dynamic Yoga *(www.amazon.com)*
- The Ashtanga Yoga Collection (*www.ashtanga.com*)
- Bikram's Beginning Yoga Class (*www.bikramyoga.com*)
- Lilias! Yoga Gets Better With Age (*www.amazon.com*)
- Power Yoga: The Total Strength and Flexibility Workout (*www.amazon.com*)
- Power Yoga—Total Body Workout (*www.amazon.com*)

For estrogen deficient-fast processors, these are my preferred resources:

- Living Yoga: P.M. Yoga for Beginners (*www.amazon.com*)
- Yoga Journal's Yoga Practice for Relaxation (*www.amazon.com*)
- Yoga Alignment and Form (*www.amazon.com*)
- Yoga Over 50 (*www.amazon.com*)
- Insight Yoga (*www.santosha.com*)

Practice Pilates

The Pilates ["pill-ought-tease"] Method was developed by a physical trainer named Joseph Pilates back in the 1920's to help dancers and athletes restore and build muscle tone and strength. It's similar to yoga in that you do a series of exercises that stretch and strengthen your muscles and joints. But while yoga is based on the flow of energy throughout your body, Pilates focuses on physical conditioning and toning.

This workout is best for estrogen dominant women and estrogen deficient-slow processors. It is a great complement to any cardiovascular exercise you are doing. It helps you build a healthy, injury-free body by using gentle and concentrated movements, with each one centering the body with breathing awareness while maintaining a dynamic flow. When you finish your workout, you'll be in better balance, both mentally and physically.

Emerging Breast Cancer Research

Pilates' research is fairly new in the U.S. While most of the research centers around flexibility and strength training, especially for the lower back (see below), there is exciting research emerging in the area of breast cancer.

The Canadian Breast Cancer Research Alliance has recently provided funding for Dr. Susan Harris and Kim Keays to conduct a study to examine the effects of Pilates on women with breast cancer. The researchers are hoping to provide information about the safety and efficacy of Pilates, especially as it related to managing the adverse physical and emotional effects commonly associated with breast cancer treatment.

Best for Back Pain

Pilates has been shown to be particularly beneficial in easing back pain. As much as your back may ache, sitting is the worst thing you can do. Gravity, coupled with a lot of sitting and slouching, compresses the lower back. This can lead to bulging of the pillow-like discs between the vertebrae, asymmetrical contraction of the muscles around the spine, and misalignment.

Instead, try the Pilates-inspired BodyBridge, a specially designed table that puts the spine into a gentle arch when you lay on it. Arching your back helps to counteract the compression of gravity. It also lengthens and stretches the spine and relaxes asymmetrically clenched muscles that pull the vertebrae out of alignment.

My family and I love our BodyBridge and have used it for nearly two decades. Not only does draping over the arch ease the spine into healthy alignment, it also feels great.

To learn more about the BodyBridge, visit *www.bodybridge.com*. Besides the table, there are various back-friendly products available, including instructional videos that show you how to do back-strengthening exercises on the table.

Similarly, if you have never tried Pilates, I recommend taking a few classes to be sure you understand the technique. Otherwise, you can try purchasing either a book, tape, or kit and do the workouts at home. You can't go wrong with the Winsor Pilates books and tapes (*www.winsorpilates.com* or 800-747-3503). When it comes to equipment (accessories and props) you can use at home, I am partial to Balanced Body Pilates (*www.pilates.com* or 800-745-2837).

Focus on Feldenkrais

One of the most effective ways to stretch is by using the Feldenkrais Method, first developed in the 1940's by Dr. Moshe Feldenkrais, a brilliant scientist, physicist, engineer, and educator. He also was a respected judo instructor and the first European to earn a black belt. He authored many books on judo, as well as other topics that he studied and researched.

Feldenkrais-based exercise has tremendous benefits for women who want to stay fit, active, and healthy because it can dramatically improve flexibility, coordination, balance, and strength. Feldenkrais exercises work by helping to re-educate the muscles, nerves, and brain to function in the most effective and beneficial manner. This helps relieve stiffness and pain and allows you to walk more effectively. And, an added bonus is that it can help prevent Alzheimer's disease and dementia, and enhance breathing, creativity, and speech.

What is the Feldenkrais Method?

Simply put, the Feldenkrais method is an educational therapy that teaches you how to move your body in a way that improves your overall mind/body functioning. In essence, the Feldenkrais method helps you reprogram the way your body and mind work (and how they work together), so that they function more effectively.

After suffering a sports-related knee injury, Dr. Feldenkrais—having been given only a 50 percent chance for full recovery—decided to take his fate and healing into his own hands. He began to rigorously study anatomy, physiology, and other scientific disciplines, and combined this new knowledge with what he already knew about martial arts, physics, and engineering.

Through years of research, experimentation, and fine-tuning, Dr. Feldenkrais developed an innovative method of healing that involved reeducating the brain and body (specifically, the nerves and muscles) to function in the most effective and beneficial manner possible. His new method not only helped heal his own knee, but also became the therapy thousands of others were searching for to help them get back to vibrant, pain-free living. Today, the Feldenkrais method is believed to be the leading technique in helping your body achieve optimal mind, nerve, and muscle control. This therapy proved so popular that many similar mind/body empowerment techniques have been developed since.

A Method to Your Movement

Dr. Feldenkrais believed that, for whatever reason, once most people come up with a movement that they feel comfortable with, they're resistant to change it. This is the reason your body gets "stuck in a rut," moving in the same manner every day. And, as you may know from experience, doing the same repetitive movement day after day can eventually lead to injury. Dr. Feldenkrais claimed that people often assume that their injuries are caused by the actual activity, when the real culprit is the way they performed that activity.

The Feldenkrais method works by reactivating the curiosity-driven, investigative learning style that is so common in toddlers when they first learn how to walk and talk. By doing so, you rediscover new ways to communicate more effectively with your body. Not to be confused with massage, T'ai Chi, yoga, chiropractic, or any other healing therapy, the Feldenkrais method goes a step beyond by incorporating your mind, along with your muscles and nerves, to recreate your everyday movements. In essence, it teaches your body a more beneficial way to move!

Pain and Stress Benefits

The Feldenkrais method has amazing benefits, including improved flexibility, coordination, balance, and strength. In a study published in the *American Journal of Pain Management*, patients with chronic headaches or musculoskeletal problems who participated in a Feldenkrais program all reported better mobility and decreased pain—both immediately after the study's conclusion, and one year later.

In another study, published in the *Journal of Occupational Rehabilitation*, 97 female industrial workers who suffered from neck and shoulder pain were randomly split into three groups—a control group, as well as physiotherapy and Feldenkrais groups. After 16 weeks, the group that practiced the Feldenkrais method showed significant decreases in shoulder and neck complaints, while the other two groups experienced no positive changes or worsening of complaints.

I also use (and highly recommend) this technique to reduce stress and to feel more relaxed and grounded. In fact, Feldenkrais can be used to help conquer a wide range of mental, learning, and developmental disabilities. A study published in the *Journal of Fluency Disorders* found that the use of Feldenkrais and other somatic education to treat stuttering may facilitate the development of new behavior patterns, therefore creating better relaxation in general.

Putting the Method to Practice

The Feldenkrais method is practiced in two formats—*awareness through movement* and *functional integration*. If you practice awareness through movement, you'll most likely be part of a class that's directed by a skilled practitioner. The sessions contain a series of slow, small movements, along with meditation and breathing exercises. Throughout the class, the teacher guides you through the movements so that, over time, you replace your old patterns of movement with new, more effective ones.

Functional integration is a more hands-on, individualized approach. The practitioner detects any patterns of resistance in your body, which usually represent the limitations that cause pain or other problems. Once the practitioner identifies your limitations, he/she then helps you reprogram your thought and movement processes to overcome them. In these sessions, the practitioner manually guides your body through very slight, subtle movements tailored to your particular situation. Movements often focus on bending, turning, and leaning.

Both formats are equally effective. And once you get the hang of it after several sessions, you can easily practice Feldenkrais on your own. Personally, I enjoy practicing Feldenkrais exercises in my own home, using CDs created by my very good friend and colleague, Barbara White, an experienced and very gifted Feldenkrais practitioner in San Francisco. I find her work to be magical in its ability to not only help me relax in the early evening, but to also help release tense and contracted muscles, and maintain my flexibility and mobility. You can learn more about Barbara or purchase her CDs by calling 877-872-4504 or by visiting her Web site at *www.SmallMovesLibrary.com*. She has two sets—one contains general Feldenkrais exercises, and her new one is for walking healthfully.

I also recommend a wonderful book by Thomas Hanna, Ph.D. called *Somatics: Reawakening the Mind's Control of Movement, Flexibility, and Health.* In 1975, Dr. Hanna directed the first Feldenkrais training course in the United States, and has since developed his own exercises based on the brilliant work of Dr. Feldenkrais. Somatic exercises are very similar to the movements you would do in an awareness-through-movement session, and his book easily outlines how to do them in the comfort of your own home. You can order Dr. Hanna's book Somatics, as well as his fantastic tapes and CDs from the Novato Institute for Somatic Research and Training (*www.somaticsed.com* or 415-897-0336).

Traditional T'ai Chi

T'ai Chi, a traditional Chinese conditioning exercise, was first practiced over 700 years ago. Literally translated as "moving life force," T'ai Chi involves controlled breathing and choreographed movements that combine to resemble a deliberate, flowing dance. The graceful motions, called forms, are performed by slowly shifting your body's weight from one foot to another while making synchronized arm, body, and leg movements.

Several studies have also shown that T'ai Chi can help you avoid falls by improving your balance. In the *Archives of Otolaryngology—Head & Neck Surgery*, researchers studied 22 people with mild balance disorders. Just eight weeks of T'ai Chi training helped to improve their balance significantly.

Similarly, in the *Journal of the American Geriatrics Society*, researchers found that 15 weeks of T'ai Chi exercise reduced the risk of falls in persons aged 70 and older. This is very helpful in preventing osteoporosis-related fractures, a major disability issue for older women.

I consider activities like T'ai Chi to be the essence of great preventive medicine. Ideally, you should practice T'ai Chi for 30 minutes three to five times a week. However, due to the low intensity and relaxing quality of the exercise, I know many women who make T'ai Chi a part of their daily lives.

If you have never tried T'ai Chi before, I highly recommend you start with a trained instructor who can supervise your posture and movements. Once you have learned how to do the forms correctly, you can practice on your own or with a small group.

You can also use instructional books and/or DVDs. I suggest T'ai Chi for Arthritis (*www.smartaichi.com* or 877-482-4241); T'ai Chi and Qigong: Prescription for the Future (*www.smartaichi.com* or 877-482-4241); and Simply T'ai Chi (*www.amazon.com*).

* * *

Clearly, all three forms of exercise—aerobic, strength training, and stretching—are critical for great hormonal balance and overall health. If you have already started an exercise routine, good for you! Just be sure you are doing those activities that are best suited to your hormonal type.

If you are just getting started, make sure you go slow and choose exercises that support your hormonal type. Soon you'll discover that once you establish exercise as a habit, you won't want to spend a day without it.

To ensure that you are choosing the right exercises for you, let's recap quickly:

Estrogen Dominant Women and Estrogen Deficient-Slow Processors

- Fast-paced aerobic activity such as jogging, race-walking, triathlons, tennis, racquetball, and ballroom dances like the tango, foxtrot, and swing.
- Weight-bearing, strength training with free weights or Nautilus equipment.
- Stretching exercises such as Pilates or Ashtanga, Bikram, or power yoga.

Estrogen Deficient-Fast Processors

- Slower, more moderate aerobic activity such as walking, biking, swimming, gardening, or ballroom dances like the waltz.
- Weight-bearing strength training, ideally with your own body weight or in the water.
- Stretching exercises such as Feldenkrais and T'ai Chi.

Section Five: Summary

In this section, we looked at how your lifestyle—namely your diet, stress, and exercise routine—can impact your hormonal health. I know it can be a lot to absorb, so I created this little cheat sheet for you (see next page). Simply look for your specific hormonal type (estrogen dominant, estrogen deficient-fast processor, or estrogen deficient-slow processor), then look for the diet, stress reduction, and exercise programs that work best for you.

	Estrogen Dominant	Estrogen Deficient-Fast Processor	Estrogen Deficient-Slow Processor
Diet	- High fiber foods - Flaxseed - Citrus fruits - Berries - All vegetables - Free-range poultry - Wild fish - Free-range beef and lamb - Game meats like venison - Soy and soy-based foods - Vinegar - Hot, spicy foods - Almonds - Walnuts	- Grains like rice, oats, and quinoa - Non-acidic vegetables like peppers, carrots, broccoli, and mushrooms - Papaya and mango - Avocado - Melon and banana - Legumes like lentils, kidney beans and pinto beans - Hummus - Soy and soy-based foods - Wild fish	- High fiber foods - Flaxseed - Citrus fruits - Berries - All vegetables - Free-range poultry - Wild fish - Free-range beef and lamb - Game meats like venison - Soy and soy-based foods - Vinegar - Hot, spicy foods - Almonds - Walnuts
Stress Reduction	- deep breathing exercises with red orange - affirmations - visualizations - meditation - prayer - positive self-talk and emotions	- deep breathing exercises with blue, violet, or green - affirmations - visualizations - meditation - prayer - positive self-talk and emotions	- deep breathing exercises with red orange - affirmations - visualizations - meditation - prayer - positive self-talk and emotions
Exercise	- Fast-paced aerobic activity (jogging, race-walking, triathlon) - Dances like the tango, foxtrot, and swing - Weight-bearing, strength training with free weights or Nautilus equipment - Pilates - Feldenkrais - Ashtanga, Bikram, or power yoga	- Slower, more moderate aerobic activity (walking, biking, or gardening) - Dances like the waltz. - Weight-bearing, strength training, ideally with your own body weight or in the water. - Feldenkrais - T'ai Chi - Hatha yoga	- Fast-paced aerobic activity (jogging, race-walking, triathlon) - Dances like the tango, foxtrot, and swing - Weight-bearing, strength training with free weights or Nautilus equipment - Pilates - Feldenkrais - Ashtanga, Bikram, or power yoga

conclusion

It has been my great honor to offer this book as my gift to you. By putting all of the research, solutions, and fabulous resources I've gathered over many years of working in my field into one book, my wish for you is that this journey helps you create vastly improved hormonal health, as well as wonderful overall health and well-being.

Remember, there is no right or wrong way to use this book. Whether you are looking to support healthy menstruation, relieve menopause symptoms, reverse osteoporosis, lose weight, treat insomnia, melt away fibroid tumors and endometriosis, or even delay menopause, my program will go a long way towards helping you feel vibrant and healthy.

Simply pick and choose from all of the different therapies I have described, and decide how you want to start your own program. Whatever you decide, start slowly and choose those therapies that most appeal to you.

Most importantly, make sure you keep your program as easy to implement as possible. Putting together a program that is too complicated, time-consuming, or expensive is a setup for failure.

Once you have seen the benefits of these changes, you'll want to make even more—you'll feel that amazing! Be proud of yourself for the changes you are making and love yourself every day. You are worth it.

I send you my love,

Susan

resource guide

I have gathered every health product I love and personally use and placed them in this practical, easy-to-use Resource Guide for your enjoyment. For your convenience, I've arranged them by the section in the book in which they were featured. I hope you find it helpful!

To learn more about Dr. Lark's products and projects, go to *www.DrLarksHormone Revolution.com.* It is a one-stop resource with information about and links to my monthly newsletter *Women's Wellness Today*; my biweekly eLetter *Women's Health Updates*; and my line of nutritional supplements, food, and skin care products. You can also find information about other books and CDs I have written, as well as my projects in the field of energy medicine.

For additional information specifically about my energy medicine projects, you can also visit *www.QuantumEducation.com* and *www.nrgcards.com.*

Section Three: Restoring the Balance

Testing:

- Genova Diagnostics—formerly Great Smokies Diagnostic Laboratory— (*www.gdx.net* or 800-522-4762)
- ZRT Laboratory (*www.zrtlab.com* or 866-600-1636)
- Life Cycles saliva test kit from Aeron Laboratories (*www.aeron.com* or 800-631-7900)
- Neurotransmitter testing from NeuroScience, Inc. (*www.neurorelief.com* or 888-342-7272)

Supplements:

- Daily Balance Alkalinizer (*www.drlark.com* or 888-314-5275)
- Standard Process Glandulars and wheat germ oil (*www.standardprocess.com*)
- Viobin wheat germ oil (*www.viobinusa.com*)
- Bioidentical hormones (estriol, progesterone, and testosterone) from Women's International Pharmacy (*www.womensinternational.com* or 800-279-5708)
- Whole World Botanicals' Royal Maca (*www.wholeworldbotanicals.com* or 888-757-6026)
- Mucuna from Natural Path Center (*www.naturalpathcenter.com* or 608-826-9076)

- Mucuna from NutriScience (*www.nutriscienceusa.com* or 203-334-3535)

Skin and Hair Care:

- BioMarine Squalane (*www.drlark.com* or 800-941-1997)
- Royal jelly from Glory Bee (*www.glorybee.com* or 800-456-7923)
- Aloe Life's whole leaf aloe juice concentrate (*www.aloelife.com* or 800-414-ALOE)
- Your Crown and Glory shampoo and conditioner (*www.yourcrownandglory.com* or 801-466-1517)
- MOOM sugaring hair removal (*www.imoom.com* or 800-492-9464)

Miscellaneous:

- Hysterectomy tips from *www.hystersisters.com*

Section Four: Energy Medicine for Healthy Hormones

Acupuncture/Acupressure:

- To find a licensed acupuncturist in your area, visit *www.acufinder.com* or the Acupuncture and Oriental Medicine Alliance (*www.aomalliance.org* or 253-851-6896)
- Dr. Sha's books, including *Soul, Mind, Body Medicine* and *Power Healing* (*www.drsha.com*)
- To purchase Chunyi Lin's Spring Forest tapes or a copy of his book, *Born a Healer*, (*www.springforestqigong.com* or 866-292-1861)

Light Therapy:

- For an ophthalmologist in your area (*www.aao*.org)
- For an optometrist in your area (*www.9.org*)
- Lazr Pulsar 4, a red light laser from Next Generation Therapeutics (*www.ngtlasers.com* or 866-918-0399)
- The NGT I from Next Generation Therapeutics (*www.ngtlasers.com* or 866-918-0399)
- X Light from the Chee Energy Company (*www.cheeenergy.com* or 888-263-9214)

- Red Light Shaker from the Light Energy Company (*www.lightenergycompany.com* or 800-544-4826)
- Photon Stimulator from LifeForms (*www.photonstimulator.com* or 800-233-1754)
- Dr. Shealy's RelaxMate II (*www.soundstrue.com* or 800-333-9185)
- emWave Personal Stress Reliever from the Institute of HeartMath (*www.heartmath.org* or 831-338-8500)
- Life Vessel of Tulsa (*www.lvtulsa.com* or 918-286-3030)
- Verilux Happy Skin light unit (*www.verilux.net* or 800-786-6850)
- Viatek HairPRO Laser Hair Treatment Brush (*www.drlark.com* or 800-941-1997)
- Alaska Northern Lights (*www.alaskanorthernlights.com* or 800-880-6953)
- Apollo Light Systems (*www.apollolight.com* or 800-545-9667)
- Enviro-Med (*www.bio-light.com* or 800-222-DAWN)
- Light Therapy Products (*www.lighttherapyproducts.com* or 800-486-6723)
- Light-A-Lux (*www.sunalite.com* or 800-339-9572)
- Photo Therapeutics (*www.phothera.com* or 800-498-5975)
- SunBox Co. (*www.sunbox.com* or 800-548-3968)
- True Sun (*www.truesun.com* or 877-878-3786)
- Verilux (*www.ergolight.com* or 203-921-2430)
- SAD, circadian rhythms, and light therapy devices from Circadian Solutions (*www.circadiansolutions.com*)

Frequency Medicine:

- Luanne Oakes' Spiritual Alchemy and Sound Health, Sound Wealth CDs, both of which are available from Nightingale Conant (*www.nightingale.com* or 800-323-3938)
- Maria Kostelas' A Time for Peace and One Heart (*www.flutesoftheworld.com* or 888-813-5883)
- Paul Scheele's Paraliminals CDs and new Sonic Access program from Learning Strategies Corp. (*www.learningstrategies.com/SonicAccess* or 866-292-1861)
    –*Tell them you learned about them from Dr. Susan Lark and give them code 607L to receive a $20 discount!*
- Robert Aviles and Intention Energy (*www.healinglullabies.com* or *lifeisgood@iegroupusa.com*)

- Healing Rhythms System from Sounds True (*www.soundstrue.com* or 800-333-9185)
- Pathway STM-10 Vaginal and Rectal Intracavity Stimulator from the Prometheus Group (*www.theprogrp.com* or 800-442-2325)
- "Myself" biofeedback to help reduce leaks caused by stress incontinence (available at many drugstore chains or at *www.dependonmyself.com*)
- "PMTx" biofeedback to help reduce leaks caused by stress incontinence (*www.biolifedynamics.com*)
- To find a qualified biofeedback therapist in your area, contact the Biofeedback Certification Institute of America (*www.bcia.org* or 303-420-2902)
- Thoughtstream biofeedback device (*www.mindplace.com*)
- For more information about EPFX-SCIO, visit *www.QuantumEducation.com* or call 888-236-9730
- For a well-trained, careful EPFX-SCIO practitioner, call Quantum Source for Life at 877-488-4359 (*www.quantumsourceforlife.com*)
- NRG cards (*www.nrgcards.com* or 888-674-8227)
- The Hidden Messages in Water by Dr. Emoto (*www.beyondwords.com* or *Amazon.com*)
- Resonant Light Technology EMT device (*www.resonantlight.com* or 250-338-4949)—they have hand-held electrodes ($850) and radio frequency device for non-contact frequency induction ($3,000)
- Alternative Technologies EMT device (336-885-6625)
- Bruce Stenulson's very sophisticated, custom-made device that uses argon gas-filled tubes that vibrate at whatever frequency you set (*www.stenulson.net/althealth* or 719-836-2489)
- EarthPulse EMT device (*www.earthpulse*.net or 772-485-9724)
- Bemer 3000 EMT device (*www.bemt.net/products.php* or 877-362-3637)
- Total Relaxation from Binaural-Beats (*www.binaural-beats.com*)

Section Five: The Optimum Lifestyle for Healthy Hormones

Diet:

- Trinity water from Paradise, Idaho (*www.trinitysprings.com*)
- hiOsilver oxygenated water (*www.hiosilver.com* or 713-937-8630).

- AlkaZone and Alkaline Booster by Better Health Lab, Inc. (*www.alkazone.com* or 800-810-1888)
- Microwater (*www.1microwaterco.com* or 740-758-5707)
- Sweet Leaf stevia (*www.sweetleaf.com*)
- Teeccino herbal coffee (*www.teeccino.com*)
- Good Karma Organic Rice Cream (dairy- and wheat-free) (*www.goodkarmafoods.com*)
- XyloSweet xylitol (*www.xylosweet.com*)
- Z Sweet erythritol (*www.zsweet.com*)
- Pamela's wheat-free products (*www.pamelasproducts.com*)
- Namaste Foods (pizza crust) (*www.namastefoods.com*)
- Foods by George (English muffins) (*www.foodsbygeorge.com*)
- Didi's Living Granola (*www.bakingforhealth.com*)
- pH Choice by pH Sciences (sprinkles take acid out of food) (*www.phsciences.com* or 877-353-2243)
- *Inflammation-Free Diet Plan* by Monica Reinagel (*Amazon.com*)
- Sproutman sprout seeds (*www.sproutman.com*)
- Glyconutrients from Ambrotose from Mannatech, Inc. (*www.glycoscience.com* or 831-476-1526, or *www.mannapages.com/ronalanda*)
- ImmunEnhancer™ from Lonza (*www.larex.com* or 201-316-9200)
- Barlean's Greens (*www.barleans.com*)
- Miss Roben's gluten- & dairy-free foods (*www.missroben.com*)
- Glutino plain or sesame bagels (*www.glutino.com*)
- Redwood Hill Farms goat yogurt (*www.redwoodhill.com*)
- Milled Flaxseed (*www.drlark.com*)
- Galaxy Foods cream cheese (*www.galaxyfoods.com*)
- Justin's Nut Butter (*www.justinsnutbutter.com*)
- SeaBear Wild Alaskan salmon (*www.drlark.com*)
- Carvalho wild-caught Albacore tuna (*www.drlark.com*)
- Vital Choice Seafood (*www.vitalchoice.com* or 800-608-4825)
- Ruth's MacaPower bars (*www.drlark.com*)
- Arico snack bars (*www.aricofoods.com*)
- Kind fruit and nut bars (*www.peaceworks.com*)

- ReBar snack bars (*www.drlark.com*)
- Native Kjalii chips and fresh salsas (*www.sfsalsa.com*)
- Luxe teas (*www.luxetea.com*)
- Zhena's Gypsy Tea (*www.gypsytea.com*)
- Sweet Leaf flavored liquid stevia (*www.sweetleaf.com*)
- Ito En bottled, unsweetened green tea (*www.itoen.com*)
- XyloSweet xylitol (*www.xylosweet.com* or *www.drlark.com*)
- La Tourangelle nut oils (*www.latourangelle.com*)
- Mac Nut oil (*www.drlark.com*)
- Organicville dressings (*www.organicvillefoods.com*)
- Japanese sea vegetables are available from Eden Foods (*www.edenfoods.com* or 888-424-3336) or from Kushi Institute (*www.kushistore.com* or 413-623-6679)

Stress Reduction:

- Institute of HeartMath tapes (*www.heartmath.com* or 800-450-9111)
- *Simple Abundance* by Sarah Ban Breathnach (*Amazon.com*)
- *The Art of Thank You: Crafting Notes of Gratitude* (*Amazon.com*)
- *Reinventing Medicine* and *Prayer is Good Medicine* by Larry Dossey, M.D
- *Forgive for Good* by Fred Luskin, Ph.D., director of the Stanford Forgiveness Project
- Linda Eastburn's book *Riding the Intuitive Wave: Learn to Listen to What Your Body Already Knows* (Endue Publishing, Springfield, MO)
- Information about Linda Eastburn and Susan Lark's CDs (*www.DrLarksHormoneRevolution.com*)
- Linda Eastburn's classes or private consultation (*www.intuitiveacademy.com* or 417-863-1377)
- *The 15-Minute Miracle* by Jacquelyn Aldana (*www.15minutemiracle.com* or 408-353-2050)
- To find a qualified BodyTalk practitioner near you, visit *www.bodytalksystem.com*.
- To contact Brooke Baggett (*www.mosaichealingarts.com* or 408-202-3444)
- Dr. Evelyn Oliver and her Savona Method: Life Management Strategies (715-343-6171 or *docoliver@charter.net*)
- To set up an appointment with Artemas Yaffe, call 650-365-3248

- Meditation support groups (*www.DrLarksHormoneRevolution.com*)
- BioSerene relaxation formula from Natural Medica (*www.drmarcuslaux.com* or 800-809-9618)

Exercise:

- For more information about David Dworkin and Conductorcise, visit *www.conductorcise.com* or call 914-244-3803. If you want to try Conductorcise at home, click on the marketplace section of his Web site for information on his Conductorcise instructional DVDs.
- Rykä footwear (Lady Foot Lockers or *www.ryka.com*)
- Gaiam Walkvest (*www.gaiam.com* or 877-989-6321)
- Ashtanga Yoga: The Definitive Step-By-Step Guide to Dynamic Yoga (*Amazon.com*)
- The Ashtanga Yoga Collection (*www.ashtanga.com*)
- Bikram's Beginning Yoga Class (*www.bikramyoga.com*)
- Lilias! Yoga Gets Better With Age (*Amazon.com*)
- Power Yoga: The Total Strength and Flexibility Workout (*Amazon.com*)
- Power Yoga—Total Body Workout (*Amazon.com*)
- Living Yoga: P.M. Yoga for Beginners (*Amazon.com*)
- Yoga Journal's Yoga Practice for Relaxation (*Amazon.com*)
- Yoga Alignment and Form (*Amazon.com*)
- Yoga Over 50 (*Amazon.com*)
- Insight Yoga (*www.santosha.com*)
- Yoga Alliance (*www.yogaalliance.org* or 877-964-2255)
- Yoga for Pregnancy by Sandra Jordan (*Amazon.com*)
- The Idiot's Guide to Yoga with Kids by Jodi Komitor (*Amazon.com*)
- For yoga tapes or DVDs, I'd recommend the Living Arts tapes and any of the tapes by Rodney Yee and Anna Forest (*Amazon.com*)
- BodyBridge (*www.bodybridge.com*)
- Winsor Pilates books and tapes (*www.winsorpilates.com* or 800-747-3503)
- Balanced Body Pilates (*www.pilates.com* or 800-745-2837)
- Stamina Products Pilates equipment (*www.staminaproducts.com* or 800-375-7520)

- Feldenkrais practitioner Barbara White's CDs (877-872-4504 or *www. smallmoveslibrary.com*)
- Dr. Thomas Hanna's book *Somatics: Reawakening the Mind's Control of Movement, Flexibility, and Health*, as well as his fantastic tapes and CDs from the Novato Institute for Somatic Research and Training (*www.somaticsed.com* or 415-897-0336).
- T'ai Chi for Arthritis (*www.smartaichi.com* or 877-482-4241)
- T'ai Chi and Qigong: Prescription for the Future (*www.smartaichi.com* or 877-482-4241)
- Simply T'ai Chi *(Amazon.com)*

Products from Dr. Susan Lark

All of the following products can be ordered from my newsletter publisher at Healthy Directions, LLC. Simply visit *www.drlark.com* or call 888-314-5275 to place your order.

Supplements:

- Daily Answer multinutrient
- Alkalinizer
- Bladder Answer for Women
- Blood Sugar Answer
- Bone Revitalizer
- CoQ10
- Daily Balance PGX™ Fiber
- EFA Complex
- Energy Vitalizer
- Harmony: Hormone Balance for Women
- Joint Answer
- L-Carnitine
- Life-Line 5-HTP capsules
- Memory Answer
- Natto BP
- Probiotic Answer
- Radiance Advanced Skin Supplement

- Sinupret Forte
- Vein Answer
- Vision Answer
- Weight Loss Booster
- Whole World Botanicals Organic Royal Maca

Skin and Hair Care:

- Blinc heated eyelash curler
- Emerita natural lubricant
- Epicurean sunscreen
- Lavera mineral makeup cosmetics
- Moom sugaring hair removal
- Moom nourishing face cocktail
- Moom dark circle reducer eye gel
- Moom rewind time wrinkle cream
- Ocean Actives Topical Deep Water Squalane (lavender scented and unscented)
- Ocean Actives Squalane Body Mist
- Ocean Actives Squalane Hydrating Cleanser
- Ocean Actives Squalane Rejuvenating Eye Cream
- Ocean Actives Squalane Ultra-Hydrating Night Cream
- Ocean Actives Squalane Daily Renewal Moisturizer
- Ocean Actives Squalane Travel Pack
- One-Minute Manicure
- Radiance skin care kit (cleansing gel, rejuvenating serum, super hydrating cream)
- Radiance Body Firming Gel
- Viatek HairPro Laser Hair Treatment Brush
- Your Crown and Glory shampoo and conditioner

Food and Beverages:

- Carvalho Wild-Caught Albacore Tuna
- Clipper tea
- Ecco Bella Chocolate

- Grains 'n Greens Bar
- Mac Nut oil
- Meal Replacement Shake (vanilla and chocolate)
- Milled Flaxseed
- Premium Gold Flax
- ReBar
- Ruth's MacaPower Bars (lemon hazelnut, ginger almond, and chocolate ginger)
- SeaBear Canned Wild-Alaskan Salmon
- Seeds 'n Greens Energy Bar
- XyloSweet (xylitol)

Lifestyle Products:

- Kegelmaster
- Seychelle Flip-Top Water Filter Bottle

Books and Newsletters:

- You can order my monthly newsletter *Women's Wellness Today* online at *www.drlark.com* or by calling 800-784-0863.

- While on the Web site, be sure to sign up for my free online *Women's Health Updates* e-Letter. You'll get solutions for your top health concerns and answer to difficult questions delivered right to your email inbox every other week.

- For a copy of my most recent book *Eat Papayas Naked*, visit *www.drlark.com.*

- To order any of my other books (see below), visit Amazon.*com.*

    > *Chronic Fatigue Self-Help Book*
    >
    > *The Estrogen Decision Self-Help Book*
    >
    > *Fibroid Tumor and Endometriosis Self-Help Book*
    >
    > *Heavy Menstrual Flow & Anemia Self-Help Book*
    >
    > *The Menopause Self-Help Book*
    >
    > *Menstrual Cramps Self-Help Book*
    >
    > *PMS Self-Help Book*
    >
    > *Stress & Anxiety Self-Help Book*
    >
    > *Women's Health Companion*

Products and Projects from Dr. Lark

The following products and projects can be accessed and ordered from Susan's Web site (*www.DrLarksHormoneRevolution.com*). If you wish to contact Dr. Lark regarding a potential project, please write to her at: Dr. Susan Lark, c/o Portola Press, 101 First Street, Suite 499, Los Altos, CA 94022-2750 or via email at *Susan@DrLarksHormoneRevolution.com*.

- Quantum Education (*www.QuantumEducation.com* or 888-236-9730)
- NRG Cards (*www.nrgcards.com* or 888-788-6651)
- Teleconferences (*www.DrLarksHormoneRevolution.com*)

Products and Services from Kimberly

All of the following products and services can be ordered from Kimberly's Web site (*www.DecadentHealth.com*).

- *Food for Thought: Quaffs and Cuisine for Decadent Health* online eLetter
- Revenir and Charmé skin care system
- Four-day and week-long diet, exercise, and lifestyle retreats
- Quarterly Decadently Healthy sample packs

bibliography

Abraham GE. 1984. Nutrition and the premenstrual tension syndromes. *J Appl Nutr* 36:103-124.

Adlercreutz, H and Hamalainen, E. 1992. Dietary phyto-oestrogens and the menopause in Japan. *Lancet* 339:1233.

Adlercreutz, H et al. 1993. Inhibition of human aromatase by mammalian and isoflavonoid phytoestrogens. *J Steroid Biochem Mol Biol* 44(2):147-153.

Adverse Drug Reactions Advisory Committee. 2006. Hepatotoxicity with black cohosh. *Australian Adverse Drug Reactions Bulletin* 25(2):2.

Akwa, Y et al. 1991. Neurosteroids: Biosynthesis, metabolism and function of pregnenolone and dehydroepiandrosterone in the brain. *J Steroid Biochem Mol Biol* 40(1-3):71-81.

Al-Watban, FAH and Andres, BL. 2000. Laser photons and pharmacological treatments in wound healing. *Laser Ther* Volume 12.

Al-Watban, FAH and Zhang, XY. Stimulation and inhibition effect of lasers for wound healing on rats. *Laser Surg Med.*

Amin, KMY et al. 1996. Sexual function improving effect of Mucuna pruriens in sexually normal male rats. *Fitoterapia.* 67(1):53-58.

Asagai, Y et al. 2000. Thermographic study of low level laser therapy for acute-phase injury. *Laser Ther* Volume 12.

Bachmann, GA. 1985. Correlates of sexual desire in post-menopausal women. *Maturitas* 7:211–216.

Bäckström, T and Carstensen, H. 1974. Estrogen and progesterone in plasma in relation to premenstrual tension. *J Steroid Biochem* 5:257–260.

Bakaliuk TG et al. 1998. Microwave resonance therapy in primary osteoarthrosis: the pathogenetic validation of its clinical use. *Patol Fiziol Eksp Ter* 4:22-25.

Baker, ER et al. 1995. Efficacy of progesterone vaginal suppositories in alleviation of nervous symptoms of patients with premenstrual syndrome. *J Assist Reprod Genets* 12(3):205–209.

Balick, L et al. 1982. Biofeedback treatment of dysmenorrhea. *Appl Psychophysiol Biofeedback* 7(4):499-520.

Band, P et al. 1984. Treatment of benign breast disease with vitamin A. *Prev Med* 13:549.

Barber, A, et al. 2000. Advances in laser therapy for bone repair. *Laser Ther* Volume 13.

Barrett-Connor, E et al. 1986. A prospective study of dehydroepiandrosterone sulfate, mortality, and cardiovascular disease. *NEJM* 315(24):1519-1524.

Bauer, M et al. 2002. Thyroid hormones, serotonin and mood: of synergy and significance in the adult brain. *Mol Psychiatry* 7:140-156.

Baulieu, E-E. 1996. Dehydroepiandrosterone (DHEA): A fountain of youth? *J Clin Endocrinol Metab* 81(9):3147–3151.

Bellipanni, G et al. 2005. Effects of melatonin on perimenopausal and menopausal women: our personal experience. *Ann NY Acad Sci* 1057:393-402.

Beral, V et al. 1997. Breast cancer and hormone replacement therapy: Collaborative reanalysis of data from 51 epidemiological studies of 52,705 women with breast cancer and 108,411 women without breast cancer. *Lancet* 350:1047–1059.

Berkman, LF et al. 1993. High, usual, and impaired functioning in community-dwelling older men and women: Findings from the MacArthur Foundation Research Network on Successful Aging. *J Clin Epidemiol* 46(10):1129–1140.

Bhasin, S et al. 1996. The effects of supraphysiologic doses of testosterone on muscle size and strength in normal men. *NEJM* 335(1):1-7.

Bhatavdekar, JM et al. 1994. Levels of circulating peptide and steroid hormones in men with lung cancer. *Neoplasma* 41(2):101–103.

Birkenhager-Gillesse, EG et al. 1994. Dehydroepiandrosterone sulfate (DHEAS) in the oldest old, ages 85 and over. *Ann NY Acad Sci* 719:543–552.

Biskind, MS and Biskind, GR. 1942. Effect of vitamin B complex deficiency on inactivation of estrone in the liver. *Endocrinology* 31:109–114.

Blomhoff, R et al. 2006. Health benefits of nuts: potential role of antioxidants. *Br J Nutr* Suppl 2:S52-60.

Bloomfield, S et al. 1993. Non-weightbearing exercise may increase lumbar spine bone mineral density in healthy postmenopausal women. *Am J Phys Med Rehab* 72:204.

Blumenthal, JA et al. 1999. Effects of exercise training on older patients with major depression. *Arch Intern Med* 159(19):2349-2356.

Bonnefoy, M et al. 1998. Physical activity and dehydroepiandrosterone sulfate, insulin-like growth factor I and testosterone in healthy active elderly people. *Age Ageing* (27):745-751.

Bowen, A. 1996. Older women may benefit from estrogen–androgen therapy. *Am Fam Physician* 53:939.

Boyne, PS and Medhurst, H. 1967. Oral anti-inflammatory enzyme therapy in injuries in professional footballers. *Practitioner* 198(S):543-546.

Brincat, M et al. 1987. A study of the decrease of skin collagen content, skin thickness, and bone mass in the postmenopausal woman. *Obstet Gynecol* 70:840-845.

Buffington, CK et al. 1993. Case report: Amelioration of insulin resistance in diabetes with dehydroepiandrosterone. *Am J Med Sci* 306(5):320–324.

Burris, AS et al. 1992. A long-term, prospective study of the physiologic and behavioral effects of hormone replacement in untreated hypogonadal men. *J Androl* 13(4):297–304.

Byers, T. 1993. Vitamin E supplements and coronary heart disease. *Nutrition Reviews* 51(11):333–336.

Cacciari, E et al. 1990. Effects of sport (football) on growth: Auxological, anthropometric and hormonal aspects. *J Appl Physiol* 61:149–158.

Campbell, A et al. 1997. Randomised controlled trial of a general practice programme on home based exercise to prevent falls in elderly women. *BMJ* 315:1065.

Campbell, D. 1997. *The Mozart Effect: Tapping the Power of Music to Heal the Body, Strengthen the Mind, and Unlock the Creative Spirit* (William Morrow & Company, New York, NY).

Carlsen, E et al. 1992. Evidence for decreasing quality of semen during past 50 years. *BMJ* 305:609–613.

Cassidy et al. 1994. Biological effects of a diet of soy protein rich in isoflavones on the menstrual cycle of premenopausal women. *Am J Clin Nutr* 60:333–340.

Castillo-Richmond, A et al. 2000. Effects of stress reduction on carotid atherosclerosis in hypertensive African Americans. *Stroke* 31:568.

Cha, KY et al. 2001. Does prayer influence the success of in vitro fertilization-embryo transfer? Report of a masked, randomized trial. *J Reprod Med* 46(9):781-787.

Chang, K et al. 1995. Influences of percutaneous administration of estradiol and progesterone on human breast epithelial cell cycle in vivo. *Fertil Steril* 63(4):785-791.

Check, JH and Adelson, HG. 1987. The efficacy of progesterone in achieving successful pregnancy: II. In women with pure luteal phase defects. *Int J Fertil* 32(2):139–141.

Chen, CC et al. 1995. Adverse life events and breast cancer: case-control study. *BMJ* 311:1527-1530.

Chen, HM and Chen, CH. 2004. Effects of acupressure at the Sanyinjiao point on primary dysmenorrhoea. *J Adv Nurs* 48(4):380–387.

Cheng, John. 1999. Tai chi chuan: A slow dance for health. *Phys Sportsmed* 27:109-110.

Choi, P and Salmon, P. 1995. Symptom changes across the menstrual cycle in competitive sportswomen, exercisers, and sedentary women. *Br J Clin Psychol* 34:447.

Chung, CJ. 1995. Estrogen replacement therapy may reduce panic symptoms. *J Clin Psychiatry* 56(11):533.

Clemetson, CAB and Blair, LM. 1962. Capillary strength of women with menorrhagia. *Am J Obstet Gyn* 10:1269-1279.

Cramer, DW et al. 2001. Carotenoids , antioxidants and ovarian cancer risk in pre- and postmenopausal women. *Int J Cancer* 94:128-134.

Croen, KD. 1993. Evidence for antiviral effect of nitric oxide: Inhibition of herpes simplex virus type 1 replication. *J Clin Invest* 91:2446–2452.

Croes, S et al. 1993. Cortisol reaction in success and failure condition in endogenous depressed patients and controls. *Psychoneuroendocrinology* 18:23-35.

Culhane, JF et al. 2001. Maternal stress is associated with bacterial vaginosis in human pregnancy. *Maternal Child Health J* 5:127-134.

D'Hooghe, T et al. 1996. The prevalence of spontaneous endometriosis in the baboon (Papio anubis, Papio cynocephalus) increases with the duration of captivity. *Acta Obstet Gynecol Scand* 75(2):98-101.

da Fonseca, EB et al. 2003. Prophylactic administration of progesterone by vaginal suppository to reduce the incidence of spontaneous preterm birth in women at increased risk: a randomized placebo-controlled double-blind study. *Am J Obstet Gynecol* 188(2):419-424.

Darbinyan, V et al. 2000. Rhodiola rosea in stress induced fatigue ñ A double blind cross-over study of a standardized extract SHR-5 with a repeated low-dose regimen on the mental performance of healthy physicians during night duty. *Phytomedicine* 7(5):365-371.

Davidson, JM et al. 1979. Effects of androgen on sexual behavior in hypogonadal men. *J Clin Endocrinol Metab* 48(6):955–958.

Davidson, JM et al. 1983. Hormonal changes and sexual function in aging men. *J Clin Endocrinol Metab* 57(1):71–77.

Davis, SR and Burger, HG. 1996. Androgens and the postmenopausal woman. *J Clin Endocrinol Metab* 81(8): 2759–2763.

Dennerstein, et al. 1985. Progesterone and the premenstrual syndrome: a double-blind crossover trial. *BMJ* 290:1617.

Deyle, GD et al 2005. Physical therapy treatment effectiveness for osteoarthritis of the knee: a randomized comparison of supervised clinical exercise and manual therapy procedures versus a home exercise program. *Phys Ther* 85(12):1301-1317.

Dias, RS et al. 2006. Effficacy of hormone therapy with and without methyltestosterone augmentation of venlafaxine in the treatmtent of postmenopausal depression: A double-blind controlled pilot study. *Menopause* Mar/Apr 13:202-211.

Dong, H et al. 2001. An exploratory pilot study of acupuncture on the quality of life and reproductive hormone secretion in menopausal women. *J Altern Complement Med* 7(6): 651-658.

Deuster, PA et al. 1999. Biological, social and behavioral factors associated with premenstrual syndrome. *Arch Fam Med* 8:122-128.

Editorial. 1995. Male reproductive health and environmental estrogens. *Lancet* 345:933–935.

Emmons, RA and McCullough, ME. 2000. Counting blessings versus burdens: An experimental investigation of gratitude and subjective well-being in daily life. *J Soc Clin Psychol.*

Enwemeka, CS. 2001. Attunuation and penetration of visible 632.8nm and invisible infrared 904nm light in soft tissues. *Laser Therapy* 13:95-101.

Enwemeka, CS and Reddy, GK. 2000. The biological effects of laser therapy and other physical modalities on connective tissue repair processes. *Laser Therapy* Volume 12:22-30.

Fahim, MS et al. 1982. Effect of panax ginseng on testosterone level and prostate in male rats. *Arch Androl* 8:261–263.

Feigl, EO. 1998. Neural control of coronary blood flow. *J Vasc Res* 35:85–92.

Ferrini, RL and Barrett-Connor, E. 1996. Caffeine intake and endogenous sex steroid levels in postmenopausal women: The Rancho Bernardo Study. *Am J Epidemiol* 144(7):642–644.

Field, B et al. 1990. Reproductive effects of environmental agents. *Semin Reprod Endocrinol* 8(1):44–54.

Flood, JF et al. 1992. Memory-enhancing effects in male mice of pregnenolone and steroids metabolically derived from it. *Proc Natl Acad Sci USA* 89:1567–1571.

Flood, JF et al. 1995. Pregnenolone sulfate enhances post-training memory processes when injected in very low doses into limbic system structures: The amygdala is by far the most sensitive. *Proc Natl Acad Sci USA* 92:10806–10810.

Foecking, MK et al. 1980. Progressive patterns in breast diseases. *Med Hypotheses* 6:659–664.

Folman, Y et al. 1983. The effect of dietary and climatic factors on fertility, and on plasma progesterone and oestradiol-17ß levels in dairy cows. *J Reprod Fertil* 34:267–278.

Fraga, CG et al. 1991. Ascorbic acid protects against endogenous oxidative DNA damage in human sperm. *Proc Natl Acad Sci USA* 88:11003–11006.

Fraser, GE. 1999. Diet as primordial prevention in Seventh-Day Adventists. *Prev Med* 29(6 Pt 2):S18-23.

Freeman, EW et al. 2005. The role of anxiety and hormonal changes in menopausal hot flashes. *Menopause* 12(3):258-266.

Fung, DT et al. 2002. Therapeutic low energy laser improves the mechanical strength of repairing medial collateral ligament. *Lasers Surg Med* 31:91-96.

Garfinkel MS et al. 1994. Evaluation of a yoga based regimen for treatment of osteoarthritis of the hands. *J Rheumatol* 21(12): 2341-2343.

George, MS. 1994. CSF neuroactive steroids in affective disorders: Pregnenolone, progesterone, and DBI. *Biol Psychiatry* 35:775–780.

Gerard, RM. 1958. *Differential Effects of Colored Lights on Psychophysiological Functions* (Ph.D. disseration), University of California at Los Angeles.

Gitlin, M et al. 2004. Peripheral thyroid hormones and response to selective serotonin reuptake inhibitors. *J Psychiatry Neurosci* 29(5):383-386.

Goldin, BR et al. 1981. Effect of diet on excretion of estrogens in pre-and post-menopausal women. *Cancer Res* 41:3771-3773.

Golub, L et al. 1958. Therapeutic exercise for teen-age dysmenorrhea. *Am J Obstet Gynecol* 76:670.

Golub, L et al. 1968. Exercise and dysmenorrhea in young teenagers: a 3-year study. *Obstet Gynecol* 32:508.

Golub, L. 1959. A new exercise for dysmenorrhea. *Am J Obstet Gynecol* 78:152.

Goodhart, DM and Anderson, TJ. 1998. Role of nitric oxide in coronary arterial vasomotion and the influence of coronary atherosclerosis and its risks. *Am J Cardiol* 82:1034–1039.

Gordon, GB et al. 1988. Reduction of atherosclerosis by administration of dehydroepiandrosterone. *J Clin Invest* 82:712–720.

Gouchie, C and Kimura, D. 1991. The relationship between testosterone levels and cognitive ability patterns. *Psychoneuroendocrinology* 16(4):323–334.

Gozan, HA et al. 1952. The use of vitamin E in treatment of the menopause. *NY State J Med* (15 May):1289–1291.

Grodstein, F. 1996. Postmenopausal estrogen and progestin use and the risk of cardiovascular disease. *NEJM* 335(7):453–461.

Guazzo, EP et al. 1996. DHEA and DHEA-S in the CSF fluid of men: Relation to blood levels and the effects of age. *J Clin Endocrinol Metab* 81:3951–3960.

Guth, L et al. 1994. Key role for pregnenolone in combination therapy that promotes recovery after spinal cord injury. *Neurobiology* 91:12308–12312.

Haag, JD et al. 1992. Limonene-induced regression of mammary carcinomas. *Cancer Res* 52:4021-4026.

Habek, D et al. 2002. Using acupuncture to treat premenstrual syndrome. *Arch Gynecol Obstet* 267(1):23-26.

Haffner, SM et al. 1994. Decreased testosterone and dehydroepiandrosterone sulfate concentrations are associated with increased insulin and glucose concentrations in nondiabetic men. *Metabolism* 43(5):599–603.

Hain, TC et al. 1999. Effects of t'ai chi on balance. *Arch Otolaryngol Head Neck Surg* 125:1191-1195.

Hakkinen, K and Pakarinen, A. 1994. Serum hormones and strength development during strength training in middle-aged and elderly males and females. *ACTA Physiologica Scandinavica* 150:211–219.

Hall, GM et al. 1993. Depressed levels of dehydroepiandrosterone sulphate in postmenopausal women with rheumatoid arthritis but no relation with axial bone density. *Ann Rheum Dis* 52:211–214.

Haman, J. 1945. Exercises and dysmenorrheal. *Am J Obstet Gynecol* 49:755.

Hammar, M et al. 1990. Does physical exercise influence the frequency of postmenopausal hot flushes? Acta Obstet Gynecol Scand 69:409.

Harel, Z et al. 1996. Supplementation with omega-3 polyunsaturated fatty acids in the management of dysmenorrhea in adolescents. *Am J Obstet Gynecol* 174:1335-1338.

Harrison, WM et al. 1985. Psychiatric evaluation of premenstrual changes. *Psychosomatics* 26:789-799.

Hayashi, T et al. 2000. Estriol (E3) replacement improves endothelial function and bone mineral density in very elderly women. *J Gerontol* 55A(4):B183-B190.

Head, KA. 1998. Estriol: safety and efficacy. *Altern Med Review* 3(2) 101-113.

Heerdt, AS et al. 1995. Calcium glucarate as a chemopreventive agent in breast cancer. *Isr Jf Med Sci* 31(2-3):101-105.

Hermsmeyer, K. 1997. Reactivity-based coronary vasospasm independent of -atherosclerosis in rhesus monkeys. *J Am Coll Cardiol* 29(1 March):671–680.

Henderson, E et al. 1950. Pregnenolone. *Endocrine Review* 10: 455–474.

Herbert, J et al. 1995. The age of dehydroepiandrosterone. *Lancet* 345:1193–1194.

Hirota, T et al. 1992. Effect of diet and lifestyle on bone mass in Asian young women. *Am J Clin Nutr* 55:1168.

Homberger, F et al. 1971. Inhibition of murine subcutaneous and intravenous benzu (rst)pentaphene carcinogenesis by sweet orange oils and d-limonene. *Oncology* 25:1-20.

Hughes, SL et al. 2006. Long-term impact of Fit and Strong! on older adults with osteoarthritis. *The Gerontologist* 46:801-814.

Isaacson, RL et al. 1995. The effects of pregnenolone sulfate and ethylestrenol on retention of a passive avoidance task. *Brain Res* 689:79–84.

Israel, R et al. 1985. Effects of aerobic training on primary dysmenorrheal symptomatology in college females. *J Am Coll Health* 33:241.

Jackson, J et al. 1992. Testosterone deficiency as a risk factor for hip fractures in men: A case-controlled study. *Am J Med Sci* 304(1):4–8.

Jankowski, CM et al. 2006. Effects of dehydroepiandrosterone replacement therapy on bone mineral density in older adults: A randomized, controlled trial. *J Clin Endocrinol Metab* 91:2986-2993.

Jarry, H et al. 1994. In vitro prolatin but not LH and FSH release is inhibited by compounds in extracts of Agnus castus: direct evidence for a dopaminergic principle by the dopamine receptor assay. *Exp Clin Endocrinol* 102(6):448-454.

Jiang, B et al. 2006. Evaluation of the botanical authenticity and phytochemical profile of black cohosh products by high-performance liquid chromatography with selected ion monitoring liquid chromatography-mass spectrometry. *J Agric Food Chem* 54(9): 3242-3253.

Jirtle, RL et al. 1993. Increased levels of M6P-IGF-II receptor and TGFB1 levels during monoterpene-induced regression of mammary tumors. *Cancer Res* 53:3849-3852.

Joffe, H and Cohen, LS. 1998. Estrogen, serotonin, and mood disturbance: where is the therapeutic bridge? *Biol Psychiatry* 44(9):798-811.

Johnson, J et al. 2004. Germline stem cells and follicular renewal in the postnatal mammalian ovary. *Nature* 428:145-150.

Jungersten, L et al. 1997. Both physical fitness and acute exercise regulate nitric oxide formation in healthy humans. *J App Physiol* 82:760–764.

Kaiser, FE and Morley, JE. 1994. Gonadotropins, testosterone, and the aging male. *Neurobiol Aging* 15(4):559–563.

Kaplan, N. 1985. Non-drug treatment of hypertension. *Ann Int Med* 102:359-373.

Karas, RH. 2004. Current controversies regarding the cardiovascular effects of hormone therapy. *Clin Obstet Gynecol* 47:489-499.

Karren, KJ et al. 2002. *Mind/Body Health: The Effects of Attitudes, Emotions and Relationships.* Benjamin Cummings, San Francisco, CA.

Kasra, M and Grynpas, MD. 1995. The effects of androgens on the mechanical properties of primate bone. *Bone* 17(3):265–270.

Kavinoky, NR. 1950. Vitamin E and the control of climateric symptoms. *Ann West Med Surg* 4(1):27–32.

Kiecolt-Glaser, JK et al. 2002. Emotions, morbidity and mortality: New perspectives from psychoneuroimmunology. *Annu Rev Psychol* (53):83-107.

Kilicdag, EB et al. 2004. Fructus agni casti and bromocriptine for treatment of hyperprolactinemia and mastalgia. *Int J Gynecol Obstet* 85:292-293.

Kim, C et al. 1976. Influence of ginseng on mating behavior of male rats. *Am J Chin Med* 4(2):163–168.

Knekt, P et al. 1994. Antioxidant vitamin intake and coronary mortality in longitundinal population study. *Am J Epidemiol* 139(2):1180–1189.

Knight, DC and Eden, JA. 1995. Phytoestrogens: A short review. *Maturitas* 22:167–175.

Knight, DC and Eden, JA. 1996. A review of the clinical effects of phytoestrogens. *Obste Gynecol* 87(5) part 2:897–904.

Koller-Strametz, J et al. 1998. Role of nitric oxide in exercise-induced vasodilation in man. *Life Sciences* 62:1035–1042.

Krakov, SV. 1942. Color vision and autonomic nervous system. *J Opt Soc Am.*

Krucoff, MW et al. 2001. Integrative noetic therapies as adjuncts to percutaneous intervention during unstable coronary syndromes: Monitoring and Actualization of Noetic Training (MANTRA) feasibility pilot. *Am Heart J* 142(5): 760-769.

Kugaya, A et al. 2003. Increase in prefrontal cortex serotonin 2A receptors following estrogen treatment in postmenopausal women. *Am J Psychiatry* 160:1522-1524.

Kulikauskas, BS et al. 1985. Cigarette smoking and its possible effects on sperm. *Fertil Steril* 44(4):526–528.

Kurzman, ID et al. 1990. Reduction in body weight and cholesterol in spontaneously obese dogs by dehydroepiandrosterone. *Int J Obes* 14:95–104.

Landers, DM. 1997. The influence of exercise on mental health. *President's Council on Physical Fitness and Sports Research Digest* 2(12).

Lee, JR. 1990. Osteoporosis reversal: The role of progesterone. *Int Clin Nutr Rev* 10(3):384–389.

Lee, JR. 1991. Is natural progesterone the missing link in osteoporosis prevention and treatment? *Med Hypotheses* 35:316–318.

Lee, PB et al. 2006. Efficacy of pulsed electromagnetic therapy for chronic lower back pain: a randomized, double-blind, placebo-controlled study. *J Int Med Res* 34(2):160-167.

Leonetti, HB et al. 1999. Transdermal progesterone cream for vasomotor symptoms and postmenopausal bone loss. *Obstet Gynecol* 94:225-228.

Liberman, J. 1991. *Light: Medicine of the Future*. Bear & Co., Santa Fe, NM.

Lindberg, S et al. 1997. Low levels of nasal nitric acid (NO) correlate to impaired mucociliary function in upper airways. *Acta Otolaryngol* 117:728–734.

Littman, AB et al. 1993. Physiologic benefits of a stress reduction program for healthy middle-aged army officers. *J Psychosom Res* 37(4):345–354.

Loch, E et al. 1990. Diagnosis and treatment of dyshormonal menstrual periods in the general practice. *Gynakol Praxis* 14(3):489-495.

Low Dog, T. 2005. Menopause: a review of botanical dietary supplements. *Am J Med* 118(12B):98S-108S.

Lu, LJ et al. 1996. Effects of soya consumption for one month on steroid hormones in premenopausal women: Implications for breast cancer risk reduction. *Cancer Epidemiol Biomarkers Prev* 5:63–70.

Luks, A and Payne, P. 1992. *The Healing Power of Doing Good*. Fawcett Columbine, New York, NY.

MacEwen, EG and Kurzman, ID. 1991. Obesity in the dog: Role of the adrenal steroid dehydroepiandrosterone (DHEA). *Am Instit Nutr* S51–S55.

Maddali, S et al. 1998. Postexercise increase in nitric acid in football players with muscle cramps. *Am J Sports Med* 26:820–824.

Maines, MD and Kappas, A. 1977. Metals as regulators of heme metabolism. *Science* 198:1215-1221.

Maines, MD et al. 1976. Cobalt inhibition of synthesis and induction of gamma-aminolevulinate synthase in liver. *Biochemistry* 73(5):1499.

Maman, F. 1997. *The Role of Music in the Twenty-First Century*. Tama-Do Press (CA).

Manyam, BV et al. 1995. An alternative medicine treatment for Parkinson's disease: results of a multicenter clinical trial. HP-200 in Parkinson's Disease Study Group. *J Altern Complement Med.* 1(3):249-255.

Mathis, C et al. 1999. Models for the study of memory and neurosteroids. *J Soc Biol* 193(3):299-306 (French).

Maxwell, AJ et al. 1998. Limb blood flow during exercise is dependent on nitric acid. *Circulation* 98:369–374.

McClure, RD et al. 1991. Hypogonadal impotence treated by transdermal testosterone. *Urology* 37(3):224–228.

McCraty, R et al. 1995. The effects of emotions on short-term power spectrum analysis of heart rate variability. *Am J Cardiol* 76:1089-1093.

McCullough, ME et al. 2002. The grateful disposition: A conceptual and empirical topography. *J Pers Soc Psychol* 82(1):112-127.

McEligot, AJ. 2006. Dietary fat, fiber, vegetable, and micronutrients are associated with oveall survival in postmenopausal women diagnosed with breast cancer. *Nutr Cancer* 55(2):132-140.

McGavack, et al. 1951. The use of Δ5-pregnenolone in various clinical disorders. *J Clin Endocrinol* 11(6):559–577.

Mechcatie, E. Blue light special for moderate acne. *Family Practice News* October 15, 2002.

Meikle, AW et al. 1990. Effects of a fat-containing meal on sex hormones in men. *Metabolism* 39:943–6.

Melchior, CL and Ritzmann, RF. 1994. Dehydroepiandrosterone is an anxiolytic in mice on the plus maze. *Pharmacol Biochem Behav* 47(3):437–441.

Meriggiola, MC et al. 1995. Testosterone enanthate at a dose of 200 mg/week decreases HDL-cholesterol levels in healthy men. *Int J Androl* 18:237–242.

Messina, M and Messina, V. 1991. Increasing use of soyfoods and their potential role in cancer prevention. *J Am Diet Assoc* 1(7):836–840.

Milewica, A et al. 1993. *Vitex agnus castus* extract in the treatment of luteal phase defects due to hyperprolactinemia: results of a randomized placebo-controlled double-blind study. *Arzneim-Forsch Drug Res* 43:752-756.

Miller. 2007. Health for Life. *Newsweek* March 26, 2007 pp. 48-55.

Minaguchi, H et al. 1996. Effect of estriol on bone loss in postmenopausal Japanese women: a multicenter prospective open study. *J Obstet Gynaecol Res* 22:259-265.

Moilanen, J et al. 1993. Vitamin E levels in seminal plasma can be elevated by oral administration of vitamin E in infertile men. *Int J Androl* 16:165–66.

Morales, AJ et al. 1994. Effects of replacement dose of dehydroepiandrosterone in men and women of advancing age. *J Clin Endocrinol Metab* 78(6):1360–1367.

Morely et al. 1993. Effects of testosterone replacement in old hypogonadal males: A preliminary study. *J Am Geriatr Soc* 41:149–152.

Morfin, R and Courchay, G. 1994. Pregnenolone and dehydroepiandrosterone as precursors of native 7-hydroxylated metabolites which increase the immune response in mice. *J Steroid Biochem Molecular Biol* 50(1/2):91–100.

Moyer, DL et al. 1993. Prevention of endometrial hyperplasia by progesterone during long-term estradiol replacement: Influence of bleeding pattern and secretory changes. *Fertil Steril* 59(5):992–997.

Mulder, JW et al. 1992. Dehydroepiandrosterone as predictor for progression to AIDS in asymptomatic human immunodeficiency virus–infected men. *J Infect Dis* 165:413–418.

Muti, P et al. 2000. Estrogen metabolism and risk of breast cancer: A prospective study of the 2:16 alpha-hydroxyestrone ratio in premenopausal and postmenopausal women. *Epidemiology* 11(6):635-640.

Nair, KS et al. 2006. DHEA in elderly women and DHEA or testosterone in elderly men. *NEJM* 355:1647-1659.

Nestler, JE et al. 1988. Dehydroepiandrosterone reduces serum low-density lipoprotein levels and body fat but does not alter insulin sensitivity in normal men. *J Clin Endocrinol Metab* 66(1):57–61.

Nestler, JE et al. 1992. Dehydroepiandrosterone: The "missing link" between hyperinsulinemia and atherosclerosis? *FASEB Journal* 6:3073–3075.

Nestler, JE et al. 1994. Effects of a reduction in circulating insulin by metformin on serum dehydroepiandrosterone sulfate in nondiabetic men. *J Clin Endocrinol Metab* 78(3):549–554.

Netter, A et al. 1981. Effect of zinc administration on plasma testosterone, dihydrotestosterone, and sperm count. *Arch Androl* 7:69–73.

Nielsen, F. 1988. Boron—an overlooked element of potential nutritional importance. *Nutr Today* Jan/Feb:4-7.

Nielsen, FH et al. 1992. Boron enhances and mimics some effects of estrogen therapy in postmenopausal women. *J Trace Elem Experimental Med* 5:237–246.

Nikula TD et al. 1992. Comparative evaluation of the efficacy of quantum methods of treatment of patients with hypertensive disease. *Lik Sprava* 10:32–35.

Nillson, PM and Solstad, K. 1995. Adverse effects of psychosocial stress on gonadal function and insulin levels in middle-aged males. *J Intern Med* 237:479–86.

O'Carroll, R et al. 1985. Androgens, behavior and nocturnal erection in hypogonadal men: The effects of varying the replacement dose. *J Clin Endocrinol* 23:527–538.

Opstad, PK. 1994. Circadian rhythm of hormones is extinguished during prolonged physical stress, sleep and energy deficiency in young men. *Eur J Endocrinol* 131:56–66.

Paulus, WE et al. 2002. Influence of acupuncture on the pregnancy rate in patients who undergo assisted reproduction therapy. *Fertil Steril* 77(4):721-724.

Petitti, DB et al. 1998. Ischemic stroke and use of estrogen and estrogen/progestogen as hormone replacement therapy. *Stroke* 29:23–28.

Phillips, GB et al. 1994. The association of hypotestosteronemia with coronary artery disease in men. *Arterioscler Thromb* 14:7001–7006.

Phillips, SM and Sherwin, BB. 1992. Effects of estrogen on memory function in surgically menopausal women. *Psychoneuroendocrinology* 17:485–495.

Phipps, WR et al. 1993. Effect of flax seed ingestion on the menstrual cycle. *J Clin Endocrinol Metab* 77(5):1215–1219.

Pincus, GP and Hoaglund, H. 1944. Effects of administration of pregnenolone on fatiguing psychomotor performance. *J Aviat Med* 15:98.

Pincus, GP and Hoaglund, H. 1945. Effects on industrial production of the administration of Δ5 pregnenolone to factory workers. *Psychosomatic Med* 7:342.

Plotnikoff, GA. 2000. Should medicine reach out to the spirit? *Postgrad Med* 108(6):19-25.

Pouresmail, Z and Ibrahimzadeh, R. 2002. Effects of acupressure and ibuprofen on the severity of primary dysmenorrheal. *J Tradit Chin Med* 22(3):205-210.

Primavera J. 1999. The unintended consequences of volunteerism: Positive outcomes for those who serve. *J Prev Intervention Comm* (18):1-2.

Prior, JC. 1990. Progesterone as a bone-trophic hormone. *Endocr Rev* 11(2):386–398.

Propping, D et al. 1987. Treatment of corpus luteum insufficiency. *Zeitscchrift Fur Allgemein* 63:932-933.

Raus, K et al. 2006. First-time proof of endometrial safety of the special black cohosh extract (*Actaea or Cimicifuga racemosa* extract) CR BNO 1055. *Menopause* 13(4):678-691.

Recker, R et al. 1992. Bone gain in young adult women. *JAMA* 268:2403.

Reichert, R. 1996. Yam and DHEA. *Quarterly Review of Natural Medicine* :257–258.

Rhee, Y and Brunt, A. 2006. Pilot study: Flaxseed supplementation was effective in lowering serum glucose and triacylglycerol in glucose intolerant people. *J Am Neutraceutical Assoc* 9(1):28-34.

Rimm, E et al. 1993. Vitamin E consumption and the risk of coronary heart disease in men. *NEJM* 328:1450–1456.

Roberts, E. 1995. Pregnenolone: From Selye to Alzheimer and a model of the pregnenolone sulfate binding site on the GABA receptor. *Biochem Pharmacol* 49(1):1–16.

Roeder, D. 1994. Therapie von Zyklusstorungen mit Vitex agnus-castus. *Zeitschr Phytother* 15:157-163.

Ros, E et al. 2004. A walnut diet improves endothelial function in hypercholesterolemic subjects: a randomized crossover trial. *Circulation* 109(19):1609-1614.

Rosen, LN et al. 1988. Psychosocial correlates of premenstrual dysphoric subtypes. *Acta Psychiatr Scand* 77:446-453.

Rudmen, D et al. 1994. Relations of endogenous anabolic hormones and physical activity to bone mineral density and lean body mass in elderly men. *J Clin Endocrinol* 40:653–661.

Rylance, P et al. 1985. Natural progesterone and antihypertensive action. *BMJ* 290:13-14.

Sahelian, R. 1996. *Pregnenolone: A Practical Guide*. Melatonin/DHEA Research Institute, Marina Del Rey, CA.

Salovey P et al. 2000. Emotional states and physical health. *Am Psychol* (55):110-121.

Sanders, SP. 1999. Asthma, viruses, and nitric oxide. *Proc Soc Experiment Biol Med* 220:123–132.

Sasame, HA and Boyd, MR. 1978. Paradoxical effects of cobaltous chloride and salts of other divalent metals on tissue levels of reduced glutathione and microsamal mixed-function oxidase components. *J Pharm Exp Ther* 205(3):718.

Saura, M et al. 1999. An antiviral mechanism of nitric oxide: Inhibition of a viral protease. *Immunity* 10:21–28.

Schachter, A et al. 1973. Treatment of oligospermia with the amino acid arginine. *J Urol* 110:311–313.

Schmidt, T et al. 1997. Changes in cardiovascular risk factors and hormones during a comprehensive residential three month kriya yoga training and vegetarian nutrition. *Acta Physiologica Scandinavica* 640 (Supp):158-162.

Shafagoj, Y et al. 1992. Dehydroepiandrosterone prevents dexamethasone-induced hypertension in rats. *Am Physiol Soc* E210–E213.

Sharpe, RM and Skakkebaek, NE. 1993. Are oestrogens involved in falling sperm counts and disorders of the male reproductive tract? *Lancet* 341:1392–1395.

Shelley, WB and Arthur, RP. 1955. Studies on cowhage (Mucuna pruriens) and its pruritogenic protease, mucunain. *AMA Arch Dermatol.* 72:399.

Sherwin, BB. 1985. Differential symptom response to parenteral estrogen and/or androgen administration in the surgical menopause. *Am J Obstet Gynecol* 151(2):153–160.

Sherwin, BB. 1990. Estrogenic effect on memory in women. *Ann NY Acad Med* 593:213–231.

Sherwin, BB and Morrie, GM. 1984. Effects of parenteral administration of estrogen and androgen on plasma hormone levels and hot flushes in the surgical menopause. *Am J Obstet Gynecol* 148:552.

Sherwin, BB et al. 1985. Androgen enhances sexual motivation in females: A prospective, crossover study of sex steroid administration in surgical menopause. *Psychosomatic Med* 47:339–351.

Shulman, LP. 2006. Androgens and menopause: More fuel for the fire. *Menopause* Mar/Apr 13:168-170.

Shute, E. 1937. Notes on the menopause. *Can Med Assoc J* October 350-357.

Siegel, JM et al. 1979. Life changes and menstrual discomfort. *Human Stress* 5:41-46.

Sieve, BF. 1942. The clinical effects of a new B-complex factor, para-aminobenzoic acid, on pigmentation and fertility. *South Med Surg* 104:135-139.

Silva Junior, AN et al. 2002. Computerized morphometric assessment of the effect of low level laser therapy on bone repair: an experimental animal study. *J Clin Laser Med Surg* 20:83-87.

Sliutz, G et al. 1993. Agnus castus extracts inhibit prolactin secretion in rat pituitary cells. *Horm Metab Res* 5(25):243-284.

Sma, RM. The lowering of lipoprotein(a) induced by estrogen plus progesterone replacement therapy in postmenopausal women. *Arch Intern Med* 153:1462–1468.

Snow, JM. 1996. Gingko biloba L. (Ginkgoaceae). *Protocol Journal of Botanical Medicine* 2(1):9–15.

Spasov, AA et al. 2000. Rhodiola root extract shows positive physical and mental activity in pilot study at low dose. *Phytomedicine* 7(2):85-89.

Spector, TD et al. 1997. Is hormone replacement therapy protective for hand and knee osteoarthritis in women? The Chingford Study. *Ann Rheum Dis* 56:432–434.

Sroka, R et al. 1997. Biomodulation effects on cell mitosis after laser irradiation using different wavelengths. *Laser Surg Med* 41-105.

Stahl, F et al. 1992. Dehydroepiandrosterone (DHEA) levels in patients with prostatic cancer, heart diseases and under surgery stress. *Exp Clin Endocrinol* 99:68–70.

Steeno, OP and Pangkahila, A. 1984. Occupational influences on male fertility and sexuality. *Andrologia* 16(1):5–22

Steiger, R et al. 1993. Neurosteroid pregnenolone induces sleep-EEG changes in man compatible with inverse agonistic GABA a-receptor modulation. *Research* 615:267–274.

Strawbridge, WJ et al. 2002. Physical activity reduces the risk of subsequent depression for older adults. *Am J Epidemiol* 156(4):328-334.

Studd, John. 1992. Gender and depression. *Lancet* 340:794.

Suleiman, S et al. 1997. Effect of calcium intake and physical activity on bone mass and turnover in healthy, white, postmenopausal women. *Am J Clin Nutr* 66:937.

Tagawa, N et al. 2000. Serum dehydroepiandrosterone, dehydroepiandrosterone sulfate, and pregnenolone sulfate concentrations in patients with hyperthyroidism and hypothyroidism. *Clin Chem* 46(4):523-528.

Tamimi, RM et al. 2006. Combined estrogen and testosterone use and risk of breast cancer in postmenopausal women. *Arch Intern Med* 166:1483-1489.

Taub, AF. 2003. Treatment of rosacea with intense pulsed light. *J Drugs Dermatol* 2(3):254-259.

Tenover, JS. 1992. Effects of testosterone supplementation in the aging male. *J Clin Endocrinol Metab* 75(4):1092–1098.

Tenover, JS. 1994. Androgen administration to aging men. *Endocrinol Metab Clin North Am* 23(4):877–892.

Thys-Jacobs, S et al. 1998. Calcium carabonate and the premenstrual syndrome: Effects on premenstrual and menstrual symptoms. *Am J Obstet Gyn* 179:444-452.

Tierra, M. 1997. Healing the liver, healing the body. *Int J Altern Complement Med* (February):23–25.

Tousoulis, D. 1997. Basal and flow-mediated nitric oxide production by atheromatous coronary arteries. *J Am Coll Cardiol* 29:1256–1262.

Tsitouras, PD and Bulat, T. 1995. The aging male reproductive system. *Endocrinol Metab Clin North Am* 24(2):297–315.

Urban, RJ et al. 1995. Testosterone administration to elderly men increases skeletal muscle strength and protein synthesis. *J Am Physiol Soc* E820–E826.

Usichenko TI and Herget HF. 2003. Treatment of chronic pain with millimetre wave therapy (MWT) in patients with diffuse connective tissue diseases: a pilot case series study. *Eur J Pain* 7:289–294.

Vashisht, A et al. 2005. A study to look at hormonal absorption of progesterone cream used in conjunction with transdermal estrogen. *Gynecol Endocrinol* 21(2):101-105.

Vassilios, AT et al. 1978. Estriol in the management of the menopause. *JAMA* 239(16):1638–1641.

Walaszek, Z et al. 1986. Dietary glucarate-mediated reduction of sensitivity of murine strains to chemical carcinogenesis. *Cancer Letters* 33:25-32.

Walaszek, Z et al. 1990. Antiproliferative effect of dietary glucarate on the Sprague-Dawley rat mammary gland. *Cancer Letters* 49:51-57.

Waring, N. 2000. Can prayer heal? A Duke cardiologist's controlled trials advance the debate. *Hippocrates* August 22-24.

Watts, NB et al. 1995. Comparison of oral estrogens and estrogens plus androgen on bone mineral density, menopausal symptoms, and lipid–lipoprotein profiles in surgical menopause. *Obstet Gynecol* 85(4):529–537.

Weiss, G et al. 2004. Menopause and hypothalamic-pituitary sensitivity to estrogen. *JAMA* 292(24):2991-2996.

Whitacre, FE and Barrera, B. 1944. War amenorrhea. *JAMA* 124(7):399–403.

Wiesel, LL et al. 1951. The synergistic action of para-aminobenzoic acid and cortisone in the treatment of rheumatoid arthritis. *Am J Med Sci* 222:243-248.

Wilbur, P. 1996. The phyto-estrogen debate (part 1). *Eur J Herbal Med* 2(2):20–26.

Wilbur, P. 1996. The phyto-estrogen debate (part 2). *Eur J Herbal Med* 2(3):19–26.

Wilcox, G et al. 1990. Oestrogenic effects of plant foods in postmenopausal women. *BMJ* 301:905–906.

Williams, DP et al. 1993. Relationship of body fat percentage and fat distribution with dehydroepiandrosterone sulfate in premenopausal women. *J Clin Endocrinol Metab* 77(1):80–85.

Wisniewski, TL et al. 1993. The relationship of serum DHEA-S and cortisol levels to measures of immune function in human immunodeficiency virus–related illness. *Am J Med Sci* 305(2):79–83.

Wolf, SL et al. 1996. Reducing frailty and falls in older persons: An investigation of tai chi and computerized balance training. *J Am Geriatr Soc* 44:489-497.

Wolkowitz, OM et al. 1997. Dehydroepiandrosterone (DHEA) treatments of depression. *Biol Psychiatry* 41:311–318.

Writing Group for the PEPI Trial. 1995. Effects of estrogen or estrogen/progestin regimens on heart disease risk factors in postmenopausal women. *JAMA* 273(3):199–208.

Wu, FS et al. Pregnenolone sulfate: A positive allosteric modulator at the N-methyl–d-aspartate receptor. *Mol Pharm* 40:333–336.

Wuttke, W et al. 2003. The *Cimicifuga* preparation BNO 1055 vs. conjugated estrogens in a double-blind placebo-controlled study: Effects on menopause symptoms and bone markers. *Maturitas* 44:S67-S77.

Wuttke, W et al. 2006. Efficacy and tolerability of the Black cohosh (*Actaea racemosa*) ethanolic extract BNO 1055 on climacteric complaints: A double-blind, placebo- and conjugated estrogens-controlled study. *Maturitas* (not yet published).

Wyon, Y et al. 1994. Acupuncture against climacteric disorders? Lower number of symptoms after menopause. *Lakartidningen* 91(23):2318-2322.

Yang, TS et al. Efficacy and safety of estriol replacement therapy for 356 climacteric women. *Zhonghua Yi Xue Za Zhi (Taipei)* 55(5):386-391.

Young, RL. 1993. Androgens in postmenopausal therapy? *Menopause Management* 21–24.

Zaborowska, E et al. 2007. Effects of acupuncture, applied relaxation, estrogens and placebo on hot flushes in postmenopausal women: an analysis of two prospective, parallel, randomized studies. *Climacteric* 10(1):38-45.

Zhdanova, IV et al. 2001. Melatonin treatment for age-related insomnia. *J Clin Endocrinol Metab* 86(10):4727-4730.

index

5-HTP
   neurotransmitter production, 222, 251
   progesterone, 86, 165–166
   serotonin production, 123–124
15-Minute Miracle, 475–476

a

acidic foods, 372–373
acidity, 349. see also pH
acne
   blue light therapy, 311–312
   testosterone level, 184–185
acupuncture/acupressure
   exceptional healers, 281–285
   medical uses, 274–275, 275–281
   overview, 271–272
   for puffy eyes, 65
adaptogens, 226
adrenal glands
   function, 439
   support program, 223–224
adrenal hormones
   glandular support, 90–91, 128, 170, 199, 224, 253
   stress, 439–440
adrenaline. see epinephrine
affirmations
   chakras, 294
   estrogen deficient-fast processor body type, 451
   estrogen deficient-slow processor body type, 452
   estrogen dominant body type, 449–450
   self love, 470–471
age spots, 107–108
alcohol
   estrogen levels, 22

hormone imbalance, 382
Aldana, Jacquelyn, 475–476
algae, 396–397
alkaline water, 377
alkalinity. see also pH
   described, 350
   green foods, 397
   post-surgery, 119
aloe vera, 106
alpha lipoic acid, 206–207
alpha waves, 341
Alzheimer's disease, 216
androstenedione
   cycle, 181
   production, 28
anger, 462–464
anxiety
   acupressure, 277, 280
   DHEA deficiency, 241
   exercise, 486
   hot flashes, 442
   music therapy, 321
   patient story, 448
   progesterone deficiency, 157
   testosterone deficiency, 184
appreciation
   healing power, 459–460
   vs. anger, 464
arthritis
   electromagnetic therapy (EMT), 343
   exercise, 490, 496
   pregnenolone deficiency, 216
   testosterone deficiency, 188
artificial sweeteners, 385
aspartame, 385
asthma, 245
auras, 289
autoimmune disease, 216
autonomic nervous system, 438
Aviles, Robert, 324

b

back pain, 501
Baggett, Brooke, 477–479
baked goods, 359
barley grass, 395–396
beans
    estrogen regulation, 375
    low-acid, 357
benign breast disease
    and estrogen dominance, 63
    patient story, 154
    progesterone deficiency, 154
beta-carotene
    adrenal support, 225
    DHEA production, 253–254
    estrogen regulation, 365
    progesterone production, 92, 171
beta waves, 341
beverages
    brand-name list, 406
    high-acid, 353
    low-acid, 356
    moderate-acid, 355
biofeedback
    devices, 330
    overview, 327–328
    research support, 328–329
bioflavonoids, 75–76, 145
bioidentical hormones, 55–56
biotin, 112
black cohosh, 140–141
blessings
    appreciation, 464
    healing power, 456
bloating, 278
blood pressure, 176
blood tests, 68–69
blue-green algae, 396–397
blue light therapy, 310–312
body scrub, 67
BodyTalk, 477–479

bone health. see osteoporosis
boron
    estrogen production, 132
    osteoporosis, 200
brain
    chemistry, 83–84, 121–122, 163–164, 192–193, 220–221, 249
    divisions, 82–83, 121, 162–163, 191–192, 220, 248–249
    wave patterns, 341–342
brain health
    DHEA, 259
Brassica vegetables. see diindolylmethane
breakfast
    brand-name list, 405
    for estrogen deficient-fast processor body type, 422–431
    for estrogen dominant body type, 410
breast cancer
    dietary considerations, 366–367
    diindolylmethane, 135–136
    exercise, 487–488
    hormone replacement therapy, 49
    infrared light, 309
    limonene, 80
    loneliness, 474–475
    Pilates, 501
    stress, 441–442
breast disease
    and estrogen dominance, 63
    patient story, 154
    progesterone deficiency, 154
breast health, 278
breathing, 445–446
burns, 263

c

C-reactive protein, 46
caffeine
    estrogen levels, 22
    hormone imbalance, 382–383
calcium

estrogen modulation, 77–78

nail health, 112

cancer

DHEA, 245, 262–263

electromagnetic therapy, 344

fermented foods, 389–390

music therapy, 322–323

red light therapy, 308–309

Rife technology, 338–339

cancer prevention, 126

cellulite, 65–67

cereal grasses, 395–396

chakras

balance, 293–295

color connection, 297

overview, 289

reading, 290–293

Western view of, 289–290

chaste tree berry. see vitex

chemotherapy

acupressure, 281

acupuncture, 275

chi (energy), 272–273

chlorella, 396

chlorophyll, 395

cholesterol

hormone precursor, 16, 213

testosterone levels, 29

cinnamon, 197

circulation

ginkgo, 204

red light therapy, 307

citrulline, 206

cloves, 197

cobalt, 134

coffee grounds, 66

color therapy

chakra connection, 297

meditation, 298

overview, 296–297

colored light therapy

devices, 315

guidelines, 312

mechanism, 303

overview, 300–301

research support, 301–302

use of, 313

condiments and seasonings. see also spices

brand-name list, 406

dietary considerations, 361

low-acid, 359

moderate-acid, 355, 356

pH chart, 360

Conductorcise, 491

constipation, 329

cooking, 407

copper, 109

cortisol

DHEA, 33, 260

function, 439–440

reduction program, 255–258

cortisone

side effects, 30–31

vs. pregnenolone, 212

d

D-glucarate, 79–80

dairy products

hormone imbalance, 383–384

low-acid, 358–359

moderate-acid, 355, 356

damiana, 202

deep breathing, 444–446

delta waves, 342

depression

acupressure, 277, 280

DHEA, 241, 259

exercise, 485–486

sunlight, 317–318

testosterone deficiency, 184

desserts

for estrogen deficient-fast processor body
type, 431

for estrogen dominant body type, 420

DHEA
    and appreciation, 460
    body effects, 33, 239, 258–263
    chemistry, 32–33
    exercise, 485
    overview, 32, 238
    patient stories, 243
    side effects, 265–266
    standard ranges, 247
    supplement forms, 263–264
    supplement guidelines, 264–266
    testosterone production, 199–200
DHEA deficiency
    check list, 246
    process, 239–240
    symptoms, 240–245
    testing, 246–247
diabetes, 244, 262
diet
    DHEA levels, 34
    effect on estrogen, 22
    perfect diet, 349
    testosterone production, 28–29
digestion
    progesterone levels, 26
    testosterone levels, 29
digestive enzymes, 381
diindolylmethane (DIM)
    breast cancer, 135–136
    estrogen breakdown, 79
    estrogen regulation, 367
dining out, 400–401
dinner, 405–406. see also main courses
dong quai, 144
dopamine
    function, 440
    maintenance, 86, 124, 166, 251
Dr. Lark, personal journey, 3–5
drinks. see beverages
dry brushing, 66
Dworkin, David, 491

e

Eastburn, Linda, 474–475
eating plans, 397–399
electrolysis, 186
electromagnetic frequency, 325–326
electromagnetic therapy (EMT)
    devices, 339–340
    overview, 337
    research support, 340–344
eleuthero root. see Siberian ginseng
emotional balance
    healing power, 453–454
    testosterone, 210
endometrial cancer
    and estrogen dominance, 63
    progesterone deficiency, 155
    progesterone protection, 173–174
endometrial hyperplasia
    and estrogen dominance, 63
    patient story, 64, 155
    progesterone deficiency, 155
endometriosis
    and estrogen dominance, 61
    stress, 441
endorphins, 83, 121–122, 163, 192, 220, 249
energy, 272–273
energy flow, 285–287
energy level, 188
energy loss, 215
energy medicine, 345
entrainment, 342
enzymes, 387. see also digestive enzymes
EPFX-SCIO
    described, 330–331
    modern view, 331
    use guidance, 333–334
epinephrine, 439
ERA trial, 47–48
essential fatty acids
    estrogen regulation, 368–369
    progesterone production, 92–93, 172

essential fatty acids (EFAs), 373

essential oils, 109

estradiol, 70

estriol
    bioidentical replacement, 56, 147–148
    overview, 145–147
    standard ranges, 70

estrogen. see also sex hormones
    age-related decline, 20
    body effects, 21, 26
    breakdown, 73, 78–82, 132–134
    chemistry, 19–20
    environmental influences, 21–23
    metabolic pathway, 135–136
    modulation, 74
    overview, 18
    serotonin level, 123
    types, 96–97

estrogen deficiency
    acupuncture/acupressure, 275, 278
    exercise, 488–489
    overview, 115
    stress, 442–443

estrogen deficient-fast processor body type
    described, 352
    exercise recommendation, 506
    pH-balanced diet, 370–377
    program summary, 507
    simple recipes, 408–409
    stress relief, 451–452
    symptoms, 9

estrogen deficient-slow processor body type
    described, 352
    exercise recommendation, 505
    exercise type, 486–487
    pH-balanced diet, 361–364
    program summary, 507
    simple recipes, 407–408
    stress relief, 452–453
    substantial recipes, 410–421
    symptoms, 8, 9

estrogen dominance

acupressure, 276

acupuncture, 274

    cosmetic effects, 64
    physical effects, 59–64
    during premenopause, 38
    stress, 441–442
    symptoms, 7, 9
    testing for, 67–70

estrogen dominant body type
    described, 352
    exercise recommendation, 505
    exercise type, 486–487
    pH-balanced diet, 361–364
    program summary, 507
    simple recipes, 407–408
    stress relief, 449–450
    substantial recipes, 410–421

exercise
    DHEA levels, 34
    overview, 484
    pain relief, 493
    preparation, 492
    progesterone levels, 26
    recommendation, 490, 494–495
    research support, 487–488, 489–490
    summary, 505–506

eye relaxation activity, 65

f

facial hair, 185

feet
    nail care, 111
    plantar fasciitis, 497

Feldenkrais method, 502–504

fermented foods, 389–390

fiber, 81–82, 369–370

fibrocystic breasts, 365

fibroid tumors
    and estrogen dominance, 60
    during premenopause, 38

fibromyalgia, 490

fight-or-flight response, 438

fish and shellfish
  low-acid, 358
  omega-3 fatty acid source, 368
flavonoids, 366–367
flaxseed
  estrogen mimic, 74–75
  progesterone production, 93, 172
fluid retention, 278
fluorescent light, 316
follicle-stimulating hormone (FSH)
  cycle, 97
  function, 37
forgiveness, 462–464
fruits
  digestive enzymes, 388
  high-acid, 354
  low-acid, 356
  moderate-acid, 355
fucose, 392–393
fungal infections, 111

g

gamma linolenic acid (GLA), 369
gaze, 65
generosity, 472–473
ginger, 198
ginkgo, 204
ginseng, Panax
  adrenal support, 227
  estrogen production, 129–131
  quality concerns, 229
  stress relief, 256–257
  testosterone production, 201
ginseng, Siberian, 228–229, 257
glandulars
  DHEA production, 252–253
  estrogen production, 127–129
  progesterone production, 89–91, 168–170
  testosterone balance, 198
glucosamine sulfate, 67
glucuronidation, 79–80

gluten, 385–386
glyconutrients
  body effects, 392
  food sources, 394
gotu kola, 67
grains
  digestive enzymes, 388–389
  estrogen regulation, 375
  low-acid, 359
grape seed extract, 67
gratitude, 459–461
green foods, 394–397

h

hair growth, 185
hair loss, 108–110
hair removal, 186–187
happiness, 467–468
"Heal the World" exercise, 285–287
heart disease
  DHEA, 243, 261
  at menopause, 100
  music therapy, 322
  progesterone deficiency, 157
  progestins, 174
  trial results, 46
HERS trial, 47, 174
high-fat diet, 28–29
high-fat foods, 364
hormone balance
  blue light therapy, 310–311
  conventional approach, 71–72
  electromagnetic therapy (EMT), 340–341
  red light therapy, 305
  stress, 441–443
hormone replacement therapy (HRT), 48
  breast cancer, 49
  cautions, 113
  clinical trials, 46–52
  osteoporosis, 48–49
  research summary, 52

tapering off, 148
untested nature, 45–46
hormone restoration, 54
hormone substitutes, 55
hormone testing
    estrogen dominance, 68
    progesterone deficiency, 160–161
hormones
    described, 15
    metabolic breakdown of, 35–36
hot flashes
    acupuncture/acupressure, 275, 278–279
    anxiety, 442
    described, 98–99
    exercise, 489
    red clover, 142
humor, 465–467
hypertension, 329
hypoglycemia, 384
hypothalamus
    hormone regulation, 84, 164, 181, 193
    neurotransmitter release, 122, 221, 250
hysterectomy
    artificial menopause, 96, 116
    patient story, 117
    rejection, 72
    surgery planning, 117–120
    testosterone after, 209

i

immune function, 244–245, 262–263
incontinence, 329
inflammation
    hormone balance, 379–381
    pregnenolone, 233–234
infrared light, 309
insomnia
    acupuncture/acupressure, 275, 279
    DHEA, 241, 260
    melatonin, 125–126
    during menopause, 99
    music therapy, 322

    patient story, 325–326, 335
    pregnenolone, 231
    progesterone deficiency, 156
Institute of HeartMath, 459–460
international cuisine, 401
iron, 112
isoflavones
    estrogen balance, 137–140
    estrogen regulation, 376
    in food, 74

j

JAMA study, 50–51
journaling, 461
juices, 390

k

Kegel exercises, 119
kidneys, 273
knee problems, 496

l

L-arginine, 205
laser hair removal, 186
lasers, 313
laughter, 465–467
lavender, 109
LEDs, 313
legumes, 388–389
libido. see sex drive
licorice root, 258
Life Vessel, 326–327
light therapy, 379
lignans, 74–75, 375
limbic brain, 83, 121, 163, 192, 220, 249
limonene, 80–81
Lin, Master Chunyi, 284–285
liquid sublingual formulations, 264
liver, 273
liver function
    estrogen breakdown, 35–36

estrogen levels, 22
progesterone levels, 26
liver spots, 107–108
love
healing power, 456–457
meditations, 457–458
of self, 469–472
visualizations, 458
lunch, 405–406. see also main courses
lutein
estrogen regulation, 365–366
progesterone production, 91, 171
luteinizing hormone (LH)
androgens, 182
function, 37
lycopene, 366
lymphodema, 306–307

m

maca
progesterone production, 88–89, 168
testosterone balance, 196–197
macular degeneration, 309–310
magnesium
adrenal support, 226
DHEA production, 255
estrogen modulation, 77
nail health, 112
main courses
for estrogen deficient-fast processor body
type, 427–430
for estrogen dominant body type, 415–419
mannose, 393
massage, 66
meal planning
dining out, 400–401
for kitchen devotees, 409–431
for non-cookers, 403–406
for occasional cooks, 407–409
and opposite body types, 402–403
meats
low-acid, 358

moderate-acid, 356
meditation
chakras, 294–295
color therapy, 298
gratitude, 461–462
love, 457–458
preparation, 444
stress relief, 447–448
melatonin, 125–126
memory
acupressure, 280
DHEA, 242, 259
fucose, 392–393
hormone influence, 18
at menopause, 101
pregnenolone, 215, 231–232
menopausal symptoms, 240–241
menopause
check list, 103
checkup recommendations, 104
cosmetic effects, 105–113
definition, 95
hormonal changes, 7–8, 37–39
natural vs. artificial, 95–96, 116
patient story, 102
physical changes, 39–40
physiology of, 96–98
progesterone deficiency, 156
symptoms, 98–102
testing for, 103–104
testosterone deficiency, 183
menstrual bleeding
acupressure, 277
and estrogen dominance, 6
fibroids, 60
menstrual cramps, 329
menstrual cycle
function, 36
hormone production, 97
phases, 76
menstrual symptoms, 487
menstruation, 25

mental clarity
    DHEA, 242
    exercise, 489
    at menopause, 101
    progesterone deficiency, 156–157
meridians, 273
microalgae, 396–397
micronized progesterone, 176
migraines
    biofeedback, 328–329
    Dr. Lark's family history, 305–306
    red light therapy, 305
minerals, 77–78
mood swings
    DHEA, 259
    electromagnetic therapy (EMT), 341–342
    at menopause, 101–102
    pregnenolone, 215, 232–233
    progesterone deficiency, 153, 157
mucuna bean, 194–195
multiple sclerosis, 216, 234
muscle strength
    DHEA deficiency, 245
    exercise, 497-498
muscle tension, 446
music therapy, 321–323

n

N-acetylgalactosamine, 393
N-acetylglucosamine, 393
N-acetylneuraminic acid, 393
nails (finger and toe), 110–113
neocortical brain, 83, 121, 163, 192, 220, 249
nerve disease, 158
nervous system, 438
neuropeptides, 83, 121, 163, 192, 220–221, 249
neurotransmitters
    balance, 85, 165
    described, 84, 122, 164, 192–193, 221, 250
    function, 84–86, 164–166
    stress, 440
    testing, 87, 125, 166, 223, 252

night sweats, 98–99
nitric oxide, 204–207
norepinephrine, 438, 439
NRG cards, 334–335
nutmeg, 198
nuts and seeds
    fatty acid source, 37, 374-375
    low-acid, 357

o

Oakes, Luanne, 324
Oliver, Evelyn, PhD, 479–481
omega-3 EFAs, 368
omega-6 fatty acids, 369
osteoporosis
    boron, 200
    DHEA, 242, 260–261
    electromagnetic therapy (EMT), 342–343
    estriol, 146–147
    exercise, 497–498
    hormone replacement therapy (HRT), 48–49
    at menopause, 100
    patient story, 158
    progesterone, 158, 179
    testosterone, 188, 210
ovarian cysts
    and estrogen dominance, 61
    patient story, 62
    progesterone deficiency, 154
ovaries
    hysterectomy, 116
    during menopause, 40
    during perimenopause, 152
    during premenopause, 38
    progesterone production, 91, 170
ovulation
    hormone cycle, 37, 151
    stimulation, 73

p

PABA (para-aminobenzoic acid)
    DHEA breakdown, 258

estrogen breakdown, 133
testosterone metabolism, 202
pain relief
electromagnetic therapy (EMT), 343–344
exercise, 493
Feldenkrais method, 503
patient story, 304
Pilates, 501
red light therapy, 306
pancreas, 273
paraliminals, 324
parasympathetic nervous system, 438
Parkinson's disease
mucuna bean, 195
qigong, 284
PEPI trial, 46, 174
perimenopause
hormonal changes, 38–39
patient story, 215
pregnenolone deficiency, 214
progesterone deficiency, 153–155
pH
body functions, 350–351
food chart (pre-consumption), 352–359
hormone balance, 351–352
overview, 349
regulation, 351
phenylalanine, 193
photodynamic therapy, 308–309
Pilates, 501–502
pilot study, 230
plantar fasciitis, 497
polycystic ovarian syndrome
exercise, 488
hormone balance, 194
positive attitude, 468
prana. see chakras
prayer, 454–455
pregnancy, 25
pregnenolone
benefits, 229
body effects, 213–214

cautions, 236–237
chemistry, 31
described, 213
overview, 30–31, 212
restoration, 219–220
side effects, 236
standard levels, 218
supplementing with, 234–235
pregnenolone deficiency
check list, 217
development, 214
symptoms, 214–216
testing for, 217–218
Premarin, 51
premenopause, 37–38
premenstrual syndrome (PMS)
acupressure, 276–277
acupuncture, 274
and estrogen dominance, 60
pregnenolone deficiency, 214
progesterone deficiency, 153
stress, 440, 441
probiotics
estrogen breakdown, 82
estrogen regulation, 367
progesterone. see also sex hormones
body effects, 21, 26, 151–152
chemistry, 24–25
described, 150–151
micronized form, 176
natural vs. synthetic, 173
overview, 24
physical effects, 175
skin cream, 176–177
standard levels, 161
supplementation, 172–178
progesterone deficiency
check list, 159–160
development, 152
during perimenopause, 153–155, 156–158
symptoms, 153–158
testing for, 160–161

progestins
    heart disease, 157
    physical effects, 174–175
    vs. progesterone, 25, 173–174
prostaglandins, 75

q

qigong, 284–285

r

raw foods, 390–391
recipes
    for estrogen deficient-fast processor body type,
        408–409, 422-431
    for estrogen deficient-slow processor body
        type, 407–408, 410–421
    for estrogen dominant body type, 407–408,
        410–421
red clover, 142
red light therapy, 303–310
reptilian brain, 83, 121, 162, 191, 220, 248–249
restaurant dining, 400–401
rheumatoid arthritis
    blue light therapy, 311
    electromagnetic therapy (EMT), 343–344
    music therapy, 322
Rhodiola rosea
    definition, 226–227
    stress reduction, 203
    stress relief, 255
Rife technology, 337–339
rosacea, 377–379
royal jelly
    estrogen balance, 143
    skin health, 106

s

saccharin, 385
SAD (seasonal affective disorder), 317–318
saffron, 144
salads

for estrogen deficient-fast processor body
        type, 423–425
    for estrogen dominant body type, 411–413
saliva testing
    described, 104, 190
    progesterone deficiency, 160–161
    vs. blood tests, 68–69
saponins
    described, 227
    stress relief, 130, 256
Scheele, Paul, 323–324
sea vegetables, 373
seeds, 388–389. see also nuts and seeds
self-talk, 468–469
serotonin
    blue light therapy, 311
    body effects, 123, 221–222
    described, 85, 164–165
    function, 440
    maintenance, 86, 123–124, 166, 251
sex drive
    acupressure, 281
    damiana, 202
    DHEA deficiency, 241
    drop at menopause, 99
    exercise, 489
    ginkgo, 204
    mucuna bean, 194–195
    nitric oxide, 204
    PABA, 133
    patient story, 242
    progesterone deficiency, 156
    spicy boosters, 197–198
    testosterone, 183–184, 209–210
sex hormones. see also estrogen; progesterone;
        testosterone
    described, 15
    production, 16
Sha, Dr Zhi Gang, 281–282
shopping list, 404
Siberian ginseng, 228–229, 257
side dishes

for estrogen deficient-fast processor body
      type, 426
   for estrogen dominant body type, 414
silicon, 112
skin creams
   DHEA, 264
   pregnenolone, 235
   progesterone, 176–178
   testosterone, 208
skin health. see also specific conditions such as
      acne; dry skin
   at menopause, 101
   support at menopause, 105–113
snacks, 406
sound therapy
   exceptional healers, 323–326
   health benefits, 319–322
soups
   estrogen deficient-fast processor body type,
      424–425
   estrogen dominant body type, 412–413
soy
   confusion resolved, 138
   estrogen balance, 137–140, 375–376
   estrogen mimic, 74
sperm count, 23
spices, 364. see also condiments and seasonings
spinal cord recovery, 216, 234
spirulina, 396
spleen, 273
sprouts, 388–389
squalene, 106–107
strains, vs. sprains, 494
stress
   adrenal hormones, 439–440
   body effects, 432–433
   check list, 435–436
   DHEA, 34, 241, 260
   electromagnetic therapy (EMT), 341–342
   hormone balance, 441–443
   messages from, 433–434
   minor tensions, 436

neurotransmitters, 440
   overview, 432
   patient story, 443
   physiology of, 438
   progesterone, 26, 157
   storage areas, 434
   testosterone, 29
stress relief
   exceptional healers, 474–482
   ginseng, 130
   music therapy, 321
   pregnenolone, 230
   qigong, 284
   Rhodiola rosea, 203
stretching, 498
stroke
   hormone replacement, 51
   at menopause, 100
stroke recovery, 307–308
sublingual formulations
   DHEA, 264
   pregnenolone, 235
   progesterone, 178
   testosterone, 209
sucralose, 385
sugar
   healing types, 391–394
   hormone imbalance, 384
sugar substitutes
   cautions, 385
   healthy alternatives, 386
sugaring, 187
sunlight, 316
support systems, 62
suppositories, 178
surgery, 117–120
sweeteners
   cautions, 385
   low-acid, 359
   moderate-acid, 355
sympathetic nervous system, 438

t

T'ai Chi, 504–505
tamoxifen, 138
tea tree oil, 185
TENS therapy, 340
tension relief, 446
testosterone. see also sex hormones
    balance program, 194–199
    body effects, 28, 182
    body production, 199–201
    breakdown, 202
    chemistry, 27–28
    described, 181–182
    excess, 188, 211
    overview, 27
    research support, 209–210
    standard ranges, 190
    supplemental, 207–209
    systemic support, 202–207
testosterone deficiency
    check list, 189
    mechanism, 182–183
    symptoms, 183–188
    testing, 189–190
theta waves, 341
thyroid hormones
    DHEA, 261–262
    glandular supplements, 90, 128, 169–170, 199
    serotonin levels, 124
    soy, 138
transdermal sprays, 178
travel, 403
Tribulus terrestris, 195–196
tryptophan, 165
tyrosine
    dopamine supplementation, 251
    neurotransmitter balance, 193
    neurotransmitter production, 222

u

urinary tract infections, 146

v

vaginal dryness
    acupressure, 280
    biofeedback, 329
    at menopause, 100
vaginal infections/vaginitis, 100, 131
vegetables
    digestive enzymes, 388
    high-acid, 354
    low-acid, 356–357
    moderate-acid, 355
vibrational healing, 319
visualizations
    for estrogen deficient-fast processor body
        type, 451–452
    for estrogen deficient-slow processor body
        type, 453
    for estrogen dominant body type, 450
    love, 458
    self love, 471–472
vitamin B complex
    adrenal support, 225–226
    DHEA production, 254
    estrogen breakdown, 78–79, 136–137
    hair growth, 109
vitamin C
    adrenal support, 225
    DHEA production, 254
    estrogen modulation, 76
    nitric oxide production, 206–207
vitamin E
    estrogen balance, 144–145
    estrogen modulation, 76–77
vitamins, 76–77
vitex, 87–88, 167

w

water
    emotional vibration, 336
    estrogen regulation, 370, 377
    before exercise, 492

waxing, 186
weight management
  cellulite reduction, 66
  DHEA, 243–244, 262
  exercise, 490, 495–496
  music therapy, 322
wheat, 385–386
wheat germ, 131–132
wheat grass, 395–396
Women's Health Initiative, 48, 50
wrinkles, 281

X

xenoestrogens, 22–23
xylose, 394

Y

Yaffe, Artemas, 481–482
yin, 143-144
yin-yang
  balance with acupuncture, 271–272
  characteristics, 8
yoga, 499–500

Z

zinc
  adrenal support, 226
  DHEA production, 254
  hair growth, 108
  nail health, 112

notes

notes

notes